Nutraceuticals Inspiring the Contemporary Therapy for Lifestyle Diseases

In today's fast-paced and modern world, our lifestyles have undergone a dramatic shift. The conveniences and comforts that accompany our technological advancements have come at a cost – an increased prevalence of lifestyle diseases. Lack of physical activity, stress, sedentary habits, and poor dietary choices have become leading causes of a spurt in varied health complications such as obesity, diabetes, and cardiovascular diseases. Various health awareness programmes organized by central/state governments, private organizations, and NGOs from time to time have generated interest among common people in exploring organic foods that are free from chemicals and full of nutraceuticals. There has been a growing interest in exploring the potential of nutraceuticals to address lifestyle diseases.

Recognizing the urgent need to address this global health crisis, this book delves into a realm of science that offers immense potential for improving our health and well-being. Nutraceuticals, which combine "nutrition" with "pharmaceuticals," offer a promising strategy for treating certain conditions caused by a particular way of life. They include a variety of bioactive substances obtained from plants, including fruits, vegetables, herbs, and marine organisms. Certain substances have therapeutic qualities and have shown significant promise in treating and even preventing certain disorders.

Features:

- The chapters in this book have been meticulously curated to provide readers with a diverse range of perspectives.
- Provides a comprehensive exploration of nutraceuticals and their potential benefits.
- Examines the impact of specific nutraceuticals on various lifestyle diseases to discuss their synergistic effects and potential adverse reactions.
- Each chapter offers valuable insights and practical guidance for healthcare professionals, researchers, and individuals seeking to enhance their overall well-being.
- A systematic overview of the state-of-the-art in nutraceuticals with recent research results.

This book will certainly be a valuable resource for researchers engaged in studies on nutraceuticals to develop a depth of understanding of the latest trends and tools in this field. Additionally, it can serve as a comprehensive textbook for graduate-level courses in food and nutrition, biomedical, and health sciences.

Nutraceuticals: Basic Research and Clinical Applications

Series Editor: Yashwant Pathak, PhD

Advances in Nutraceutical Applications in Cancer: Recent Research Trends and Clinical Applications
Edited by *Sheeba Varghese Gupta, Yashwant Pathak*

Flavor Development for Functional Foods and Nutraceuticals
M. Selvamuthukumaran and Yashwant Pathak

Nutraceuticals for Prenatal, Maternal and Offspring's Nutritional Health
Priyanka Bhatt, Maryam Sadat Miraghajani, Sarvadaman Pathak, Yashwant Pathak

Bioactive Peptides: Production, Bioavailability, Health Potential and Regulatory Issues
Edited by *John Oloche Onuh, M. Selvamuthukumaran, Yashwant Pathak*

Nutraceuticals for Aging and Anti-Aging: Basic Understanding and Clinical Evidence
Edited by *Jayant Lokhande, Yashwant Pathak*

Marine-Based Bioactive Compounds: Applications in Nutraceuticals
Edited by *Stephen T. Grabacki, Yashwant Pathak, Nilesh H. Joshi*

Applications of Functional Foods and Nutraceuticals for Chronic Diseases: Volume I
Edited by *Syam Mohan, Shima Abdollahi, and Yashwant Pathak*

Flavonoids and Anti-Aging: The Role of Transcription Factor Nuclear Erythroid 2-Related Factor2
Edited by *Karam F.A. Soliman and Yashwant Pathak*

Molecular Mechanisms of Action of Functional Foods and Nutraceuticals for Chronic Diseases: Volume II
Edited by *Shima Abdollahi, Syam Mohan and Yashwant Pathak*

Plant Food Phytochemicals and Bioactive Compounds in Nutrition and Health
Edited by *John O. Onuh, Yashwant V. Pathak*

Anxiety, Gut Microbiome, and Nutraceuticals: Recent Trends and Clinical Evidence
Edited by *Yashwant V. Pathak, Sarvadaman Pathak, and Con Stough*

Wealth out of Food Processing Waste: Ingredient Recovery and Valorization
Edited by *M. Selvamuthukumaran*

Nutraceuticals Inspiring the Contemporary Therapy for Lifestyle Diseases
Edited by *Mala Trivedi, Sachidanand Singh, Parul Johri, Pedro Lopez-Sanchez*

For more information about this series, please visit: https://www.crcpress.com/Nutraceuticals/book-series/CRCNUTBASRES

Nutraceuticals Inspiring the Contemporary Therapy for Lifestyle Diseases

Edited by
Mala Trivedi,
Sachidanand Singh,
Parul Johri, and
Pedro López-Sánchez

CRC Press
Taylor & Francis Group
Boca Raton London New York

CRC Press is an imprint of the
Taylor & Francis Group, an **informa** business

Designed cover image: Getty Images

First edition published 2024
by CRC Press
2385 NW Executive Center Drive, Suite 320, Boca Raton FL 33431

and by CRC Press
4 Park Square, Milton Park, Abingdon, Oxon, OX14 4RN

CRC Press is an imprint of Taylor & Francis Group, LLC

ISBN: 978-1-032-49270-4 (hbk)
ISBN: 978-1-032-49271-1 (pbk)
ISBN: 978-1-003-39293-4 (ebk)

DOI: 10.1201/9781003392934

Typeset in Times New Roman
by MPS Limited, Dehradun

Contents

Preface

We have the honour of working with a group of respected professionals in the disciplines of clinical research, pharmacology, nutrition, and medicine who have freely contributed their knowledge and experience to our project. Their input has been crucial in transforming this book into a trustworthy and knowledgeable resource for comprehending and utilizing the power of nutraceuticals. We, the editors, hope that readers who are curious about the potential of nutraceuticals for treating lifestyle disorders will find this book to be a useful resource. We sincerely believe that by implementing the ideas presented in these pages, we may take significant steps towards a healthy future.

We would like to express our sincere appreciation to the authors, editors, and hardworking staff at our publishing company for their constant support and dedication to this undertaking. We would also like to thank the readers for inspiring us to establish this extensive resource because of their curiosity and need for information.

Let's explore the incredible potential of nutraceuticals to alter our lives and overcome the obstacles provided by lifestyle diseases as we set off on a journey of empowerment and discovery together.

Editors

Mala Trivedi, Sachidanand Singh,
Parul Johri, Pedro López-Sánchez

Editor Biography

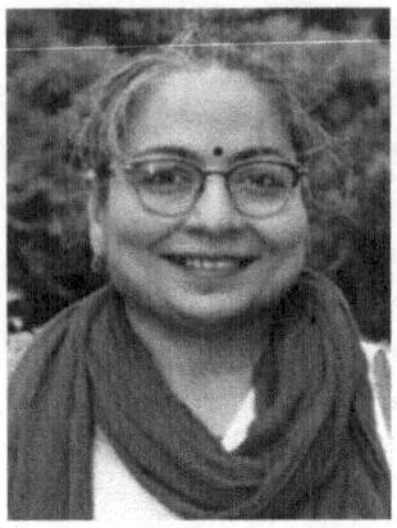

Dr. Mala Trivedi, Professor, Amity Institute of Biotechnology, Head, Directorate of Research and Publications, Amity University Uttar Pradesh, Lucknow. She is a recipient of a double Gold Medal from University of Allahabad during her M.Sc. in 1993. She did her PhD in Plant Genetics and Breeding from Central Institute of Medicinal and Aromatic Plants, (CIMAP) (CSIR), Lucknow. She was a Research Associate at the Institute of Cell Biology, School of Life Sciences, Lanzhou University, Lanzhou, PR China. She has good experience in plant transgenics. She has published more than 60 research papers in leading journals of National and international repute. Dr. Trivedi has published two books and several book chapters with international publishers. She has five Indian and two US patents to her credit. She is a member of many prestigious societies. She was also visiting faculty at the University of Lanzhou, Lanzhou, PR China. Currently, she is involved in mass multiplications of economically important plants (horticulture and medicinal plants). She is PI of a DBT-funded project and has supervised 12 PhD scholars so far.

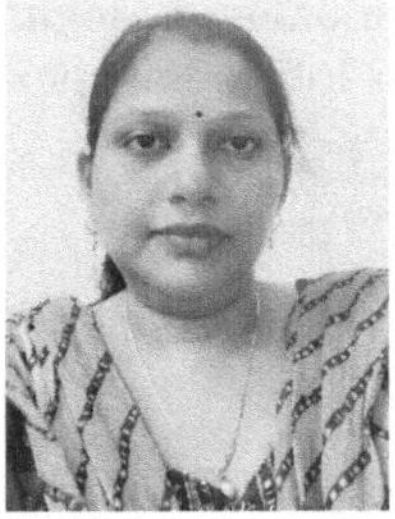

Dr. Parul Johri, Faculty, **Department of Biotechnology, Dr. Ambedkar Institute of Technology for Handicapped**, Kanpur, Uttar Pradesh, India. She is a recipient of a Gold Medal from Padmashree Dr. D. Y. Patil University Navi Mumbai, Maharashtra. She did her PhD at Amity University Uttar Pradesh. Her expertise includes bioinformatics, genomics, proteomics, biostatistics, and metagenomics. She has published more than **20 research papers** in various journals of National and International repute. Dr. Johri has edited a book and has written more than **15 book chapters** with various National and International publishers. She has **two Indian patents** to her credits. She has received various funds like the **DBT CTEP, NCW, ATAL AICTE** for conducting Lecture series, Sensitization Programs, and FDPs. Currently, she is involved in algorithm development for protein secondary structure prediction.

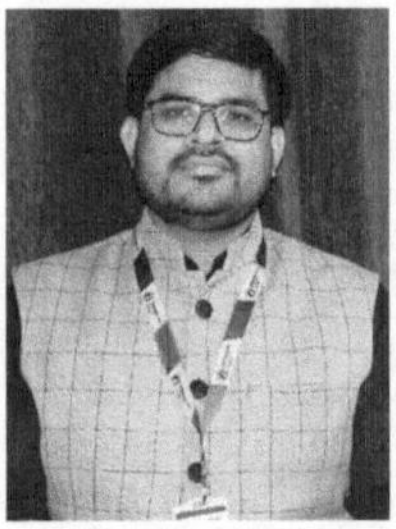

Dr. Sachidanand Singh, Associate Professor and Head, Department of Biotechnology, School of Energy Technology, Pandit Deendayal Energy University, Gandhinagar, Gujarat, India. He has completed B.Tech Biotechnology, M.Tech Bioinformatics, and PhD in Bioinformatics. He has a postdoctoral research experience from the college of Pharmacy, Ohio State University, USA. **His specialization area includes plant biotechnology, systems biology, and drug design**. He has more than 12 years of research and academic experience.

He has served for a decade in the School of Biotechnology and Health Sciences, Karunya University, Coimbatore, Tamil Nadu, India. He also worked as a consultant for the college of pharmacy, Ohio State University as a Statistical Genetics during the year 2018. He has published more than 38 research articles in peer-reviewed journals and completed one SERB, Govt of India funded project, and two University research grant projects. He has received several awards in his area of research and for his teaching strategies. He has organized different conferences and workshops and received Govt. funds for the same. He has shared his area of expertise with different colleges and universities as an invited speaker at different conferences and workshops. He has guided 36 B.Tech and 10 M.Tech projects. Presently 6 PhD students are enrolled under him and 2 PhD completed are working in the field of herbal products, drug design, and integration with network biology.

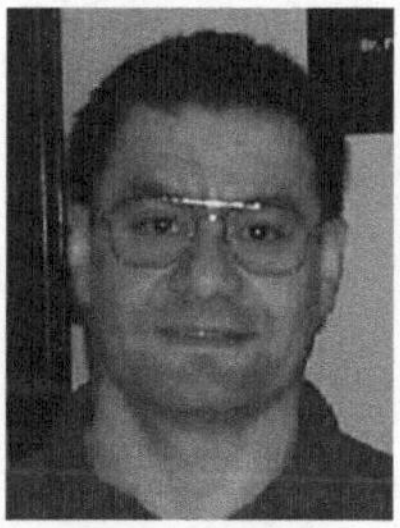

Dr. Pedro López Sánchez, MD, MSc, and PhD in Pharmacology. Dr. López made a three-year postdoctoral stance at Vanderbilt University, USA. He is a specialist in chronic degenerative illnesses, having more than 20 years studying diabetes mellitus, hypertension, and pregnancy-related hypertensive disorders, both in clinical and animal research. Renin-angiotensin aldosterone system has been his interest for the last 15 years. Dr. López has conducted several research projects sponsored by the National Council of Science and Technology. He has published more than 60 research papers. He has patented several drug delivery systems based on nanoparticles. Dr. López has more than 25 years as a senior lecturer in pharmacology lectures at the National Polytechnic Institute School of Medicine. He is a founding professor of the pharmacology MSc and the PhD program, coordinating both programs in 2009–2012 and 2012–2015, respectively. He is a senior lecturer in molecular pharmacology in both programs. He is a member of several societies: Mexican Pharmacology Association, Mexican Society of Physiological Sciences, National Sciences Academy, American Society of Pharmacological and Experimental Therapeutics, and American Physiological Society. Dr. López is a regular reviewer of several reputed journals published by Elsevier, Taylor & Francis, Springer Nature, Oxford University Press, PLOS, John Wiley & Sons, and Spandidos.

Contributors

Ankita Acharya
Department of Pharmaceutical Technology, JIS University
Agarpara, Kolkata, India

Mustansir Bhori
School of Biotechnology and Bioinformatics, D.Y. Patil Deemed to be University
Navi Mumbai, India

Manas Bhowmik
Department of Pharmaceutical Technology, Jadavpur University
Kolkata, India

Dimple Chauhan
Shoolini University of Biotechnology and Management Sciences
Solan, India

Sonam Chawla
Department of Biotechnology, Jaypee Institute of Information Technology
Noida, India

Dinesh Kumar Chellappan
Department of Lifesciences, School of Pharmacy, International Medical University
Kuala Lumpur, Malaysia

Dheeraj Chitara
Department of Science, Biyani Girls Colleges
Jaipur, India

Trudi Collet
Indigenous Medicines Group, Institute of Health & Biomedical Innovation, Queensland University of Technology
Brisbane, Australia

Sanchita Das
Department of Pharmaceutical Technology, JIS University
Agarpara, Kolkata, India

Shreya Das
School of Biotechnology and Bioinformatics, D.Y. Patil Deemed to be University
Navi Mumbai, India

Ameyota De
School of Biotechnology and Bioinformatics, D.Y. Patil Deemed to be University
Navi Mumbai, India

Hiral S. Desai
Smt. S.S Patel Nootan Science and Commerce College, Department of Biotechnology, Sankalchand Patel University
Visnagar, India

S. Diksha
Department of Pharmaceutical Technology, University College of Engineering (BIT Campus), Anna University
Tiruchirappalli, India

Aaysha Gupta
Department of Biotechnology, Jaypee Institute of Information Technology
Noida, India

Pramodkumar P. Gupta
School of Biotechnology & Bioinformatics, D.Y. Patil Deemed to be University
CBD-Belapur, Navi Mumbai, India

Arpita Gupte
School of Biotechnology and Bioinformatics, D.Y. Patil Deemed to be University
Navi Mumbai, India

Smita Jadhav
Department of Biotechnology, HVPSs Ramniranjan Jhunjhunwala College of Arts, Commerce and Science
Ghatkopar, Mumbai, India

Tanvi Jain
Faculty of Biotechnology, Institute of Biosciences and Technology, Shri Ramswaroop Memorial University
Lucknow, India

Swati Joia
Department of Food Technology, Eternal University
Baru Sahib, India

S. N. Jegasubramaniam
Department of Pharmaceutical Technology, University College of Engineering (BIT Campus), Anna University
Tiruchirappalli, India

Parul Johri
Department of Biotechnology, Dr. Ambedkar Institute of Technology for Handicapped
Kanpur, India

Aayushi Kadam
Department of Food and Human Nutritional Sciences, University of Manitoba
Winnipeg, Canada

Anjali Kembhavi
Müller UK and Ireland, Shrewsbury Road
Market Drayton, UK

Vaishnavi Kesarkar
School of Biotechnology and Bioinformatics, D.Y. Patil Deemed to be University
Navi Mumbai, India

Noopur Khare
Department of Food Technology, Bhai Gurdas Institute of Engineering and Technology
Sangrur, India

Pragati Khare
Department of Pharmacy, Bhagwant University
Ajmer, Rajasthan

Anuja Kulkarni
School of Biotechnology and Bioinformatics, D.Y. Patil Deemed to be University
Navi Mumbai, India

Akash Kumar
Department of Food Technology, SRM University
Sonepat, India

Prashant Kumar
Department of Bioinformatics, Kalinga University
Raipur, India

S. Meganathan
Department of Pharmaceutical Technology, University College of Engineering (BIT Campus), Anna University
Tiruchirappalli, India

Mala M. Parab
School of Biotechnology & Bioinformatics, D.Y. Patil Deemed to be University
CBD-Belapur, Navi Mumbai, India

K. A. Pavithran
Department of Pharmaceutical Technology, University College of Engineering (BIT Campus), Anna University
Tiruchirappalli, India

Pratik Pawar
School of Biotechnology and Bioinformatics, D.Y. Patil Deemed to be University
Navi Mumbai, India

S. Lakshmana Prabu
Department of Pharmaceutical Technology, University College of Engineering (BIT Campus), Anna University
Tiruchirappalli, India

Bhupendra G. Prajapati
Shree S. K. Patel College of Pharmaceutical Education and Research, Ganpat University
Kherva, India

Jhilam Pramanik
Department of Food Technology, ITM University
Raipur, India

A. Prabitha Priyadharshini
Department of Biotechnology, Alagappa College of Technology, Anna University
Tiruchirappalli, India

A. Puratchikody
Department of Pharmaceutical Technology, University College of Engineering (BIT Campus), Anna University
Tiruchirappalli, India

S. Barath Raj
Department of Chemical Engineering, Alagappa College of Technology, Anna University
Tiruchirappalli, India

Amit Kumar. Shrivastava
Department of Pharmacology, Universal College of Medical Sciences
Bhairahawa, Rupandehi, Nepal

Kavita Srivastava
Faculty of Biotechnology, Institute of Biosciences and Technology, Shri Ramswaroop Memorial University
Lucknow, India

Lily Srivastava
Department of Law, Sri J.N.M.P.G College, Associated College of Lucknow University
Lucknow, India

Garima Singh
Department of Oral & Maxillofacial Pathology, Mahatma Gandhi University of Medical Science and Technology
Jaipur, India

Sachidanand Singh
Department of Biotechnology, School of Energy Technology, Pandit Deendayal Energy University
Gandhinagar, Gujarat, India

Rajju Priya Soni
CSK Himachal Pradesh Krishi Vishwavidyalaya
Palampur, India

Sheetal. Sonawdekar
School of Biotechnology & Bioinformatics, D.Y. Patil Deemed to be University
CBD-Belapur, Navi Mumbai, India

S. Sowntharya
Department of Pharmaceutical Technology, University College Of Technology, Anna University
Tiruchirappalli, India

M. Dhivya Sree
School of Health and Health-Related Research, University of Sheffield
England, UK

Ashish Thakur
Department of Prosthodontics, Command Military Dental Centre
Jaipur, India

KanchanlataTungare
School of Biotechnology and Bioinformatics, D.Y. Patil Deemed to be University
Navi Mumbai, India

R. Thirumurugan
North Carolina State University
Raleigh, USA

Rajesh K. Tiwari
Amity Institute of Biotechnology, Amity University Uttar Pradesh
Lucknow, India

Yamini Tiwari
Department of Food science and nutrition, National Institute of Medical Sciences (NIMS)
Jaipur, India

A. Umamaheswari
Department of Pharmaceutical Technology, University College of Engineering (BIT Campus), Anna University
Tiruchirappalli, India

M. Vijayalakshmi
Department of Pharmaceutical Technology, University College of Engineering (BIT Campus), Anna University
Tiruchirappalli, India

1 Overview of Nutraceuticals for Management of Lifestyle Diseases

Noopur Khare, Pragati Khare, Hiral S. Desai, Mala Trivedi, Parul Johri, and Sachidanand Singh

1.1 INTRODUCTION

Since the beginning of time, mankind has created medicine from the extracts of natural materials and employed it for a variety of functions. The word "Nutraceuticals" was first used by Dr. Stephen in 1989 and refers to a mix of pharmaceuticals and nutrition. Since a new trend in companion animal care and related changes in the human population arose in the 1990s, nutraceuticals have advanced significantly. The definition of nutraceuticals has been expanded to cover vitamins, minerals, herbs and other botanicals, amino acids, and dietary substances for human use as a supplemental diet since the Dietary Supplement Health and Education Act of 1994 was passed (Stauffer 1999). The term "nutraceutical" is not widely recognised by regulatory systems around the world; dietary supplements are thought to be more prominent. Currently, there are more than 470 nutraceutical and functional food items with documented health benefits (Brower 1999). The art of harmonising the effects of one type of food with another so that they all complement one another is largely responsible for the success of traditional therapies. Medical professionals are currently thought of as a magic wand that can cure disease. According to a recent survey, 70% of patients normally see a doctor before or during traditional therapy, indicating that natural therapy is not preferred (Kessler et al. 2001). Patients are, however, quite aware of the adverse effects and contraindications brought on by chemical agents in both short- and long-term therapy. The trend of using alternative remedies, especially with the aid of nutritional methods, was sparked by the desire to prevent medicine from all minor illnesses. This chapter will give an overview of nutraceuticals and the role of nutraceuticals in prevention and treatment of diverse diseases along with their importance.

1.2 CONCEPT OF NUTRACEUTICALS

Recent epidemiological research has demonstrated that diet is the most effective means of preserving a state of wellbeing and preventing many ailments. Nutrition

DOI: 10.1201/9781003392934-1

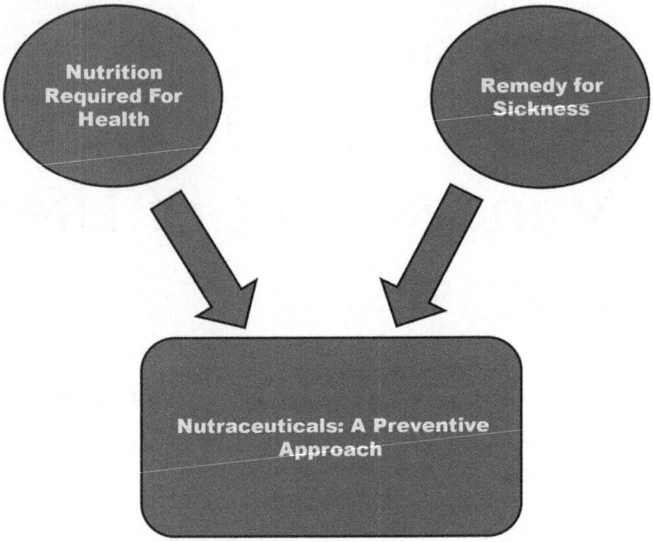

FIGURE 1.1 Concept of nutraceuticals.

has a progressive relationship with a number of degenerative, autoimmune, and neoplastic disorders, and the interaction between nutrients and organisms may reveal the balance between health and sickness (Calvani et al. 2020). Natural bioactive compounds known as nutraceuticals provide both nutritional value and advantageous therapeutic effects for a variety of disorders. It benefits human health by either treating or avoiding disorders. In 1989, Dr. Stephen DeFelice distinguished between nutrients and pharmaceuticals by using the word "Nutraceuticals" (Ranzato et al. 2014). A food or component of a diet that promotes and nourishes health in addition to its nutritional value is referred to as a nutraceutical. They are either dietary supplements or active ingredients derived from plants or animals. When properly provided, they can produce a highly effective therapeutic toolbox to aid with and prevent many ailments (Santini et al. 2017) (Figure 1.1).

1.3 NUTRACEUTICALS FOR HEALTHY LIFESTYLE

Nutrition is provided through food. Mostly plant and animal sources are used to acquire it. Fungal origins can also be used to produce food. According to Wikipedia, food typically contains proteins, carbs, fats, vitamins, and minerals. Fast food is very popular these days. That is why there are so many terrible diseases that we have to deal with, including cancer, diabetes, obesity, and cardiovascular disease. A balanced diet is crucial for overcoming these issues. In contrast to "diet food" (or "dietetic food"), which refers to any food or drink consumed to decrease fat and/or carbohydrates in a special programme or diet, diet is the amount of food consumed by a person or other living organism (https://en.wikipedia.org/wiki/Diet_(nutrition)).

Nutraceuticals include fortified dairy products like milk, citrus fruits like orange juice, garlic, soyabeans, and others (Cencic and Chingwaru 2010). Functional foods,

TABLE 1.1
Diseases and Their Nutraceuticals

Disease	Nutraceuticals
Cardiovascular diseases	Anti-oxidants, Dietary fibres, Omega-3 polyunsaturated fatty acids, Vitamins, minerals for prevention and treatment of CVD.
	Polyphenol(in grape) prevent and control arterial diseases [96]
Diabetes	Lipoic acid, an antioxidant, for treatment of diabetic neuropathy [97].
	Dietary fibres from psyllium have been used for glucose control in diabetic patients and to reduce lipid levels in hyperlipidemia [98]
Cancer	Lycopene concentrates in the skin, testes, adrenal, and prostate where it protects against cancer [99].
	Saponins (found in peas, soybeans, some herbs, spinach, tomatoes, potatoes, alfalfa, and clover) contain antitumor and antimutagenic activities [100].
	Curcumin (diferuloylmethane) which is a polyphenol of turmeric possesses anticarcinogenic, antioxidative, and anti-inflammatory properties [101].
	Top of Form Beetroots, cucumber fruits, spinach leaves, and turmeric rhizomes, were reported to possess anti-tumour activity [102].
Osteoarthritis	Glucosamine (GLN) and chondroitin sulphate (CS) alleviate symptoms of O.A. [103].

such as fruits and vegetables, are nutrient-dense foods that have been fortified with vitamins, minerals, probiotics, and fibre to provide health advantages above and beyond their nutritional value (Souyoul et al. 2018). Foods designed for functional purposes have higher dietetic value. To improve health, dietary supplements are made from food, separated nutrients, or food-like ingredients. A category of dietary supplements called nutraceuticals promotes health by using only whole foods (Sachdeva et al. 2020) (Table 1.1).

1.4 POLYPHENOLS AS NUTRACEUTICALS OF MODERN LIFE

Global economic expansion and globalisation have both contributed to an increase in the prevalence of lifestyle diseases. The impact of the agricultural and industrial revolutions on alterations in human lifestyle has increased life expectancy and expanded medicine, substantially altering ecological interactions and patterns of population sickness (Maria et al. 2018). Human population growth and environmental climate change have a significant impact on people's everyday lives, which results in shortcomings that must be addressed by battling various lifestyle problems. Developing habits that prevent people from exercising and encourage a sedentary lifestyle can lead to a variety of health issues, including chronic non-communicable diseases with potentially fatal outcomes. The customers' frustration with their disease-treating strategy with contemporary medicine has narrowed them towards complementary medicines due to worries about healthcare administration and treatment costs (Burger and Fristoe 2018). The effectiveness of functional foods and food items currently falls short of local knowledge. This gap has been closed recently with the rise of nutraceutical concepts based on pre-clinical circumstances.

1.5 ROLE OF NUTRACEUTICALS IN THE TREATMENT AND PREVENTION OF CANCER

Due to the quick change in modern lifestyles and the lack of time for physical care, exercise, and desk jobs, the significance of a healthy diet as a fundamental need has increased over the past two decades. The criteria that are most important when choosing what to eat have changed as people's concerns about their health have increased. In order to reduce their chance of developing chronic diseases, more and more people are focusing on eating more food than is recommended by the RDA (Ahmed and Haboubi 2010). Obesity, diabetes, high blood pressure, stress, allergies, cardiovascular disease, and cancer are common problems nowadays. According to the new health and wellness paradigm, eating well will help individuals live longer. To better themselves, people aim for a healthier body and a more youthful appearance. A wide range of health concerns, including those affecting women's health, skin, eyes, joints, mental health, bone health, sleep quality, cancer prevention, weight management, and athletic performance, can be improved by natural healing ingredients (Cencic and Chingwaru 2010). Nature teaches us to approach health from a more comprehensive perspective. Customers are more worried about their health, thus businesses must support their promises about new bioactive compounds and cutting-edge administration techniques with scientific data.

1.6 NUTRACEUTICALS FOR CANCER MANAGEMENT

Cancer has been ranked as the most prevalent disease in the globe among all other diseases. More than half of the 10 million people who are diagnosed with cancer each year around the world die from it. In many countries, cancer is the second most common cause of death. In many parts of the world, it has already surpassed cardiovascular disease as the major cause of death, and this expansion is predicted to continue. Population ageing, which is a major worldwide health issue because elderly people are most susceptible to cancer, is continuing in many countries (Ma and Yu 2006). Visits with oncology healthcare professionals are essentially required in order to address the patient's psychological, social, and economical needs as well as to provide information regarding the patient's malignancy, prognosis, treatment goals, and options. Doctors must pay great attention to cancer patients and communicate clearly with them in order to deliver an effective treatment that also addresses their emotional sensitivity. Higher-quality care, more appropriate medical decisions, and better health outcomes have all been linked to patient and provider communication. In terms of how information is conveyed between the doctor and patients, oncology appointments are distinct from other contexts for receiving medical care (ElKefi and Asan 2021). The mortality data from 1930 can be found at the National Centre for Health Statistics (NCHS) (Wingo et al. 2003; Murphy et al. 2015).

1.7 ROLE OF NUTRACEUTICALS IN THE TREATMENT OF DIABETES THROUGH PREBIOTICS

Diabetes is a "chronic disease caused by either ineffective insulin use by the body or insufficient insulin production by the pancreas" (World Health Organization. *Diabetes.* https://www.who.int/news-room/fact-sheets/detail/diabetes (accessed 2023-02-15)). Type 1 diabetes, type 2 diabetes, and gestational diabetes are all diabetes subtypes (Cole and Florez 2020). In the world, diabetes is the fifth most common cause of death, having contributed to 1.6 million deaths (Roglic et al. 2005). Studies show that those with type I and type II diabetes have a 15% higher chance of dying and a 10- and 20-year shorter life expectancy, respectively (Tancredi et al. 2015). According to the International Diabetes Federation (IDF) for 2017, 8.8% of adults aged 20 to 79 have diabetes globally (International Diabetes Federation. IDF Diabetes Atlas, 8th Ed.; International Diabetes Federation: Brussels, Belgium, 2017). Diabetes, one of the diseases with the highest global growth rates, is predicted to affect 693 million people by 2045 (Cole and Florez 2020). In 2014, statistics showed that 422 million individuals worldwide have diabetes (World Health Organization. Global Report on Diabetes; World Health Organization: Geneva, Switzerland, 2016). Consequently, a recent estimate states that there will be at least 592 million cases of diabetes worldwide in 2035 (Forouhi and Wareham 2014).

1.8 NUTRACEUTICALS FOR HORMONAL IMBALANCE MANAGEMENT

All living things use hormones, sometimes known as biochemical emissaries or stimulants, in a variety of metabolic activities. Without these signals, a child's growth may be stunted, fertility may be reduced, sleep patterns may become irregular, and metabolic diseases may develop (YussraElobidi et al. 2022). Hormones are a broad category of chemicals that can be categorised. Eicosanoids (such as prostaglandins and thromboxanes), steroids (such as oestrogen and brassinosteroid), amino acid derivatives (such as epinephrine and auxin), proteins or peptides (such as insulin and CLE peptides), and gases (such as ethylene and nitric oxide) are among the biometabolites that can be considered hormones (Hiller-Sturmhöfel and Bartke 1998).

1.9 ROLE OF DIET ON HORMONAL IMBALANCE AND RELATED METABOLIC DISORDERS

A high intake of fatty foods that contributes to obesity and an increased conversion of testosterone to oestrogen in the presence of the enzyme aromatase are two factors that have been linked to hyperestrogenism. Additionally, hyperinsulinism, which is characterised by uncontrolled insulin secretion and may cause mild to severe hypoglycemia, could be the cause (Collison et al. 2011). Additionally, it increases ovarian testosterone production and decreases sex hormone-binding globulins, which raises blood levels of free oestrogen. As a result, food considerably affects the production, metabolism, and receptor function of oestrogen (Malik Aubead 2021). Alcohol use also raises blood levels of estradiol and hinders the liver's ability to detoxify oestrogen. Breast cancer could result from elevated estradiol levels (Deshpande N. Hormonal imbalance in breast cancer. Elsevier; 1976: https://linkinghub.elsevier.com/retrieve/pii/B9780080196824500962). Another major health worry for many is the presence of an oestrogenic chemical in dairy products and other foods.

1.10 ROLE OF NUTRACEUTICALS IN MANAGEMENT OF HYPERTENSION

Products made from food or food components, isolated nutrients, or any dietary supplements with a medicinal or physiological purpose are referred to as nutraceuticals. Based on the functional chemicals they contain, they have a variety of effects on health, either being preventative or curative. Concern over studies examining the protective health effects of these functional meals against various chronic diseases has grown. This has led us to take a chance on fully comprehending its function in the management and prevention of hypertension, a significant cause of cardiovascular diseases (CVD) (Stenvinkel 2010). A chronic illness condition known as hypertension (HTN) is characterised by persistently high blood pressure in arteries. Its multifactorial aetiology includes numerous pathophysiological, environmental, and genetic variables, many of which are intricately intertwined. Many functional compounds have been confirmed to contain the potential to control the disturbances happening in numerous physiological systems in this situation. numerous functional compounds have been characterised to examine its anti-hypertensive impact. This may involve reducing oxidative stress, inhibiting the renin-angiotensin-aldosterone system (RAAS), blocking calcium channel activity, inhibiting sympathetic activity, promoting diuresis, producing NOS, activating the signalling pathways for hydrogen sulphide and nitric oxide, stimulating vasodilation, and managing inflammatory stress (Akhmedov and Sharipov 2023).

1.11 CONCLUSION

Many nutraceuticals, functional foods, and naturally occurring substances that have been researched and documented in several studies showed that these products are incredibly active, have tremendous effects on cell metabolism, and frequently have few negative effects. It makes sense that people's attention is turning towards proactive methods of disease prevention in order to maintain their health. The scientific field of nutraceuticals has been developed all over the world. Nutraceuticals frequently outperform the synthetic medications being developed by the pharmaceutical sector. Novel pharmacological activity is what has attracted interest because of their potential clinical applications, which could aid in the prevention and treatment of many diseases. The majority of pharmaceutical businesses frequently lack the drive to confront these challenges in securing patents. It is hoped that government organisations and academic institutions will support additional nutraceutical research.

REFERENCES

About cancer - Surveillance, Epidemiology. https://seer.cancer.gov/data/citation.html [Accessed on 01.01.2023]

Ahmed, T., & Haboubi, N. (2010 Aug 9). Assessment and management of nutrition in older people and its importance to health. *Clinical Interventions in Aging*, 5, 207–216.

Akhmedov, A.T., & Sharipov, Z.R. (2023 Mar 31). The role of cytokines in the development of arterial hypertension. *International Journal of Medical Sciences and Clinical Research*, 3(03), 59–67.

Baradaran, A., Madihi, Y., Merrikhi, A., Rafieian-Kopaei, M., & Nasri, H. (2013). Serum lipoprotein (a) in diabetic patients with various renal function not yet on dialysis. *Pakistan Journal of Medical Sciences*, 29(Suppl), 354–357.

Brower, V. (1999). Nutraceuticals: poised for a healthy slice of the healthcare market. *Nature Biotechnology*, 16, 728–731.

Burger, J.R., & Fristoe, T.S. (2018). Hunter-gatherer populations inform modern ecology. *Proceedings of the National Academy of Sciences of the United States of America*, 115(6), 1137–1139.

Calvani, M., Pasha, A., & Favre, C. (2020). Nutraceutical boom in cancer: Inside the labyrinth of reactive oxygen species. *International Journal of Molecular Sciences*, 21(6), 1936.

Cencic, A., & Chingwaru, W. (2010 Jun 1). The role of functional foods, nutraceuticals, and food supplements in intestinal health. *Nutrients*, 2(6), 611–625.

Cole, J.B., & Florez, J.C. (2020). Genetics of diabetes mellitus and diabetes complications. *Nature Reviews Nephrology*, 16(7), 377–390. 10.1038/s41581-020-0278-5.

Collison, K.S., Zaidi, M.Z., Saleh, S.M., Inglis, A., Mondreal, R., Makhoul, N.J., et al. (2011 Jul 28). Effect of trans-fat, fructose and monosodium glutamate feeding on feline weight gain, adiposity, insulin sensitivity, adipokine and lipid profile. *British Journal of Nutrition*, 106(2), 218–226. Available from: https://www.cambridge.org/core/product/identifier/S000711451000588X/type/journal_article

Deshpande, N. (1976). Hormonal imbalance in breast cancer. In *Proceedings of the Fourth International Congress on Hormonal Steroids [Internet]*. Elsevier, pp. 735–741. Available from: https://linkinghub.elsevier.com/retrieve/pii/B9780080196824500962

ElKefi, S., & Asan, O. (2021). How technology impacts communication between cancer patients and their health care providers: A systematic literature review. *International Journal of Medical Informatics*, 149, 104430.

Elobidi, Y., Ashour, M., AteiaElmabsout, A., &ID (2022). Women hormonal imbalance: Risk factors, clinical characteristics, and nutritional status. *International Journal of Research Publication and Reviews*, 3(1), 219–230. Available from: https://ijrpr.com/uploads/V3ISSUE1/IJRPR2303.pdf

Forouhi, N.G., & Wareham, N.J. (2014). Epidemiology of diabetes. *Medicine (United Kingdom)*, 42(12), 698–702. 10.1016/j.mpmed.2014.09.007.

Gulcin, I., Mshvildadze, V., Gepdiremen, A., et al. (2006). The antioxidant activity of a triterpenoid glycoside isolated from the berries of Hedera colchica: 3-O-(B-dglucopyranosyl)-hederagenin. *Phytotherapy Research*, 20, 130–134.

Hardy, G. (2000). Nutraceuticals and functional foods: Introduction and meaning. *Nutrition*, 16, 688–689.

Hiller-Sturmhöfel, S., & Bartke, A. (1998). The endocrine system: an overview. *Alcohol Health and Research World*, 22(3), 153–164. Available from: http://www.ncbi.nlm.nih.gov/pubmed/15706790

International Diabetes Federation (2017). *IDF Diabetes Atlas*, 8th Ed. International Diabetes Federation, pp. 9–44.

Kessler, R.C., Davis, R.B., Foster, D.F., et al. (2001). Long term trends in the use of complementary and alternative medical therapies in the United States. *Annals of Internal Medicine*, 135(4), 344–351.

Ma, X., & Yu, H., (2006). Global burden of cancer. *Yale Journal of Biology and Medicine*, 79(3-4), 85–94.

Malik Aubead, N. (2021). Role of sex hormones in human body. In C. Marsh (ed.) *Reproductive Hormones [Internet]*. IntechOpen. Available from: https://www.intechopen.com/books/reproductive-hormones/role-of-sex-hormones-in-human-body

Maria, G.V.G., Vera, E.C., Vilma, M.J., & Carla, H.A.S. (2018). Impact of human aging and modern lifestyle on gut microbiota. *Critical Reviews in Food Science and Nutrition*, 58(9), 1557–1564.

Murphy, S.L., Kochanek, K.D., Xu, J., & Heron, M. (2015). Deaths: Final data for 2012. *National Vital Statistics Reports*, 63(9), 1–117.

Ranzato, E., Martinotti, S., Calabrese, C., & Giorgio, C. (2014). Role of nutraceuticals in cancer therapy. *Journal of Food Research*, 3(4), 18–25.

Roglic, G., Unwin, N., Bennett, P.H., Mathers, C., Tuomilehto, J., Nag, S., Connolly, V., & King, H. (2005). The burden of mortality attributable to diabetes realistic estimates for the year 2000. *Diabetes Care*, 28(9), 2130–2135. 10.2337/DIACARE.28.9.2130.

Sachdeva, V., Roy, A., & Bharadvaja, N. (2020 Aug 1). Current prospects of nutraceuticals: A review. *Current Pharmaceutical Biotechnology*, 21(10), 884–896.

Santini, A., Tenore, G.C., & Novellino, E. (2017). Nutraceuticals: A paradigm of proactive medicine. *European Journal of. Pharmaceutical Sciences*, 96, 53–61.

Souyoul, S.A., Saussy, K.P., & Lupo, M.P. (2018 Mar). Nutraceuticals: a review. *Dermatology and Therapy*, 8, 5–16.

Stauffer, J.E. (1999). Nutraceuticals. *Cereals Food World*, 44(2), 115–116.

Stenvinkel, P. (2010 Nov). Chronic kidney disease: a public health priority and harbinger of premature cardiovascular disease. *Journal of Internal Medicine*, 268(5), 456–467.

Tancredi, M., Rosengren, A., Svensson, A.-M., Kosiborod, M., Pivodic, A., Gudbjörnsdottir, S., Wedel, H., Clements, M., Dahlqvist, S., & Lind, M. (2015). Excess mortality among persons with type 2 diabetes. *New England Journal of Medicine*, 373(18), 1720–1732. 10.1056/NEJMOA1504347/SUPPL_FILE/NEJMOA1504347_DISCLOSURES.PDF.

Wingo, P.A., Cardinez, C.J., Landis, S.H., Greenlee, R.T., Ries, L.A.G., & Anderson, R.N., et al. (2003). Long-term trends in cancer mortality in the United States, 1930–1998. *Cancer*, 97(12), 3133–3275.

World Health Organization. *Diabetes*. https://www.who.int/news-room/fact-sheets/detail/diabetes (accessed 2023-02-15).

World Health Organization (2016). *Global Report on Diabetes*. World Health Organization.

2 Nutraceuticals for Healthy Lifestyle

Before the Drugs Beyond the Diets

Sanchita Das, Manas Bhowmik, and Ankita Acharya

2.1 INTRODUCTION

Food is administered for nutrition. It is mainly obtained from plant and animal sources. Food may be obtained from fungal origin also. Food generally contains proteins, saccharides, fats, micronutrients, and minerals (Rahman and McCarthy 1999). Nowadays, people are fonder of fast foods. That's why we are facing so many dreadful diseases like cardiovascular disease, cancer, diabetes, obesity, etc. To overcome these problems, a healthy diet is essential. Diet is the amount of food consumed by a person or other living organism whereas "diet food" (or "dietetic food") denotes any food or drink consumption to decrease fat and/or carbohydrates in a special programme or diet.

Assessment by the U.K., Germany, and France, the idea of "nutraceutical" ascended first (https://www.worldnewsnaturalsciences.com). In these places, the diet was valued for good health (Pandey et al. 2010). The name "nutraceutical" was derived from "nutrition" and "pharmaceutical" by Stephen De Felice in 1989 (Maddi et al. 2007).

It is a food or food component that has therapeutic properties and is used for treatment or to prevent diseases. A nutraceutical is a substance that may contain different nutrients or medicinally active compounds such as omega-3 fatty acids of salmon and other cold-water fish.

Milk, orange juice, garlic, soyabean, etc., are examples of nutraceuticals (Avrelija and Walter 2010).

Functional foods are nutrient-rich and foods fortified with vitamins, minerals, probiotics, and fibre that offer health benefits beyond their nutritional values including fruits and veggies (Souyoul et al. 2018).

Functional foods are tailored for superior dietetic value (Figure 2.1 and Figure 2.2). Dietary supplements are prepared from foodstuff, isolated nutrients, or food-like substances to supplement health. Nutraceuticals are edible supplements made of foods to boost physical condition (Sachdeva et al. 2020).

DOI: 10.1201/9781003392934-2

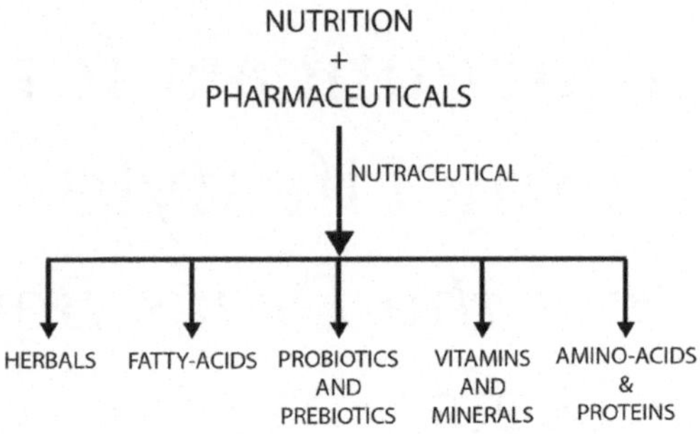

FIGURE 2.1 Classification of nutraceuticals.

Source: Developed by authors from primary material.

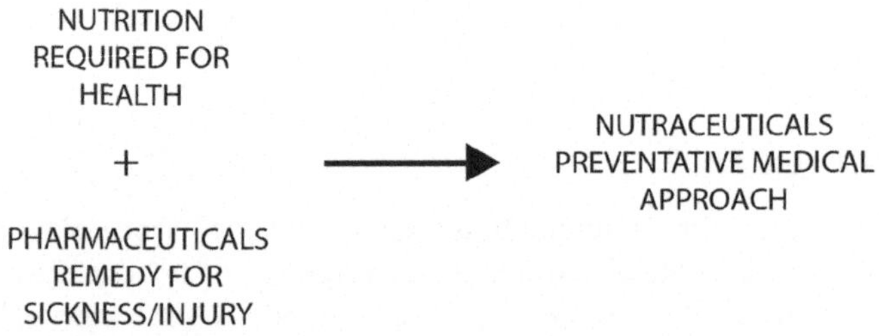

FIGURE 2.2 Nutraceuticals: Approach for nutrition and health benefit.

Source: Developed by authors from primary material.

2.2 CLASSIFICATION OF NUTRACEUTICAL

Nutraceuticals are divided into four categories according to the following (Espín et al. 2007):

i. Their food source (Table 2.1)
ii. Their mechanism of action (Table 2.2)
iii. Their chemical nature (Table 2.3)
iv. Their higher content in specific food items (Table 2.4).

TABLE 2.1
Food Source-Based Nutraceuticals

Food Source	Examples
Plant	Gallic acid, quercetin, potassium, pectin, etc.
Animal	Conjugated Linoleic Acid (CLA), Docosahexaenoic acid (DHA), Coenzyme Q10, etc.
Microbe	*Saccharomyces boulardii, Lactobacillus acidophilus,* etc.

Source: Developed by authors from primary material.

TABLE 2.2
Nutraceuticals According to Mechanism of Action

Category	Examples
Anticancer	Capsaicin, curcumin, lutein, ellagic acid, etc.
Antioxidant	Ascorbic acid, Lycopene, catechin, gingerol, etc.
Anti-inflammatory	Quercetin, curcumin, DHA, linoleic acid, etc.
Bone protective	Soy protein, inulin, calcium, CLA, etc.
Antibacterial	Curcumin, garlic, etc.

Source: Developed by authors from primary material.

TABLE 2.3
Nutraceuticals According to Chemical Nature

Component		Source	Potential Benefits
Carotenoids	i. Zeaxanthin	Eggs, citrus fruits, and corn.	Helps to maintain healthy vision.
	ii. α-carotene	Carrots	Neutralises free radicals which are responsible for cell damage.
	iii. Lycopene	Tomato	Reduces the possibility of prostate cancer.
Soy protein		Soybeans, soy-based foods.	Reduces possibility of heart disease (25 gm/day)
Saponins		Soybeans, soy-protein-containing foods.	Decrease LDL cholesterol, prevent cancer.
Tannins and proanthocyanidins		Cranberries, cranberry products, cocoa	Improve UT health and decrease the chance of CVDs.
Phenols	i. Caffeic acid ii. Ferulic acid	Fruits, vegetables.	Helpful for eye disease, degenerative disease, heart disease. Used as an antioxidant.
Dietary fibre	i. Insoluble fibre	Wheat bran	Lower the chance of colon or breast carcinoma.
	ii. Soluble fibre	Psyllium	Reduce susceptibility of CVDs.
	iii. Whole grains	Cereal grains	Reduce vulnerability of CVDs.
Fatty acids	i. Omega-3-fatty acids	Tuna fish and marine oils	Reduce risk of CVDs, enhances vision and responsiveness.
	ii. CLA	Cheese and meat products	Decrease the risk of certain cancers.
Flavonoids	i. Anthocyanidins	Fruits	Anticancer and antioxidant.
	ii. Catechins	Tea	Anticancer and antioxidant.
	iii. Flavanones	Citrus	Anticancer and antioxidant.
	iv. Flavones	Fruits and vegetables	Anticancer and antioxidant.

Source: Developed by authors from primary material.

TABLE 2.4
Nutraceuticals According to Their Higher Content in Specific Food Items

Nutraceutical Substances	Foods of Remarkably High Content
Allyl sulphur compounds	Onion and garlic
Quercetin	Onion extract, red grapes, lemon and orange, broccoli, Italian yellow squash.
Lycopene	Tomato
FPA and DHA	Fish oils
Isoflavones	Soybeans and other legumes.
β- carotene	Citrus fruits, carrots, squash, pumpkin.
Catechins	Tea, berries, apples, grapes.

Source: Developed by authors from primary material.

2.3 MARKETED NUTRACEUTICALS

Nutraceuticals can be categorised on the basis of foods or supplements already marketed.

2.3.1 Traditional Nutraceuticals

Traditional nutraceuticals are simply natural foods where no changes have occurred. These foods are rich in several components as well as general nutrition which includes Lycopene, omega-3 fatty acids, and saponins in salmon, tomatoes, and soy respectively are examples of traditional nutraceuticals (Rajasekaran et al. 2008).

2.3.2 Chemical Constituents

2.3.2.1 Nutrients

Essential Nutrients like Vitamins, Minerals along with Amino Acids, fatty acids, milk products, meat, poultry are capable of producing beneficial effects in the treatment of diseases like Diabetes, Arthritis, Cardiac stroke, etc. Some mineral extracts present in plant, animal, and milk-derived products are useful in treating bone diseases and anaemia, and they can strengthen bones, muscles, teeth, and help maintain cardiac rhythm and optimum nerve impulse (Mistry 2021).

Omega-3 PUFAS adequately present in flaxseed and salmon are responsible for controlling inflammatory pathways, maintaining nervous responsiveness, and reducing lipid deposition (Sasi 2017).

2.3.2.2 Herbals

Herbs or botanical products are used as concentrated extracts.

2.3.2.3 Supplements

With the help of different types of herbal supplements, nutraceuticals hold great promise to improve living and prevent chronic disease states (Andlauer and Fürst 2002). Willow bark (*Salix nigra*) is used to prevent inflammation, reduce severe pain, reduce raised body temperature, prevent bleeding by precipitation of proteins, and treat arthritis due to the presence of salicin. Flavonoids (apiol and psoralen)-enriched parsley (*Petroselinum cripsum*) is used to treat renal diseases, reduce flatulence, and treat fever. Peppermint (*Mentha piperita*) cures common cold and flu infections because of menthol. Lavender (*Lavandula angustifolia*) is a good example of an herbal medicine from which antidepressant, hypotensive, stress reliever, and common cold protective effects can be achieved. Cranberries (*Vaccinium erythrocarpum*) are found to be useful in the treatment of cancer, ulcer-related complications, and mostly abolishing urinary tract infections due to proanthocyanidin (Augustin and Sanguansri 2015).

2.3.2.4 Phytochemicals

These are one type of nutraceuticals.

Carotenoids (isoprenoids) present in a large group of fruits, vegetable sources, and egg yolks have been observed to be useful in Cancer treatment. They can trigger NK immune cells and safeguards the cornea against UV light.

Non-carotenoids found in legumes (chickpeas and soybeans), grains, and palm oil are responsible for removing cholesterol, and they are also anticarcinogenic. Flavonoid-enriched fruits, berries, vegetables, and leguminous plants are very potent antioxidants and plant estrogen products, and they are important nutraceuticals in the prevention of carcinoma of prostate and breast, and diabetes management.

Non-flavonoid polyphenolics are found in dark grapes, raisins, berries, and peanuts. Turmeric roots work to prevent inflammation, stop cell damage, and exhibit blood thinner properties, and they can lower lipid profiles. Phenolic acids, found in blueberries, tomatoes, and bell peppers and having preventive activity towards cell damage, are responsible for reducing the induction of mutations by polycyclic aromatic hydrocarbons. Seeds of *Barbarea verna and* broccoli have antitumorigenic activity because of isothiocyanates (glucosinolates) (Alagawany et al. 2021).

2.3.3 Probiotic Microorganisms

Probiotics are living microorganisms that can be found in dairy products such as A/B-culture yoghurts, sour milk, and so on. It stands for life and living organisms, which, when uptaken in sufficient quantities, have a positive influence on the host. These are good absorbents of nutrients thereby serving as digestion-friendly microbes (Chintale et al. 2013).

2.3.3.1 Sources of Probiotic Microorganisms

Milk: *Lactobacillus acidophillus*, *Lactobacillus lactis*, *Propioni bacterium freudenreichli.*

Yoghurt: *Stretococcus thermophilus*, *L. delbrueckii* subp *bulgaricus*, *Bifido bacterium adolescentis.*

Fermented products: *Lactobacillus casei*, *Lactobacilluscellobiosus*, *Lactobacilluscurvatus*, *Lactobacillusfermentum*, *Lactobacillushelviticus*, *Lactobacillusfarciminis*, *B.* thermophilum, *B. animalis.*

Human breast milk: *Lactobacillus salivarius*, *Lactobacillus reuteri*, *B. infantis*, *B.* longum, B. *breve*, *B. lactis*.

GIT: *E. coli* Nissle 1917, *Lactobacillus gassert*, *Lactobacillus johnsoni*.

Vegetables/grains/fruits: *Lactobacillus brevis*, *Lactobacillus plantarum*, *Saccharomyces cerevisiae*, *Saccharomyces boulardii*, Mushrooms.

2.3.4 Nutraceutical Enzymes

Enzymes are biological catalysts that occur naturally as proteins. Without enzymes, our bodies are unable to perform critical functions. There are so many enzymes that are used as nutraceuticals (Mistry 2021).

Microbial enzymes/ Source: Hemicellulase (Microorganisms and mushrooms), Catalase, amyloglucosidase (Ascomycetes), glucoamylase, cellulase, etc.

Plant enzymes/ Source: Hemicellulase (plant walls), Pectinase (cell wall), α-Galactosidase (mostly present in beans, cabbage, Brussels sprouts, broccoli, asparagus, and whole grains), β-Amylase (higher plants), Bromelain (pineapple), etc.

Animal enzymes/ Source: Oxbile (Ox), Trypsine (Pancreatic juice), Pancrelipase (Pancreatic juice), α-Amylase (saliva), Lysozyme (abundant in saliva, tears, egg white, and many animal fluids), pepsin (Animal tracheal secretion), etc. (Prabu et al. 2012).

2.4 NON-TRADITIONAL NUTRACEUTICALS

These are man-made foods created with the application of biotechnology. Non-traditional nutraceuticals are classified as fortified nutraceuticals and recombinant nutraceuticals.

2.4.1 Fortified nutraceuticals include protected foods from agricultural rearing or with nutrients in excess quantity.

2.4.2 Recombinant nutraceuticals include energising foods like bread, alcohol, yoghurt, cheese, vinegar, etc. (Gul et al. 2016).

2.5 NUTRACEUTICAL PRODUCTS AVAILABLE IN THE GLOBAL MARKET

The global nutraceutical market is categorised depending on the following different criteria.

2.5.1 Based on Type of Edibles

2.5.1.1 Food

It includes snacks, products from confectionery, bakery, dairy.

2.5.1.2 Beverages

It includes health drinks, energy drinks, and juices.

2.5.1.3 Dietary Supplements

These include tablets, liquids, powders, and other products like soft gels, gummies, and chewable products.

2.5.2 Based on Distribution Channel Stores

2.5.2.1 Conventional Stores

These include regular grocery stores, mass merchandisers and retailers available online.

2.5.2.2 Speciality Stores

These include stores like bakery, gourmet, confectionery, cosmetic and health centres.

2.5.3 Based on Sources

The Market classification of Nutraceuticals based on source are as follows probiotics, proteins, amino acids, phytochemicals and plant extracts, fibres, omega-3 fatty acids, vitamins, prebiotics, carotenoids, minerals, and others.

2.5.4 Based on Region

The Market classification of Nutraceuticals based on region are as follows North America, Europe, Asia-Pacific, South America, Africa, and the Middle East (Da Costa 2017).

2.6 NEW DEVELOPMENT AND NUTRACEUTICAL PRODUCT MANUFACTURERS

The industry of Nutraceuticals is an exponentially developing market in the world. Adding to this, the rise of awareness of health protection, population growth, and massive changes in daily habits are stimulating their development.

The complete list of Top Nutraceutical Manufacturers being superior in their manufacturing quality, effectiveness and long-lasting Nutraceuticals for the benefit of Humankind are mentioned below. The details include some of the product lists of companies, which are given in Table 2.5.

2.7 HEALTH BENEFITS OF NUTRACEUTICALS

There are countless advantages of Nutraceuticals, and still extensive research is going on to get another bunch of benefits from it (Figure 2.3). Starting from Physical to Mental health, there are plenty of disease conditions to be

TABLE 2.5
Lists of Some Marketed Products and Manufacturers

Sl. No.	Manufacturer	Product Name
1	United Laboratories	• Softgel capsules • Digestive supplements • Derma products • Cardiology medicines • Gynecology medicines
2	Bionova Lifesciences	• CARDL-NRG tablet • Garciniacambogia capsules
3	Lactonova Nutripharm	• Banana leaf extract • Soy lsoflavones
4	Sydler remedies	• Nutrisyd stress & anxiety care formula • Nutrisyd male support formula • Fortimune tablets • Nutrisyd female support formula
5	Neiss Wellness (India) Ltd.	• Tracewell • Cranwell • Fracpro • Protein kids • Ten Q plus • Niswell women
6	KD Chem-Pharma	• A Balanced Combination of Proprietary Pea And Rice Protein With Added BCAAs • Bioactive Pure Whey Protein With Naturally Occurring Immunoglobulins
7	Agati Healthcare Pvt Ltd.	• Lcololipid-Lg • Buffalo Colostrum Powderwhole Powder Granules
8	Premier Nutraceuticals Pvt Ltd (Pnpl)	• Coral calcium • Coral calcium D3 • Superantioxidant
9	Kraft Heinz	• FRUITLOVE It is available in different flavours, like blend and strawberry banana twirl.
10	Conagra Company	• EVOL a new product called Modern Nutrition Bowls. It consists of breakfast bowls with vitamins and nutrients
11	Amway India Enterprises Pvt. Ltd.	• Nutrilite Milk Thistle Plus Tablet • Nutrilite Natural B with Yeast Tablet • Nutilite Vasaka, Mulathi and Surasa Tablet • Nutilite All Plant Protein Powder • Nutilite Daily

Source: Developed by authors from primary material.

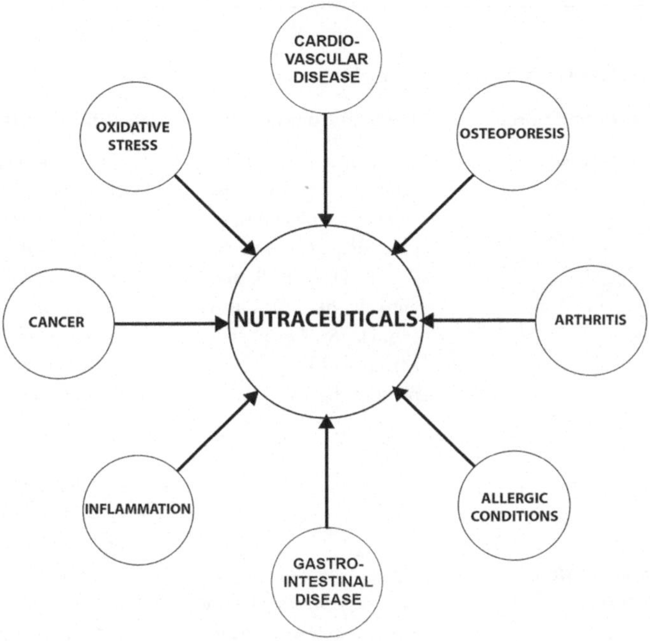

FIGURE 2.3 Health benefits of nutraceuticals.

Source: Developed by authors from primary material.

controlled by them. Nutraceuticals have major applications in (Gupta et al. 2010):

- Promotes healthier livelihood
- Makes active
- Provides quietness
- Assist clear thoughts
- Sustain profound and lengthy nap
- Eradicate persistent symptoms
- Removes drug dependence
- Anti-ageing consequence
- Increases living duration
- Supervise and manage functions of the body.

Currently, ongoing studies revealed that Nutraceuticals are equally effective in the treatment of major diseases like Carcinoma, Diabetes, Parkinson's disease, Alzheimer's, or maybe in conditions like obesity (Wang and Weller 2006). In Table 2.6, a list of plants, their chemical active constituents as nutraceutical and health benefits are summarised.

In cancer prevention, polyphenols, quercetin, resveratrol, epigallocatechin-3-gallate (EGCG), vitamins, and minerals are very helpful (Ruchi 2017). The sources of these are given below.

TABLE 2.6
List of Plants Used as Nutraceuticals

Sl. No	Drug's Name/Source	Chemical Compounds	Health Benefits
1	*Medicago sativa* (Alfalfa)	Carotenoids, triterpenes, saponins, isoflavonoids, coumarins, alkaloids, glycosides, vitamins A, B_6, B_{12}, C, D, K, E, P, and nutrients like Cu, Ca, K, Mg, Na, Si, Fe, etc.; hormones like phytoestrogens.	1. Useful in lowering cholesterol levels, improving metabolic health, relieving menopausal symptoms, strengthening the digestive system, and controlling blood sugar levels. 2. Antioxidant 3. People also take it for its high content of vitamins C and K, copper, folate, and magnesium. 4. Alfalfa is also extremely low in calories.
2	*Cichorium intybus* (Chicory)	Aliphatic compounds and their derivatives, chicoric acids, inulin with sugar, various sesquiterpene lactones and glycosides, coumarins, cinchorin, esculetin, esculin, umbelliferone, vitamin B_6, Mn, scopoletin.	1. Hepatoprotective, anti-inflammatory, antioxidant, sedative, anticancer, gastro-protective, antidiabetic, tonic, and laxative. 2. Vitamin B_6 and manganese help to maintain brain health. 3. Effective in rheumatoid arthritis and gout.
3	*Zingiberofficinale* (Ginger)	Volatile oil like bisaboline, zingiberene, zingiberol, oleo- resin, citral, geraniol, α-curcumene, β-bisabolene.	1. Carminative, flavouring agents, spice, stomachic. 2. Useful in treating asthma, sore throats, colds and coughs, and motion sickness. 3. Used in various beverages, liquors, mouthwashes, and gargles.
4	*Allium sativum* (Garlic)	Allin, Volatile oil, mucilage, albumin.	1. Spice, carminative, expectorant, antibacterial agent, aphrodisiac and stimulant. 2. Used in dysentery, indigestion, hypertension, colds, flu, fever, sore throat, etc. 3. Helpful in lowering blood cholesterol.

TABLE 2.6 (Continued)
List of Plants Used as Nutraceuticals

Sl. No	Drug's Name/Source	Chemical Compounds	Health Benefits
5	*Apismellifera*, *Apis indica*, or *Apis florae* (Honey)	Mixture of dextrose, glucose, fructose, and water; sucrose, dextrin, volatile oil, wax, pollen grain, and formic acid; and small amounts of enzymes, vitamins, and minerals.	1. Sweetening agent, demulcent, antiseptic, and antioxidant. 2. Nutrients for patients and infants. 3. Used in burns and wounds. 4. Used for the preparation of candies, lotion, and creams. 5. Used in cough mixtures, cough syrups, and as a vehicle for many Ayurvedic preparations.
6	*Withania somnifera* (Aswagandha)	Alkaloids like withasomnine, withanin, anahygrine, and anaferine, and steroidal lactones like withaferin A and withanolides.	1. Sedative, aphrodisiac, bacteriostatic, anticancer. 2. Used in epilepsy, bradycardia, and rheumatism.
7	*Emblica officinalis* (Amla)	Vitamin C, pectin, tannins, glucose, minerals (Iron, Phosphorus, Calcium).	1. Used for the treatment of scurvy, this is caused by a deficiency of vitamin C. 2. Useful in diabetes and liver disease. 3. Anti-viral, antifungal, and antibacterial. 4. Used in the treatment of anaemia, jaundice, and cough (dried form).
8	*Trigonella foenum-graecum* (Fenugreek)	Steroidal saponinlike Diosgenin; Furostanol glycoside like trigofoenoside A, B, C, D, E, F and G; trigonelloside C; yamogenin; yamogenin tetroside B and C; gitogenin, etc.; Sitosterol; mucilage, protein, alkaloids like trigonelline; lipids like linoleic acid and linolenic acid; flavouring agents, flavonoids like quercetin, luteolin, vicenin 1 and 2; 4-hydroxyisoleucine.	1. Anticancer, emollient, demulcent, febrifuge, expectorant, carminative, laxative, antioxidant, tonic, and a condiment. 2. Used in the synthesis of sex hormones, oral contraceptives. 3. Used in the treatment of inflammation and ulcers of the stomach and intestine. 4. Helps induce labour and increase breast milk production. 5. Lowers blood cholesterol and regulates blood sugar levels.

(*Continued*)

TABLE 2.6 (Continued)
List of Plants Used as Nutraceuticals

Sl. No	Drug's Name/Source	Chemical Compounds	Health Benefits
9	*Panax ginseng* (Korean ginseng), *Panax notoginseng* (Chinese ginseng), *Panax japonica* (Japanese ginseng)	Chikusetsusaponin, ginsenosides, and panaxosides; polysaccharides such as glycans; acetylenic compounds such as panaxynol and panaxydol; sesquiterpenes like - elemene; panasinsanol A, B, and ginsenol; vitamin A and D; sterols; amino acids; minerals (zinc).	1. Immunomodulator, adaptogenic, aphrodisiac, and tonic. 2. Used to improve appetite, memory, and concentration. 3. Used in gastritis and exhibits demulcent properties. 4. It is used to treat menopausal symptoms by increasing oestrogen levels. 5. Used to treat neurasthenia.
10	*Spirulina platensis* (Spirulina)	Protein, γ-linoleic acid, heptadecanoic acid, linoleic acid, oleic acid, palmitic acid, and palmitoleic acids; glycogen, rhamnose; β-carotene, vitamins B_1, B_2, B_3, B_6, B_{12} and E_3; phycocyanin; Superoxide dismutase (SOD); Ca, Mg, crude fibres, ash.	1. Stimulates the proliferation of bone marrow stem cells, macrophages, and T cells and also increases their activity. 2. Anti-HIV, anti-viral, anticancer 3. Lowers the cholesterol level 4. Helps suppress the appetite 5. Used to treat cataracts, diabetes, arthritis, atherosclerosis, the ageing process, and emotional stress (Kuppusamy et al. 2014)

Source: Developed by authors from primary material and elaboration.

2.7.1 Polyphenols

They are found in various vegetables, tea, cocoa, wines, etc. Polyphenols containing groups like flavonoids, phenolic acids, stilbene, and curcuminoids play a critical function in inhibiting the initiation of carcinogenic action and in suppressing the progression of cancers (Santini et al. 2017).

2.7.2 Resveratrol

It occurs as stilbene. It acts as a phytoalexin (plant antibiotic) with natural antiproliferative activity and other bioactivities such as anticarcinogenic, anti-inflammatory, and anticancer effects.

2.7.3 Vitamins and Minerals

Vitamin A, Vitamin C, and Vitamin E, as well as minerals like selenium, a trace element, have been found to be effective in cancer prevention.

2.7.4 EGCG

EGCG is a catechin found in green tea. It plays a vital activity in the prevention of cancer due to its antitumor activities (Nasri et al. 2014).

2.7.5 Quercetin

It occurs in various fruits and vegetables. It also shows low bioavailability upon oral administration. It shows the following anticancer effects:

i. Prevention of induced colon carcinogenesis
ii. Inhibition of growth, invasion, and metastatic potential of melanoma.

REFERENCES

Alagawany, M., Elnesr, S.S., Farag, M.R., Abd El-Hack, M.E., Barkat, R.A., Gabr, A.A., & Dhama, K. (2021). Potential role of important nutraceuticals in poultry performance and health-A comprehensive review. *Research in Veterinary Science*, 137, 9–29.

Andlauer, W., & Fürst, P. (2002). Nutraceuticals: a piece of history, present status and outlook. *Food Research International*, 35(2-3), 171–176.

Augustin, M.A., & Sanguansri, L. (2015). Challenges and solutions to incorporation of nutraceuticals in foods. *Annual Review of Food Science and Technology*, *6*(1), 463–477.

Avrelija, C., & Walter, C. (2010). The role of functional foods, nutraceuticals, and food supplements in intestinal health. *Nutrients*, 2, 611–625.

Chintale Ashwini, G., Kadam Vaishali, S., Sakhare Ram, S., Birajdar Ganesh, O., & Nalwad Digambar, N. (2013). Role of nutraceuticals in various diseases: A comprehensive review. *International Journal of Research in Pharmacy and Chemistry*, 3, 290–299.

Da Costa, J.P. (2017). A current look at nutraceuticals–Key concepts and future prospects. *Trends in Food Science and Technology*, 62, 68–78.

Espín, J.C., García-Conesa, M.T., & Tomás-Barberán, F.A. (2007). Nutraceuticals: facts and fiction. *Phytochemistry*, 68(22), 2986–3008.

Gul, K., Singh, A.K., & Jabeen, R. (2016). Nutraceuticals and functional foods: the foods for the future world. *Critical Reviews in Food Science and Nutrition*, 56(16), 2617–2627.

Gupta, S., Chauhan, D., Mehla, K., Sood, P., & Nair, A. (2010). An overview of nutraceuticals: current scenario. *Journal of Basic and Clinical Pharmacy*, 1(2), 55–62.

Rahman, S.M., & McCarthy, O.J. (1999). A classification of food properties. *International Journal of Food Properties*, 2(2), 93–99.

Mistry, S. (2021). Classification of nutraceuticals. https://solutionpharmacy.in/classification-of-nutraceuticals/ (accessed February 12, 2023)

Kuppusamy, P., Yusoff, M.M., Maniam, G.P., Ichwan, S.J.A., Soundharrajan, I., & Govindan, N. (2014). Nutraceuticals as potential therapeutic agents for colon cancer: a review. *Acta Pharmaceutica Sinica B*, 4(3), 173–181.

Maddi, V.S., Aragade, P.D., Digge, V.G., & Nitaliker, M.N. (2007). Importance of nutraceuticals in health management. *Pharmacognosy Reviews*, 1, 377–379.

Nasri, H., Baradaran, A., Shirzad, H., & Rafieian-Kopaei, M. (2014). New concepts in nutraceuticals as alternative for pharmaceuticals. *International Journal of Preventive Medicine*, 5(12), 1487–1499.

Pandey, M., Verma, R.K., & Saraf, S.A. (2010). Nutraceuticals: new era of medicine and health. *Asian Journal of Pharmaceutical and Clinical Research*, 3, 11–15.

Prabu, S.L., Suriya Prakash, T.N.K., Kumar, C.D., Suresh Kumar, S., & Ragavendran, T. (2012). Nutraceuticals: A review. *Elixir Pharma*, 46, 8372–8377.

Rajasekaran, A., Sivagnanam, G., & Xavier, R. (2008). Nutraceuticals as therapeutic agents: A review. *Research Journal of Pharmacy and Technology*, 1(4), 328–340.

Ruchi, S. (2017). Role of nutraceuticals in health care: A review. *International Journal of Green Pharmacy*, 11(03), S385–S394.

Sachdeva, V., Roy, A., & Bharadvaja, N. (2020). Current prospects of nutraceuticals: A review. *Current Pharmaceutical Biotechnology*, 21(10), 884–896.

Santini, A., Tenore, G.C., & Novellino, E. (2017). Nutraceuticals: A paradigm of proactive medicine. *European Journal of Pharmaceutical Sciences*, 96, 53–61.

Sasi, S. (2017). Nutraceuticals–a review. *International Journal of Industrial Biotechnology and Biomaterials*, *3*(1), 25–29.

Souyoul, S.A., Saussy, K.P., & Lupo, M.P. (2018). Nutraceuticals: a review. *Dermatology and Therapy*, 8(1), 5–16.

Wang, L., & Weller, C.L. (2006). Recent advances in extraction of nutraceuticals from plants. *Trends in Food Science and Technology*, 17(6), 300–312.

3 Polyphenols as Nutraceuticals of Modern Life

S. Lakshmana Prabu, A. Umamaheswari, S. N. Jegasubramaniam, N. Tamilselvan, and R. Thirumurugan

3.1 BACKGROUND

Globally, the prevalence of lifestyle illnesses has increased in tandem with economic growth and globalization. The agricultural and industrial revolutions' influence on human lifestyle modifications has furthered life expectancy and advanced medicine, which has fundamentally changed ecological interactions and population illness patterns (Maria et al. 2018).

Fostering habits that hinder people from exercising and encourage a sedentary lifestyle may create different health illnesses, as well as chronic non-communicable diseases with potentially fatal consequences.

The recent rise in nutraceutical concepts based on pre-clinical conditions has reduced the gap between local knowledge and the effectiveness of functional foods.

Higher prescription costs and the reluctance of some individuals to cover the costs of modern medicines have focused human beings on nutraceuticals and established its position in the world market for treatment of the diseases as therapeutic agents. Thus, the increased demand paves the way for nutritional supplements to be considered an alternative medicine and provide therapeutic effects for various diseases by interfacing between drugs and food.

Thus, the need for watchful medicine has increased in priority in this fast-moving allopathic generation. The growth of nutraceuticals is significant because of its dire to adhere towards lavish lifestyle.

3.2 INTRODUCTION

Internationally, the market of nutraceuticals and functional foods has become a multi-million-dollar industry, and it is certain to grow exponentially. The selection of medicinal phytochemical constituents is limited, which has paved the way for the opening of nutraceuticals. Stephen DeFelice has coined the most descriptive term: "Nutraceuticals," which are defined as any material that can be classified as a food or a component of a food and has health and medical benefits,

DOI: 10.1201/9781003392934-3

such as the ability to avoid or alleviate disease. Nutritional and other health benefits of dietary supplements can fall into the category of *"before the drug, beyond the diet"* (Lakshmana Prabu et al. 2012).

The focus of the researchers has shifted towards this nutraceutical field which supports a preventive medical approach and also provides remedies for various sicknesses and illnesses.

The clinical test for the assessment of the therapeutic effectiveness of newly formulated pharmaceuticals can be bypassed as the result of utilizing this dietary nutrition as the constituent in the formulations.

3.3 POLYPHENOLIC COMPOUNDS

It has been reported that the literature survey on polyphenolic compounds comprising over 20000 published papers in this field showed that these Polyphenolic compounds have antioxidant, anti-inflammatory antibacterial, antifungal, anti-diabetic, antitumor activities, and for other chronic diseases (Tungmunnithum et al. 2018). Eight thousand phenolic compounds have been successfully identified from different plants in the last decade (Pandey et al. 2009).

The primary and foremost function of PC is the protection of plants or plant protection. A well-known antioxidant property of the polyphenol needs to be certified by the amount and frequency of consumption, chemical nature, bioavailability, and its metabolic pathways involved. The occurrence of Cardiovascular diseases tends to be lower in nations where the consumption of PC is higher. Dietary changes must be taken into account as part of a comprehensive approach to lowering the prevalence of these diseases.

The consumption of polyphenols via dietary complement remains strong in establishing good health.

3.4 POLYPHENOLS: AN ELIXIR FOR LONGEVITY

Polyphenols are secondary metabolites containing phenolic rings with two or more hydroxyl groups. Both phenols and polyphenols share common biosynthetic pathways such as shikimic acid and acetyl-CoA (Lacroix et al. 2015). The biosynthetic pathway is shown in Figure 3.1.

Acetate-derived phenols (Polyketides) typically have a meta-hydroxylation pattern, while shikimate-derived metabolites generally have a single hydroxyl group or poly-hydroxyl functions in para to the side-chain function (Chi et al. 2022).

3.4.1 Polyphenols as Nutritional Supplement

Compounds are exclusively derived from the shikimate/polyketide pathway with no nitrogen-based functions with more phenolic groups. "*L*-phenylalanine" is considered a key source of the polyphenol derivatives from nutritional supplements (Gollucke et al. 2015).

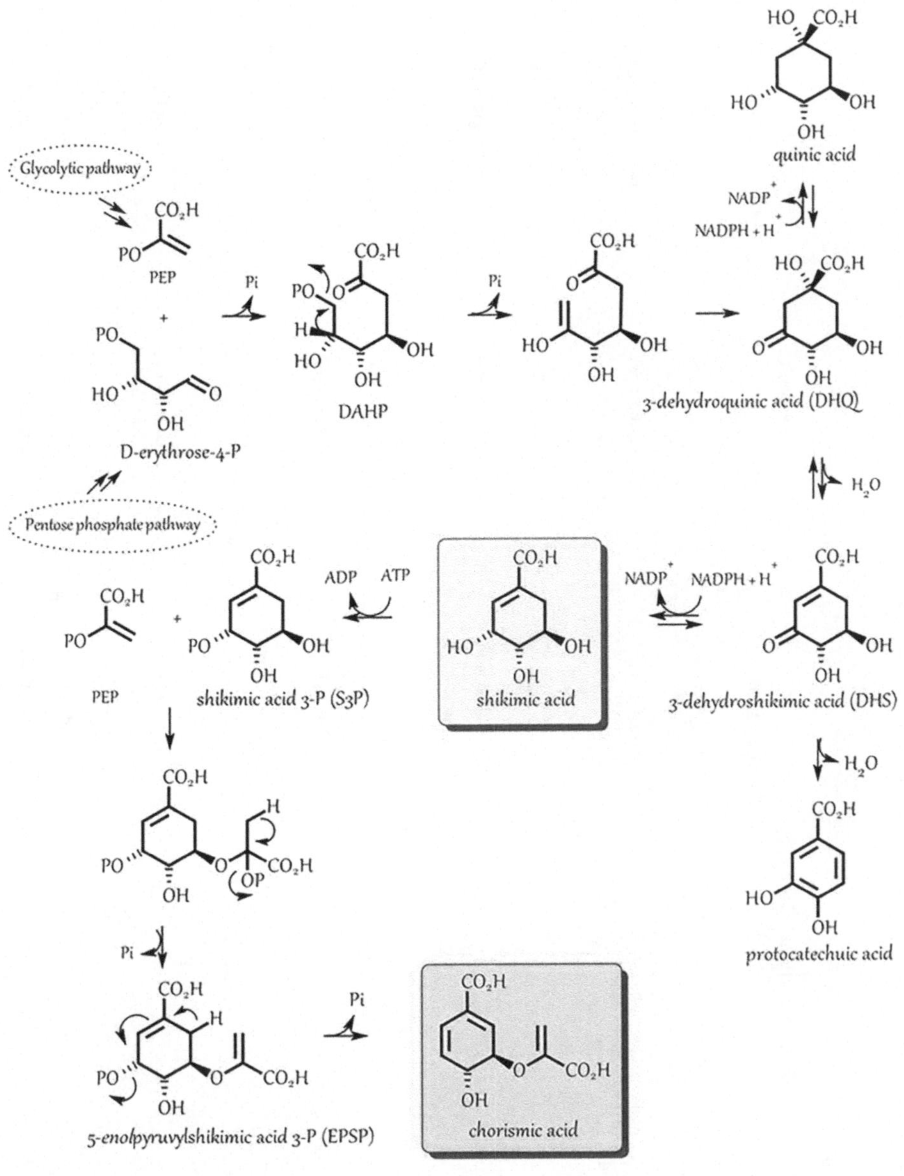

FIGURE 3.1 Shikimic acid pathway – Biosynthesis of phenolic compounds.

3.4.2 Classification

PCs are classified under different categories based on the position of the carbon in the main chain nucleus and their cyclization pattern. Classification of polyphenols is shown in (Chairez et al. 2001; Zhou et al. 2016; Marta et al. 2017; Silveira et al. 2019; Alotaibi et al 2021) Table 3.1.

TABLE 3.1
Classification of Polyphenols

S. No	Classification	Basic Functional Group	Examples		
			Phenolic Acids		
1	Hydroxycinnamic acid	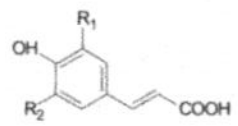	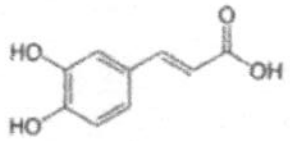 Caffeic acid	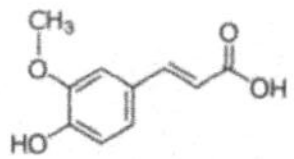 Ferulic acid	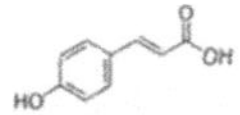 p-coumaric acid
2	Hydroxybenzoic acid	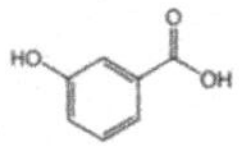	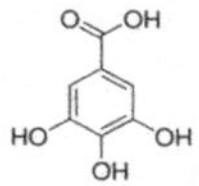 Gallic acid	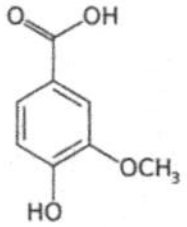 Vanillic acid	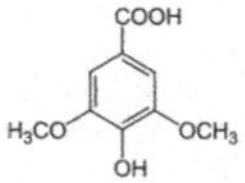 Syringic acid
			Flavonoids		
3	Flavanones	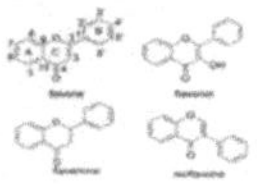	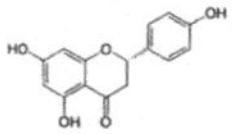 Naringenin	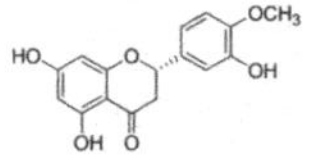 Hesperetin	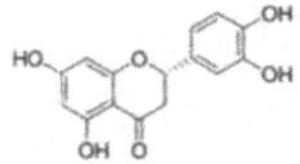 Eriodictyol
4	Flavones	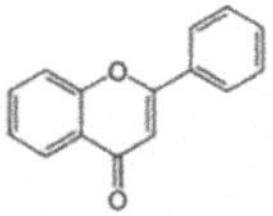	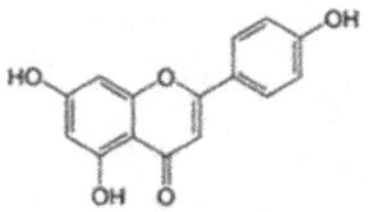 Apigenin	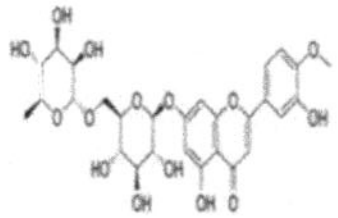 Diosmin	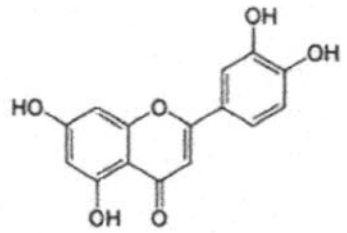 Luteolin
5	Isoflavones	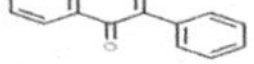	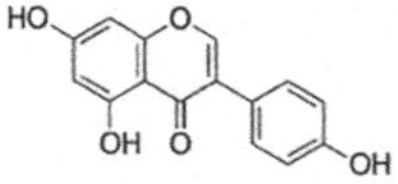 Genistein	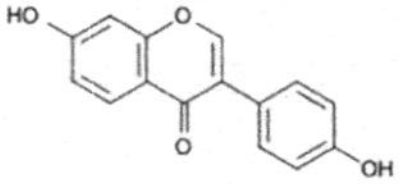 Daidzein	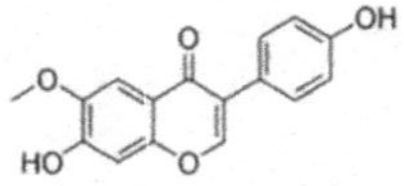 Glycitein

6	Flavonols	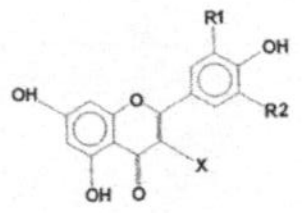	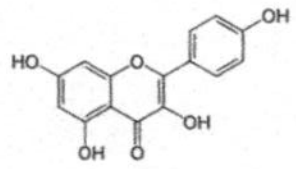 Kaempferol	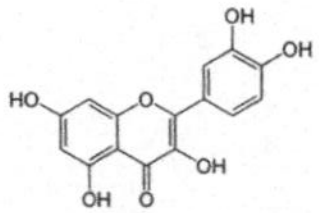 Quercetin	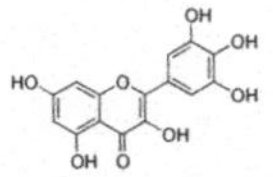 Myricetin
			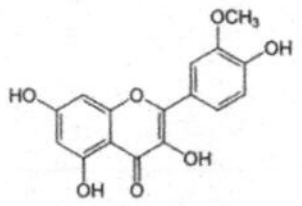 Isorhamnetin	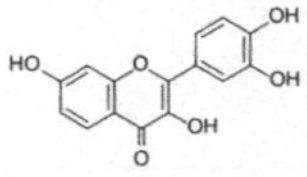 Fisetin	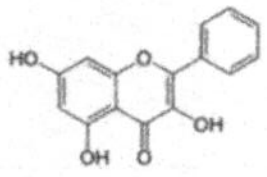 Galangin
7	Flavanols	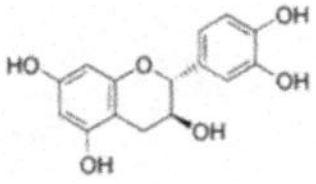	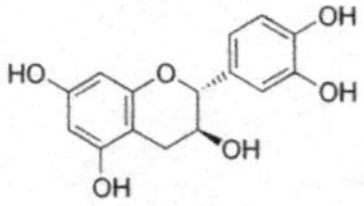 Catechin	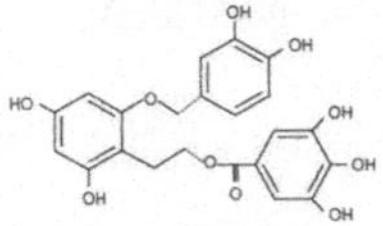 Epicatechins	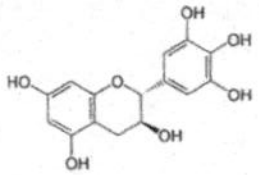 Gallocatechin
			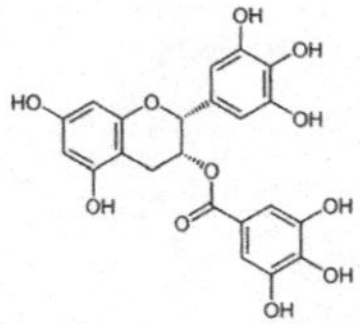 Epigallocatechin	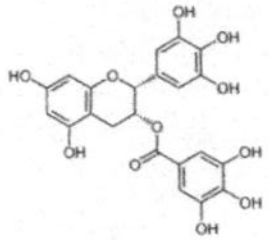 Epigallocatechin gallate	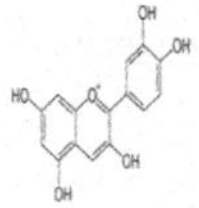 Cyanidin
8	Anthocyanidins	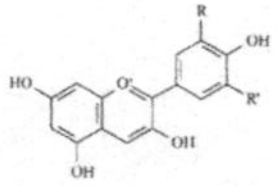	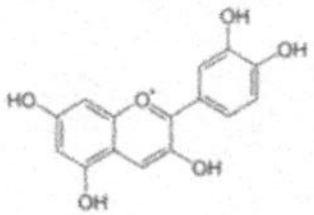 Cyanidin	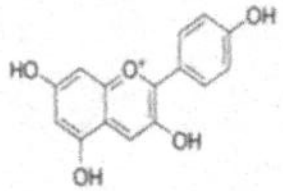 Pelargonidin	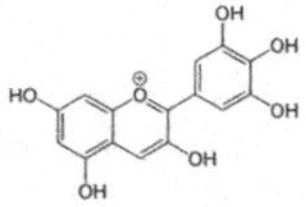 Delphinidin

(*Continued*)

TABLE 3.1 (Continued)
Classification of Polyphenols

			Non-Flavonoids		
9	Stilbenoids	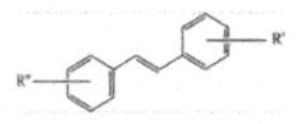	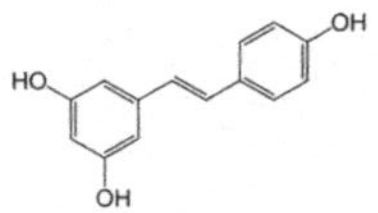 Resveratrol	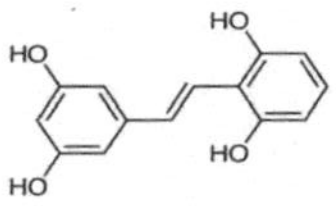 Gnetol	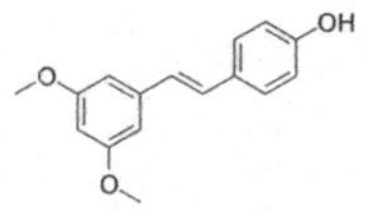 Pterostilbene
10	Lignans	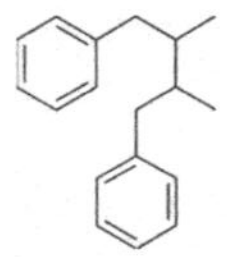	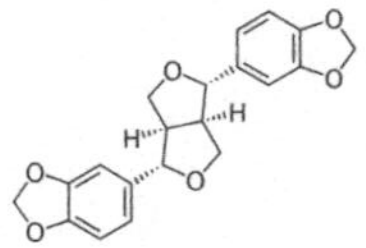 Sesamin	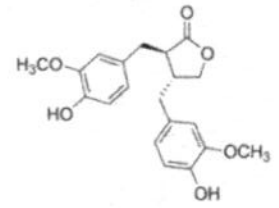 Matairesinol	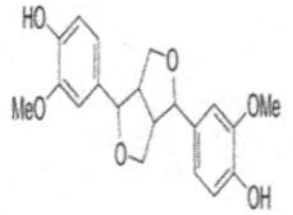 Pinoresinol
11	Tannins		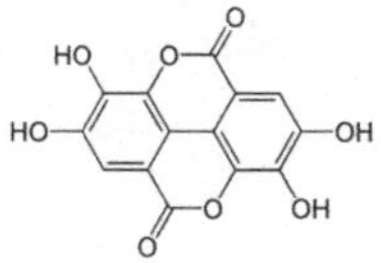 Ellagic acid	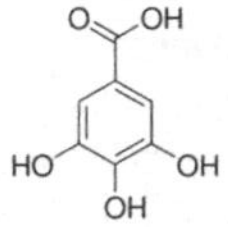 Gallic acid	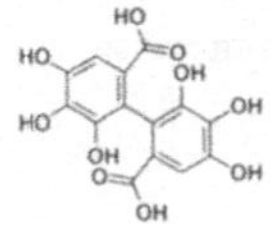 hexahydroxydiphenic acid

3.4.3 Importance of Microbiota Modulation in Polyphenol

The microbes in the gut have a significant role in modulation as well as the generation of bioactive metabolites. Huge proportions of dietary polyphenols remain unabsorbed in the GI tract due to their high molecular weight and complicated structure. Polyphenols maintain the healthy microbes in the gut region and also modulate the intestinal microbe's composition. These intestinal microbes metabolize the polyphenols into low-molecular-weight phenolic metabolites, which are bioactive and improve their bioavailability and bioactivity (Rodríguez et al. 2021).

3.5 CELLULAR MECHANISM – AN OVERVIEW

It is becoming more and more obvious that even though polyphenols can serve as generalized free-radical scavengers, the cellular mechanism behind its activities in human health may reside in three different areas:

a. Effect on gene expression in human cells
b. Effect on the gut microbiota
c. Ability to maintain mitochondrial health.

Polyphenols are secondary metabolites which are present abundantly in fruits, vegetables, nuts, and seeds.

As dietary supplements, polyphenols relieve many symptoms of metabolic syndrome (MtS), including obesity, dyslipidemia, atherosclerosis, and inhibit the genesis of pathophysiological perturbations in redox circuitry, elevated blood sugar, accelerating aging, liver intoxication, hypertension, and cancer by maintaining optimal cellular functions (Zhang et al. 2021).

However, the mechanism for its biological activities is mainly based on its:

1. Antioxidant
2. Anti-inflammatory.

3.5.1 Antioxidant

Intrinsic antioxidant properties of these compounds have been considered to inhibit diseases related to oxidative stress by giving an electron or preventing the lipoperoxidation chain reaction due to its ability to nullify, neutralize, or suppress free radicals (Fawole et al. 2016).

3.5.2 Anti-Inflammatory

Most second messengers (Protein kinases, cAMP, cCMP), transcription factors (NF-κB, AP-1 and proto-oncogenes) as well as other enzymes and substances (COX-2, iNOS), cytokines (IL-1, TNF-), neuropeptides, and proteases, are known to play a significant role in the regulation of inflammation (Yao et al. 2020).

Polyphenols have been found to inhibit inflammatory enzymes such as PLA2, COX-1, COX-2 and LOX, which leads to reduced proliferation of cells, angiogenesis, and immobilization of leukocytes and decreased 5-lipoxygenase enzyme activities. In addition, polyphenols' activation of PPAR-gamma, a peroxisome proliferator-activated receptor, is linked to their anti-inflammatory effects. Moreover, it suppresses the activity of cyclooxygenase 2 (COX2), prevents the formation of prostaglandin E2 (PGE2), and prevents (IκBα) degradation leading to NF-κB inactivation (Kim et al. 2003).

3.6 ROLE OF POLYPHENOLS IN MODERN LIFESTYLE DISORDERS

3.6.1 Anticancer

3.6.1.1 Prevalence of Cancer

In 2020, worldwide, about ten million deaths were recorded due to cancer. The American Cancer Society expects that in 2040, the global burden of new cancer cases will be around 27.5 million and cancer deaths around 16.3 [Global Cancer Facts & Figures].

Mechanisms for its anti-cancer activities are as follows:

- Cell adhesion and migration
- Arresting the cell cycle
- Regulating carcinogen metabolism and ontogenesis expression.

Polyphenols and phenolic-compound-rich dietary compounds or food supplements are significant in exerting antitumor activity. Briguglio et al. summarized the activity of polyphenols on various cancers such as colon cancer, prostate cancer, breast cancer, lung cancer, bladder cancer, skin cancer, pancreatic cancer, and Leukemia (Briguglio et al. 2020). They disrupt signaling pathways that prevent inflammation and cell proliferation, which leads to cell cycle arrest and cellular mortality.

In vitro studies have highlighted that these compounds activate Nrf2 and NF-κB in cells and can considerably impact the function of MAPK and PI3K in cells (Pacifico et al. 2016). Carnosol is a polyphenol that has cancer cell inhibition properties. An in vivo investigation study in a BC cell line showed that this substance decreases proliferation and prevents metastasis and invasion (Zhang et al. 2015).

The polyphenols having anti-cancer activities are Delphinidin, cyanidin, procyanidins, naringenin, chrysin, luteolin, genistein, myricetin, gallic acid, naringenin, ellagic acid, daidzein, xanthohumol, sesamin, pterostilbene, piceatannol, and Hesperetin (Chairez et al. 2001; Zhou et al. 2016; Vladu et al. 2022; Maleki et al. 2022).

3.6.2 Anti-Diabetic

3.6.2.1 Prevalence of Diabetes

A major cause of mortality and shorter life expectancy is diabetes mellitus. In 2019, about 437.9 million worldwide were affected by Type 2 diabetes. Prevalence based on an age-standardized point showed 5282.9 cases per 100,000 people, which is an increment of 49% since 1990 (Safiri et al. 2022).

Mechanisms for its anti-diabetic activity are as follows:

- Dietary polyphenols inhibit glucose absorption
- Inhibit digestive enzymes
- Regulate insulin secretion by stimulating the pancreas
- Protection of pancreatic islet cells
- Attenuate oxidative stress
- Blockage of glucose absorption (Kim et al. 2008; Aryaeian et al. 2017).

In Type 2 diabetes mellitus (T2DM), cAMP is crucial for maintaining the general health of pancreatic cells as well as glucose and incretin-stimulated insulin production. Dietary polyphenols from plant-based foods including fruits, vegetables, whole grains, coffee, tea, and nuts are used to reduce the risk of T2DM. Polyphenols as antioxidants have a beneficial role in improving the health effects against diabetes in view of ROS,. production of ROS by inducing hypoxia at the electron transport chain in mitochondria, which leads to inflammatory response activation.

Polyphenols having anti-diabetic activity are quercetin, kaempferol, myricetin, hesperetin, and naringenin luteolin, quercetin, genistein, and gallic acid, Curcumin, Resveratrol, flavanols that contain catechin (C), epicatechin (EC), gallocatechin (GC), epigallocatechin (EGC), and their gallates (Silveira et al. 2019; Aryaeian et al. 2017; Da Porto et al. 2021; Nie et al. 2021).

3.6.3 Cardiovascular Disease

3.6.3.1 Prevalence of Cardiovascular Diseases

In 2019, WHO stated that cardiovascular diseases were the leading cause of death globally and estimated the fact that approximately about 17.9 million people died, which represented 32% of all global deaths. This statistical evidence says that cardiovascular diseases are the most prominent among lifestyle diseases. The mechanisms for protection against cardiovascular diseases are as follows:

- Improve endothelial function
- Inhibit platelet aggregation.

There is strong evidence that polyphenols are effective, limit the occurrence of coronary heart diseases, and act at the molecular level to enhance endothelial function and prevent the aggregation of platelets. These substances play an essential role in the prevention and treatment of cardiovascular disease due to their antithrombic, anti-aggregative, and anti-inflammatory properties. The relationship between the consumption of polyphenol and the incidence of cardiovascular illnesses was investigated and the results show that polyphenols exert antithrombotic effects by inhibiting platelet aggregation, which leads to reducing the risk of CVD.

Polyphenols used to reduce the risk of CVDs are resveratrol, epigallocatechin gallate (EGCG), curcumin, and quercetin (Alotaibi et al. 2021; Michalska et al. 2010; Vita et al. 2005).

3.6.4 Anti-Obesity

3.6.4.1 Prevalence of Obesity

In 2025, WHO projects that 167 million people will be less healthy due to obesity, which is about 39 million, 650 million, 760 million, and 1 billion children. Sedentary lifestyles and less healthy diet consumption have made obesity reach the pandemic dimension due to a triplicate rise in the last two to three decades.

Anti-obesity of these polyphenols is associated with action on enzymes.

Mechanisms for its anti-obesity are as follows:

- Energy expenditure
- Appetite suppression
- Adipocyte differentiation
- Lipid metabolism.

Polyphenols that have anti-obesity activity include catechin, chlorogenic acid, coumaric acid, gallic acid, quercetin, resveratrol, rutin, curcumin, epigallocatechin-3-gallate, genistein, Isoflavones, ellagitannins, Proanthocyanidin, piceatannol, and epigallocatechin-3-gallate (Singh et al. 2020; Clodoveo et al. 2021; Wang et al. 2014; Boccellino et al. 2020). Different polyphenols that are used in treating modern lifestyle diseases are shown in (Chairez et al. 2001; Vladu et al. 2022; Aryaeian et al. 2017; Da Porto et al. 2021; Nie et al. 2021; Vita et al. 2005; Meydani et al. 2010; Singh et al. 2020; Clodoveo et al. 2021; Wang et al. 2014; Dasha et al. 2018) Table 3.2.

3.7 TOXICITY

Recent awareness about polyphenol's biological benefits among human beings helped some consume plant-based foods and beverages in their diet regularly. However, a few investigational studies highlighted that some of the polyphenols are not absorbed effectively due to their high molecular weight and toxicity. Hence, optimum amounts of PP need to be utilized to get the health promoting benefits effectively. Examining the toxicity potential of these polyphenolics has been considered an important parameter.

Earlier toxicity studies highlighted that a high dose of some polyphenols can have genotoxic effects due to their prooxidant properties (Snyder et al. 2002; Catterall et al. 2000). *In vivo* animal studies on 2% of caffeic acid outlined that it induces kidney and forestomach tumors (Hagiwara et al. 1991). Estradiol may induce renal tumors by postulating the catechol estrogens. Whereas quercetin increases 2- and 4-hydroxyestrodiol in the kidney by preventing the O-methylation of catechol estrogens, which leads to redox catechol estrogens cycling. In addition,

TABLE 3.2
Polyphenols in Modern Lifestyle Disorders

		Anti-Cancer	
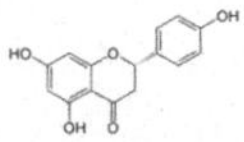	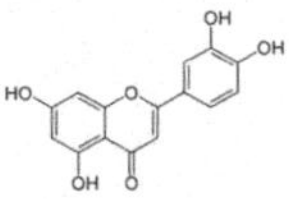	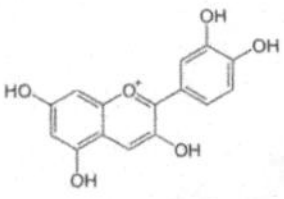	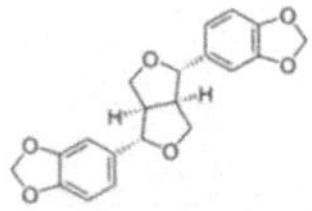
Naringenin	**Luteolin**	**Procyanidins**	**Sesamin**
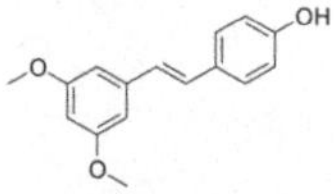	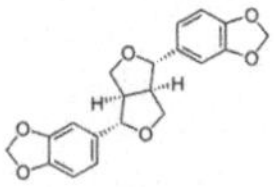	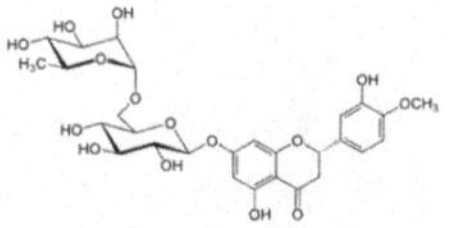	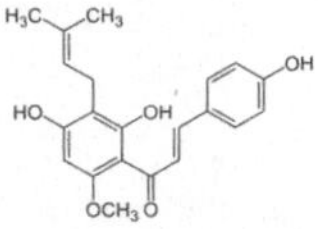
Pterostilbene	**Sesamin**	**Hesperidin**	**Xanthohumol**
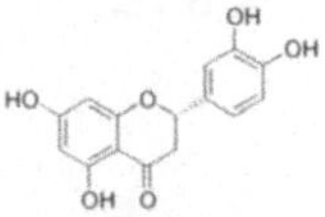	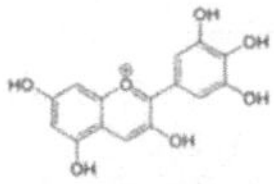	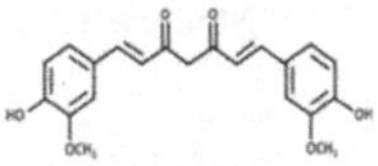	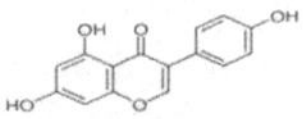
Eridictyol	**Delphinidin**	**Curcumin**	**Genistein**
		Anti-Obesity	
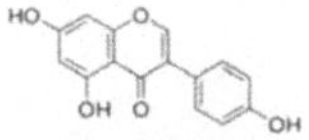	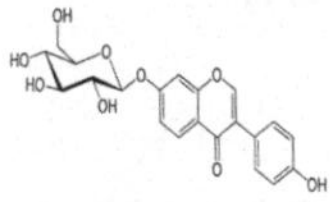	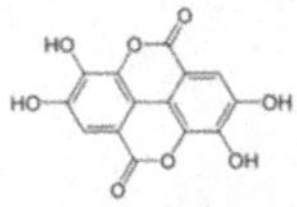	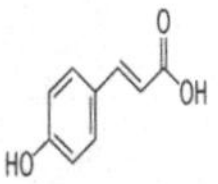
Genistein	**Daidzein**	**Ellagic Acid**	**Coumaric Acid**
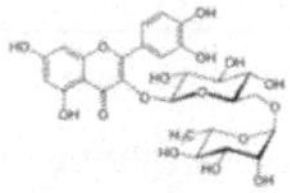	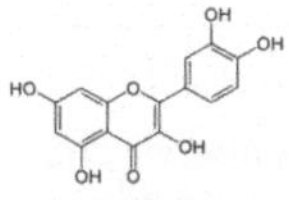	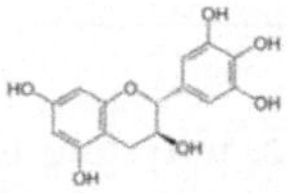	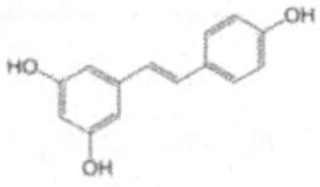
Rutin	**Quercetin**	**Gallocatechin (GC)**	**Resveratrol**
		Cardiovascular Disease Management	
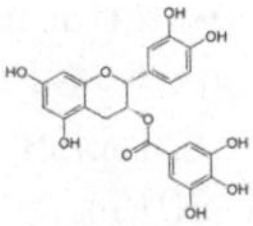	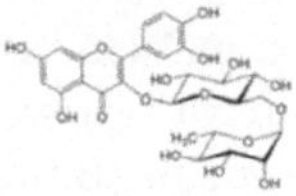	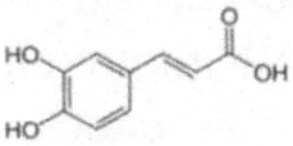	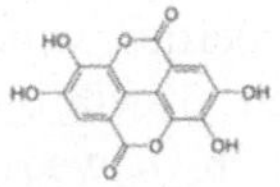
Epicatechin	**Rutin**	**Caffeic Acid**	**Ellagic Acid**
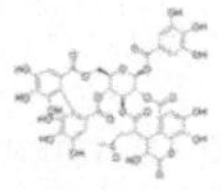	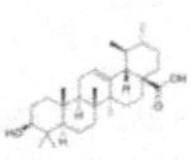	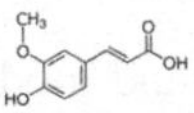	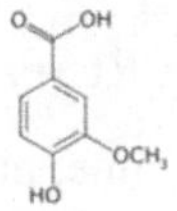
Chebulagic Acid	**Ursolic Acid**	**Ferulic Acid**	**Vanillic Acid**
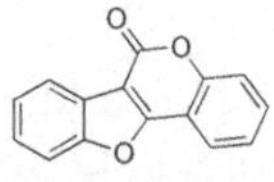	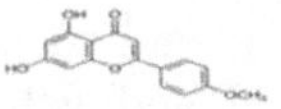	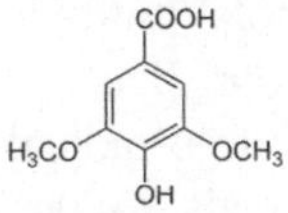	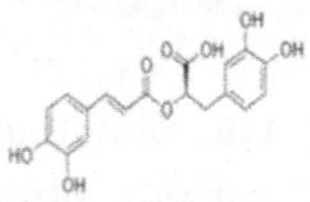
Cousmestan	**Acacetin**	**Syringic Acid**	**Rosmarinic Acid**

(Continued)

TABLE 3.2 (Continued)
Polyphenols in Modern Lifestyle Disorders

	Anti-Diabetic		
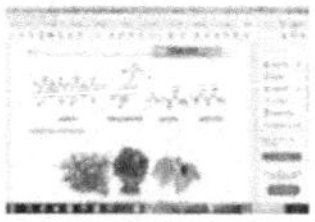	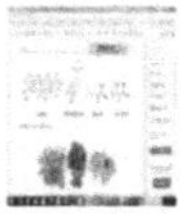	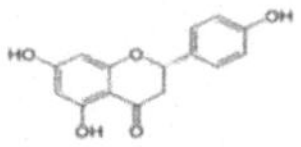	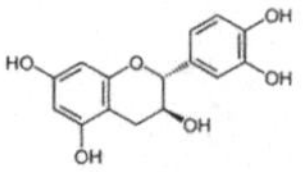
Acarbose	**Andrographolide**	**Naringenin**	**Catechin**
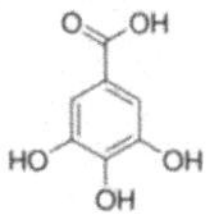	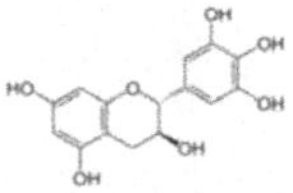	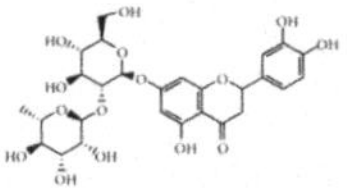	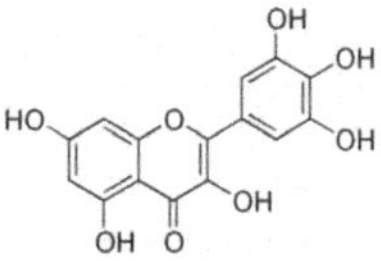
Gallic Acid	**Gallocatechin**	**Naringeni Luteolin**	**Myricetin**
	Modern Lifestyle Disorders		
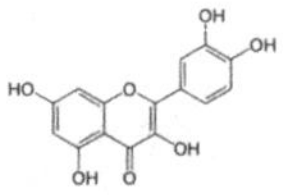	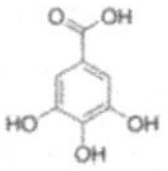	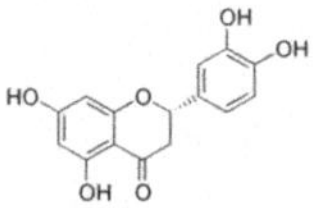	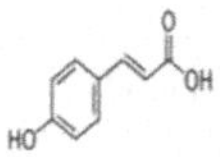
Quercetin	**Gallic Acid**	**Eridictyol**	**Coumaric Acid**
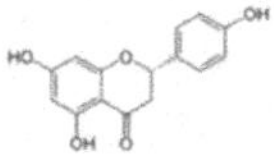	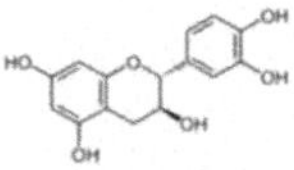	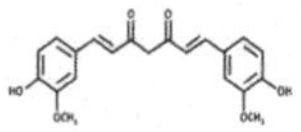	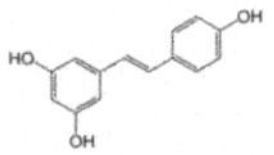
Naringenin	**Catechin**	**Curcumin**	**Resveratrol**

quercetin has prooxidant toxicity due to the presence of rich oxidative enzymes in tissues (Zhu et al. 1996). Few flavonoids under polyphenol restrict the biosynthesis of thyroid hormone by preventing thyroid peroxidase (Doerge and Chang 2002). In animal nutrition, Proanthocyanidin and ellagitannins are considered anti-nutritional properties, which inhibit several enzyme activities that lead to digestion as well as their growth by interaction with proteins. Kaempferol is a well-known polyphenol which showed cytotoxicity on mitochondria and nuclei (Boncler et al. 2017).

3.8 RESEARCH NECESSITY

Over time, more researchers and food manufacturers have developed a huge interest in polyphenols and its natural sources. The key driver of this interest is the understanding of polyphenols' antioxidant qualities and the substantial portions in which they are present in our diets.

The abundance of the free-radical-scavenging and metal-chelating activities of various polyphenols needs to be investigated and validated thoroughly for effectiveness. Cooking vegetables can damage the polyphenol properties due to diffusion into the surrounding media, which may lead to poor stability and bioavailability that drastically reduce their effectiveness (Santangelo et al. 2007). Cooking has a damaging effect on polyphenols in vegetables, resulting in a huge loss of polyphenols, likely due to diffusion into boiling water.

In the near future, isolation of polyphenols by complementary methods, and its investigational studies in humans, need to be performed to understand their bioavailability, safety, efficacy, and the mechanism for therapeutic benefits in humans to bridge the gap between nutraceuticals and their therapeutic health benefits.

3.9 CONCLUSION

From ancient times, human beings both actively and passively devoured natural products as a part of their regular diet. Rapid industrialization, advancement, environmental pollution, and lifestyle changes played an important role in the progress of several health disorders among human beings. Lately, there has been increased consumption of natural foods that have expressively reduced several health disorders. Different natural foods, understanding abundance knowledge, and the effectiveness of polyphenols have been recognized for the treatment and management of certain chronic diseases. Hence, Polyphenolic food and beverages have been consistently taken in their day-to-day life as a regular diet.

The majority of polyphenols are present in nutritious, plant-based foods like vegetables and fruits, therefore, recommendations for consumption need to be integrated with existing programs in nutrition education and advice for promoting a balanced diet.

The main mechanism behind health benefits is the reduction of oxidative stress due to antioxidant activity, either direct or indirect. The nutraceutical products are considered a complimentary therapy which is reliable and useful as a supplementary supportive therapy in preventing various modern lifestyle disorders. The growth of interest in medicinal and aromatic plants among human beings can be fulfilled by chemical profiling using advanced techniques to share new knowledge about these polyphenol compositions and their therapeutic benefits.

At last, *"healthy lifestyle and proper balanced diet are essentially needed for the effective wellbeing with health promoting benefits."*

REFERENCES

Alotaibi, B.S., Ijaz, M., Buabeid, M., Kharaba, Z.J., Yaseen, H.S., & Murtaza, G. (2021). Therapeutic effects and safe uses of plant-derived polyphenolic compounds in cardiovascular diseases: A review. *Drug Design, Development and Therapy*, 15, 4713–4732.

Aryaeian, N., Khorshidi Sedehi, S., & Arablou, T. (2017). Polyphenols and their effects on diabetes management: A review. *Medical Journal of the Islamic Republic of Iran (MJIRI)*, 26(31), 134.

Aryaeian, N., Sedehi, S.K., & Arablou, T. (2017). Polyphenols and their effects on diabetes management: A review. *Medical Journal of The Islamic Republic of Iran (MJIRI)*, 26(31), 134.

Boccellino, M., & Angelo, S.D. (2020). Anti-obesity effects of polyphenol intake: Current status and future possibilities. *International Journal of Molecular Sciences*, 21(16), 5642.

Boncler, M., Golanski, J., Lukasiak, M., Redzynia, M., Dastych, J., & Watala, C. (2017). A new approach for the assessment of the toxicity of polyphenol-rich compounds with the use of high content screening analysis. *PLoS One*, 12(6), e0180022.

Briguglio, G., Costa, C., Pollicino, M., Giambo, F., Catania, S., & Fenga, C. (2020). Polyphenols in cancer prevention: New insights (Review). *International Journal of Functional Nutrition*, 1, 9.

Cardiovascular diseases (CVDs). World Health Organization. https://www.who.int/news-room/fact-sheets/detail/cardiovascular-diseases-(cvds) (accessed January 12, 2023).

Catterall, F., Souquet, J.M., & Cheynier, V. (2000). Differential modulation of the genotoxicity of food carcinogens by naturally occurring monomeric and dimeric polyphenolics. *Enviromental and Molecular Mutagenesis*, 35, 86–98.

Chairez, M.H., Cruz, K.G., & García, A. (2001). Polyphenols as antitumor agents targeting key players in cancer-driving signaling pathways. *Frontiers in Pharmacology*, 12, 710304.

Chi, I.V., Thirumurugan, R., Marvin, M., & Slavko, K. (2022). All polyphenols are not created equal: Exploring the diversity of phenolic metabolite. *Journal of Agricultural and Food Chemistry*, 70, 2077–2091.

Clodoveo, M.L., Cariello, M., Amato, G.D., Franchino, C., Faienza, M.F. et al. (2021). Polyphenols and obesity prevention: critical insights on molecular regulation, bioavailability and dose in preclinical and clinical settings. *Critical Reviews in Food Science and Nutrition*, 61(11), 1804–1826.

Da Porto, A., Cavarape, A., Colussi, G., Casarsa, V., Catena, C., & Sechi, L.A. (Apr 24 2021). Polyphenols rich diets and risk of type 2 diabetes. *Nutrients*, 13(5), 1445.

Dasha, M., Aneta, P., Iordanka, A., Albert, K., & Anna, L. (2018). Polyphenols as suitable control for obesity and diabetes. *The Open Biotechnology Journal*, 12, 219–222.

Doerge, D.R., & Chang, H.C. (2002). Inactivation of thyroid peroxidase by soy Isoflavones, *in vitro* and *in vivo*. *Journal of Chromatography B: Analytical Technologies in the Biomedical and Life Sciences*, 777, 269–279.

Fawole, O.A., & Opara, U.L. (2016). Stability of total phenolic concentration and antioxidant capacity of extracts from pomegranate co-products subjected to *in vitro* digestion. *BMC Complementary and Alternative Medicine*, 16, 358.

Global Cancer Facts & Figures. American Cancer Society. https://www.cancer.org/research/cancer-facts-statistics/global.html (accessed January 10, 2023).

Gollucke, A.P., Peres, R.C., Odair, A., & Ribeiro, D.A. (2015). Polyphenols: a nutraceutical approach against diseases. *Recent Patents on Food, Nutrition & Agriculture*, 5(3), 214–219.

Hagiwara, A., Hirose, M., Takahashi, S., Ogawa, K., Shirai, T., & Ito, N. (1991). Forestomach and kidney carcinogenicity of caffeic acid in F344 rats and C57BL/6N C3H/HeN F1 mice. *Cancer Research*, 51, 5655–5660.

Kim, C.S., Kawada, T., Kim, B.S., Han, I.S., Choe, S.Y., Kurata, T., et al. (2003). Capsaicin exhibits anti-inflammatory property by inhibiting IkB-a degradation in LPS-stimulated peritoneal macrophages. *Cellular Signaling*, 15(3), 299–306.

Kim, Y.S., Young, M.R., Bobe, G., Colburn, N.H., & Milner, J.A. (2008). Bioactive food components, inflammatory targets, and cancer prevention. *Cancer Prevention Research*, 2(3), 200–208.

Lacroix, S., Lauria, M., Scott, M.P., Marchetti, L., Priami, C., & Caberlotto, L. (2015). Systems biology approaches to study the molecular effects of caloric restriction and polyphenols on aging processes. *Genes & Nutrition*, 10(6), 1–10.

Lakshmana Prabu, S., Suriyaprakash, T.N.K., Dinesh Kumar, C., Suresh Kumar, S., & Ragavendran, T. (2012). Nutraceuticals: A review. *Elixir Pharmacy*, 46, 8372–8377.

Maleki, P., Sadoughi, F., Asemi, Z., & Yousefi, B. (2022). The role of polyphenols in overcoming cancer drug resistance: A comprehensive review. *Cellular & Molecular Biology Letters*, 27(1). https://doi.org/10.1186/s11658-021-00301-9

Maria, G.V.G., Vera, E.C., Vilma, M.J., & Carla, H.A.S. (2018). Impact of human aging and modern lifestyle on gut microbiota. *Critical Reviews in Food Science and Nutrition*, 58(9), 1557–1564.

Marta, G.F., Jordi, M., Qi, S., Montse, F., & Jordi, S.S. (2017). Dietary polyphenols, mediterranean diet, prediabetes, and type 2 diabetes: A narrative review of the evidence. *Oxidative Medicine and Cellular Longevity*, 1–16. 10.1155/2017/6723931

Meydani, M., & Hasan, S.T. (2010). Dietary polyphenols and obesity. *Nutrients*, 2(7), 737–751.

Michalska, M., Gluba, A., Mikhailidis, D.P., Nowak, P., Bielecka, A., Rysz, J., & Banach, M. (2010). The role of polyphenols in cardiovascular disease. *Medical Science Monitor: International Medical Journal of Experimental and Clinical Research*, 16(5), 110–119.

Nie, T., & Cooper, G.J.S. (2021). Mechanisms underlying the antidiabetic activities of olyphenolic compounds: A review. *Frontiers in Pharmacology*, 2021, 12.

Pacifico, S., Piccolella, S., Papale, F., Nocera, P., Lettieri, A., & Catauro, M.A. (2016). Polyphenol complex from *Thymus vulgaris* L. plants cultivated in the Campania Region (Italy): New perspectives against neuroblastoma. *Journal of Functional Foods*, 20, 253–266.

Pandey, K.B., & Rizvi, S.I. (2009). Plant polyphenols as dietary antioxidants in human health and disease. *Oxidative Medicine and Cellular Longevity*, 2(5), 270–278.

Rodríguez, M.C., Mateos, E.C.P., Meilleur, J.L., Guyonnet, D., Desjardins, Y., & Roy, D. (2021). Polyphenol-mediated gut microbiota modulation: Toward prebiotics and further. *Frontier in Nutrition*, 8, 689456.

Safiri, S., Karamzad, N., Kaufman, J.S., Bell, A.W., Nejadghaderi, S.A., Sullman, M.J.M. et al. (2022). Prevalence, deaths and disability-adjusted-life-years (DALYs) due to type 2 diabetes and its attributable risk factors in 204 countries and territories, 1990–2019: Results from the global burden of disease study 2019. *Frontiers in Endocrinology*, 13, 838027.

Santangelo, C., Vari, R., Scazzocchio, B., Benedetto, R., Filesi, C., & Masella, R. (2007). Polyphenols, intracellular signaling and inflammation. *Annali dell Istituto Superiore di Sanita*, 43(4), 394–405.

Silveira, A.C., Dias, J.P., Santos, V.M., Oliveira, P.F., Alves, M.G., Rato, L., et al. (2019). The action of polyphenols in diabetes mellitus and Alzheimer's disease: A common agent for overlapping pathologies. *Current Neuropharmacology*, 17(7), 590–613.

Singh, M., Thrimawithana, T., Shukla, R., & Adhikari, B. (2020). Managing obesity through natural polyphenols: A review. *Future Foods*, 1–2, 100002.

Snyder, R.D., & Gillies, P.J. (2002). Evaluation of the clastogenic, DNA intercalative, and topoisomerase II-interactive properties of bioflavonoids in Chinese hamster V79 cells. *Environmental and Molecular Mutagenesis*, 40, 266–276.

Tungmunnithum, D., Thongboonyou, A., Pholboon, A., & Yangsabai, A. (2018). Flavonoids and other phenolic compounds from medicinal plants for pharmaceutical and medical aspects: An overview. *Medicines (Basel)*, 5(3), 93.

Vita, J.A. (2005). Polyphenols and cardiovascular disease: effects on endothelial and platelet function. *The American Journal of Clinical Nutrition*, 81(1), 292S–297S

Vladu, A.F., Ficai, D., Ene, A.G., & Ficai, A. (2022). Combination therapy using polyphenols: An efficient way to improve anti tumoral activity and reduce resistance. *International Journal of Molecular Sciences*, 23, 10244.

Wang, S., Moustaid, N., Chen, L., Mo, H., Shastri, A., Su, R., et al. (2014). Novel insights of dietary polyphenols and obesity. *The Journal of Nutritional Biochemistry*, 25(1), 1–18.

Yao, Y., Wang, H., Xu, F., Zhang, Y., Li, Z., Ju, X., et al. (2020). Insoluble-bound polyphenols of adlay seed ameliorates H_2O_2 induced oxidative stress in HepG2 cells via Nrf2 signaling. *Food Chemistry*, 325, 126865.

Zhang, B., Ge, C., Yao, J., Liu, Y., Xie, H., & Fang, J. (2015). Selective selenol fluorescent probes: Design, synthesis, structural determinants, and biological applications. *Journal of the American Chemical Society*, 137(2), 757–769.

Zhang, S., Xu, M., Zhang, W., Liu, C., & Chen, S. (2021). Natural polyphenols in metabolic syndrome: Protective mechanisms and clinical applications. *International Journal of Molecular Sciences*, 22(11), 6110.

Zhou, Y., Zheng, J., Li, Y., Xu, D.P., Li, S., Chen, Y.M., et al. (2016). Natural polyphenols for prevention and treatment of cancer. *Nutrients*, 8(8), 515.

Zhu, B.T., & Liehr, J.G. (1996). Inhibition of catechol O-methyltransferase-catalyzed O-methylation of 2- and 4-hydroxyestradiol by quercetin: possible role in estradiol-induced tumorigenesis. *Journal of Biological Chemistry*, 271, 1357–1363.

4 Nutraceuticals for Cancer Management

A. Umamaheswari, A. Puratchikody, K. A. Pavithran, S. N. Jegasubramaniam, and Dinesh Kumar Chellappan

4.1 INTRODUCTION

Among the different diseases, cancer has been considered the most common disease in the world. Worldwide, tens of millions of people have cancer detected every year, and more than half of those individuals succumb to the disease. In many countries, cancer is the second-most prevalent cause of death. Anticancer medications have side effects that affect early detection of cancer, survival, and recovery. Lifestyle modification, including dietary supplements, could prevent over two-thirds of human cancer cases. Natural bioactive compounds contain anticancer properties which can produce better efficacy when used with conventional drugs (Sherman et al. 2020). Developed nations are recognizing and rapidly increasing the use of complementary and alternative medicine (CAM) for cancer patients due to the high mortality and long-term morbidity associated with surgery and chemotherapy.

4.2 NUTRACEUTICALS

Nutraceuticals are natural bioactive products with both food value and therapeutic activities for various diseases, enhancing human health by curing or preventing them. The term "Nutraceuticals" was coined by Dr. Stephen DeFelice in 1989 (Ranzato et al. 2014). "A food or part of a food that grants and nourishes health as well as its nutritional content" is what the term "nutraceutical" refers to (Santini et al. 2017). Bioactive compounds directly (acting on molecular targets) or indirectly (influencing metabolic pathways) mediate the health benefits (Ranzato et al. 2014).

Particularly, nutraceuticals can act on the cancer cell in three ways:

i. inhibition of cell proliferation
ii. antioxidant activity
iii. anti-inflammatory activity (Maiuolo et al. 2021).

The common pathogenesis of cancer and the different cancer inhibition mechanisms (Bagchi et al. 2015) are shown in Figures 4.1 and 4.2 respectively.

DOI: 10.1201/9781003392934-4

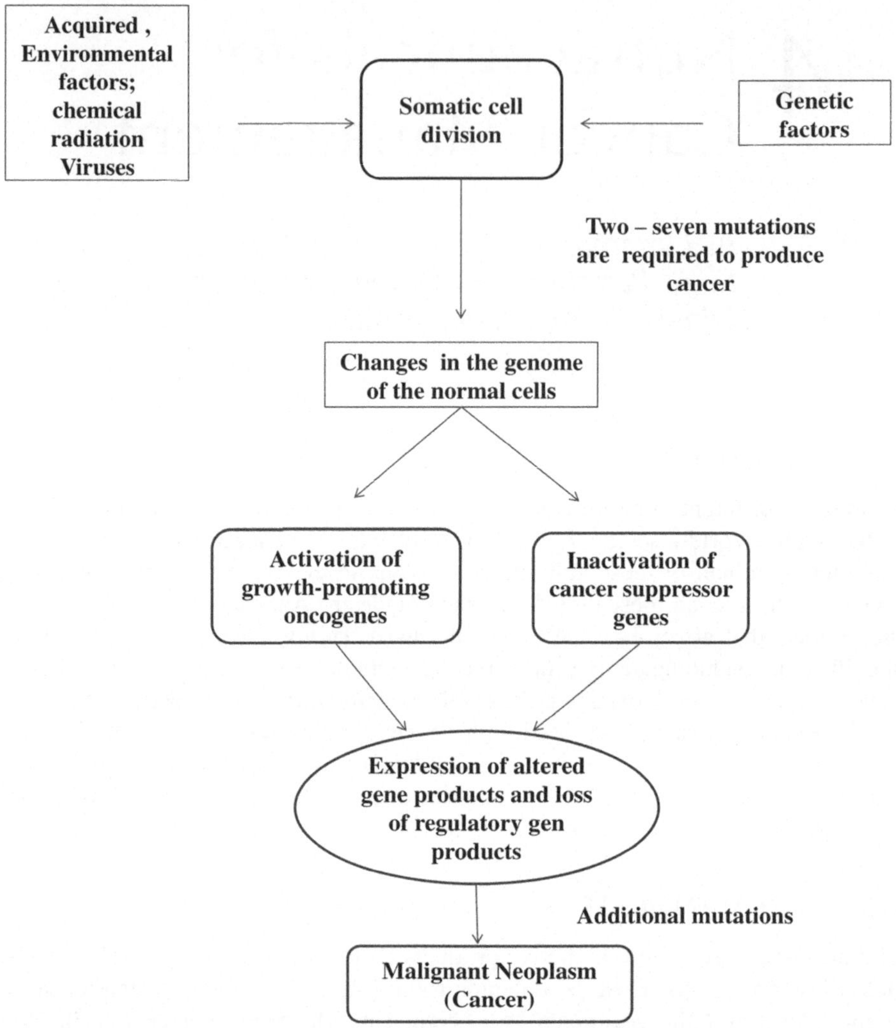

FIGURE 4.1 Common pathogenesis of cancer.

Several nutraceutical compounds have anticancer activity through different molecular targets are summarized in Tables 4.1 and 4.2.

4.3 CONTRIBUTION – PHYTOCHEMICALS AS NUTRACEUTICALS

Over 60% of permitted anticancer drugs are from natural sources that possess multitarget action and low toxicity. Phytochemicals are identified as anticancer modulators in different cellular signalling pathways. Understanding the phytoconstituents effectiveness is essential during specific medication by nutraceuticals (González-Vallinas et al. 2013).

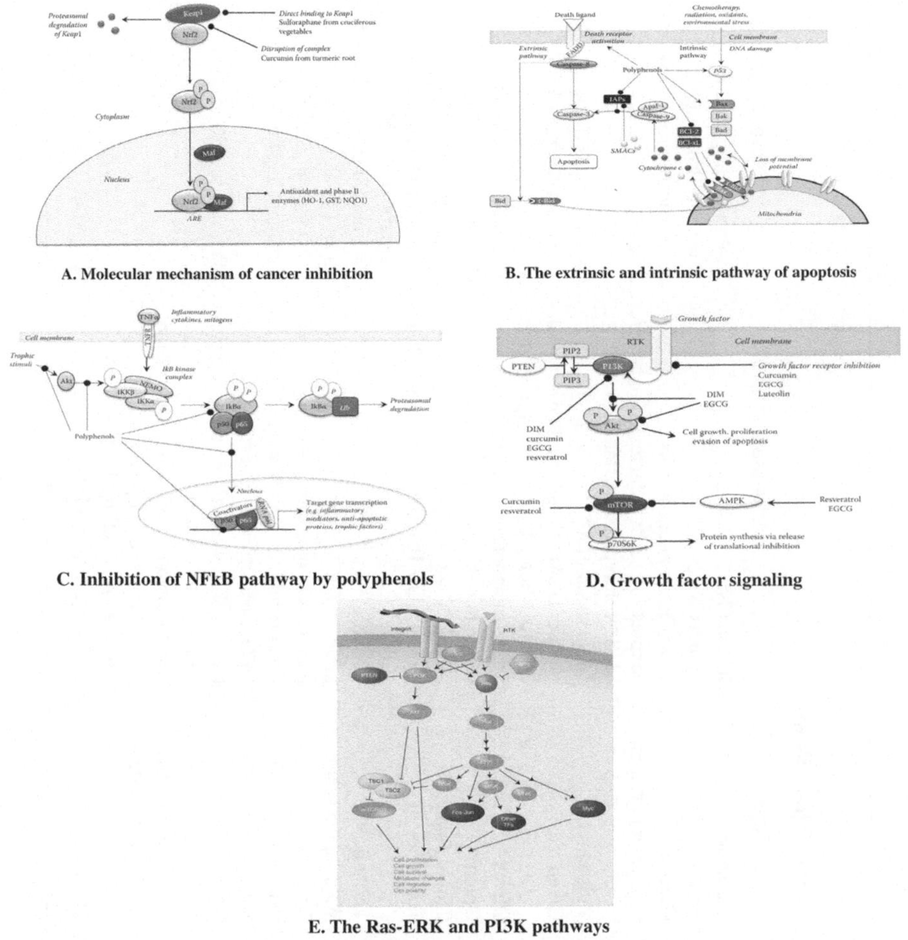

FIGURE 4.2 Nutraceuticals – Molecular targets of cancer regulation.

Phytoconstituents exhibit anticancer properties and prevent cancer cells at various stages such as cell proliferation, apoptosis, invasion and metastasis, angiogenesis, immortality, inflammation, genomic instability, mutation, cell energetics, and metabolism (Maiuolo et al. 2021).

4.4 POLYPHENOLS

Polyphenols are bioactive molecules found in fruits and vegetables. They include Anacardic acid, Caffeic acid, Chlorogenic acid, Ellagic acid, Gallic acid, and Rosmarinic acid, which are used for cancer treatment and anti-nutrients (González-Vallinas et al. 2013).

Study results highlighted that polyphenolic compounds significantly contribute to the proliferation of cancer cells by modulating Nrf2 and NF-B activation in cells.

TABLE 4.1
Molecular Targets of Nutraceuticals Compounds and Their Role

S.No	Molecular Target	Compound	Source	Mechanisms	Reference
1.	Oxidant and Xenobiotic Defence	Curcumin	Turmeric	Inhibits Nrf2, stat3	Sever and Brugge (2015)
		Sulforaphane	Broccoli	Inhibits Nrf2	Sever and Brugge (2015)
2	Apoptosis	Polyphenols	Green tea	↑ Bcl-2 in malignant cells	Sever and Brugge 2015)
		Gossypol	Gossypiumhirsutum-L.	↑expression of BCL2 interacting protein 3, TNF receptor superfamily 9	Alharbi et al. (2022)
		Resveratrol	Vitis vinifera	Suppression of TNF-α and IL-17	Calvani et al. (2020)
3	Epigenome	Polyphenols	Green tea	Inhibits DNMT1, 3a, and 3b expression, ↓ hats and alters miRNA expression	Sever and Brugge (2015)
		Oleuropein	Olives	Modifies apoptosis gene expression	Maiuolo et al. (2021)
		Quercetin	Onion	Reversion of epigenetic alterations	Calvani et al. (2020)
4	Inflammatory signalling	Eugenol	Clove, cinnamon	Inhibits COX-2	Aggarwal et al. (2009)
		Curcumin	Turmeric	NF-κb and AP-1 activation, ↓TGF-β and COX-2	Calvani et al. (2020); Alharbi et al. (2022)
5	Growth factor signalling	Curcumin	Turmeric	↓ EGFR	Shanmugalingam et al. (2016)
		Betulinic acid	Wild jujube seeds	Inhibits VEGF signalling	Alharbi et al. (2022)
6	Angiogenesis	Curcumin	Turmeric	Promotes tumour suppressor p53	Calvani et al. (2020)
		Omega-3 pufas	Flaxseed	Downregulating angiopoietin-2 (Ang-2)	Shanmugalingam et al. (2016)
		Genistein	Soy	VEGF, MMPS, and EGFR	
7	Cell proliferation	Resveratrol	Vitis vinifera	Inhibits Wnt β-catenin pathway, suppress S phase accumulation	Alharbi et al. (2022)
		Protocatechual-dehyde	Salvia miltiorrhiza	Antiproliferative, β-catenin suppression	
		Baicalin	Scutellariabaicalensi	↓ nf-κb-p65 protein production, disruption of cell cycle in g1/S phase	
		Curcumin	Turmeric	↓ PPARγ, ↓ cyclin D1	Sung et al. (2012)

TABLE 4.2
Molecular Targets and Their Role in Cancer

S.NO	Molecular Targets	Role in Cancer	References
1	EGFR	Drives tumorigenesis	Shanmugalingam et al. 2016
2	IGF1R	Inhibits apoptosis stimulates cell proliferation and promotes non-cancerous cells to malignant transformation	Shanmugalingam et al. 2016; Yuan et al. 2018
3	VEGFR	Promotes neovascularization to keep the tumour growth	Li et al. 2016
4	5-LOX	Promotes growth of cancer cells	Zhou et al. 2015
5	COX-2	Enhances apoptotic resistance, proliferation, inflammation, and metastasis of cancer cells.	Goradel et al. 2019
6	TNF-α	Stimulates growth, proliferation, invasion, and metastasis of cancer cell	Wang and Lin 2008
7	AP-1	Mediates migration and proliferation of cancer cells	Ibrahim et al. 2018
8	NF-kb	Involves tumour-cell proliferation and angiogenesis	Xia et al. 2018
9	Ras/Raf	Controls cell cycling, proliferation, and prevents apoptosis	Kelley 2016
10	STAT3	Regulates cellular proliferation, invasion, migration, angiogenesis, tumour growth and metastasis	Kamran et al. 2022
11	AMPK	Blocks cancer proliferation and growth	Li et al. 2015
12	PI3K	Regulates carcinogenesis, proliferation, invasion, and metastasis of tumour cells	Rascio et al. 2021
13	mTOR	Contributes to cell proliferation, autophagy, and apoptosis	Zou et al. 2020; Tian et al. 2019
14	NFE2	Control of redox balance	Smolková et al. 2020

Additionally, natural polyphenols like apigenin, resveratrol, genistein, luteolin, and quercetin induce apoptosis in malignant cells (Huang et al. 2010).

4.4.1 Ellagic Acid

Ellagic acid (EA), a natural polyphenolic compound found in berries, pomegranates, and dried fruits, has strong antioxidant and anticancer properties, primarily linked to its direct antiproliferative and apoptotic effects. EA induces apoptosis by stimulation of mitochondrial pathways, cytochrome C release, downregulation of caspase activation, and it regulates cell proliferation via inhibition of CDK-6 enzyme (Yousuf et al. 2020).

4.4.2 Flavonoids

Flavonoids are polyphenolic secondary metabolites that give colour and aroma to flowers, leaves, and fruits. They also contribute to the plants' survival from threats like insect attacks, and bacterial and viral infestations. Chelating metal ions or scavenging free radicals is the mechanism behind its antioxidant property, which plays an immense role in cancer by neutralization of free radicals (Yousuf et al. 2020).

4.4.3 Quercetin

Quercetin, an antioxidant found in various foods and supplements, protects against ageing, diseases, and some cancers. Quercetin has been considered a potential anticancer agent, because it can induce apoptosis, cellular senescence, inhibition of cell proliferation, and angiogenesis. The mechanism behind its anticancer activity is activating caspases, inhibiting Akt phosphorylation, cell cycle arrest in the G1 phase (Boots et al. 2008).

4.4.4 Stilbenes

Stilbenes are known as diarylethene phytoalexins, which are nonflavonoid phytochemicals of polyphenolic structure that contain a 1,2-diphenylethylene nucleus produced by over 70 plant species. By interfering with molecular events at every stage of carcinogenesis, including the initiation, promotion, and progression stages, stilbenes have demonstrated the ability to decrease the incidence of cancer (Sirerol et al. 2016).

4.4.5 Resveratrol

Resveratrol (trans-3,4,5-trihydroxystilbene), a natural stilbene, is well-known as phytoestrogen and owns antioxidant, anti-inflammatory, cardioprotective, and anticancer properties (Ko et al. 2017). Beverages and foods such as mulberries, peanuts, grapes, and red wine are rich sources of resveratrol, which exhibits anticancer activity (Sirerol et al. 2016).

The anticarcinogenic mechanism induced by the stilbene is shown in Figure 4.3.

4.4.6 Curcuminoids

Curcuminoids are phenolic compounds that exhibit numerous biological actions, including anti-inflammatory, anticancer, anti-microbial, neuroprotective, cardioprotective, and radioprotective effects (Amalraj et al. 2017).

4.4.7 Curcumin

Curcumin is a major natural polyphenol, chemically it is (1,7-bis(4-hydroxy-3-methoxyphenyl)-1,6-heptadiene-3,5-dione), also called diferuloylmethane. Antiproliferative actions of curcumin include cell cycle arrest at the G2/M phase via

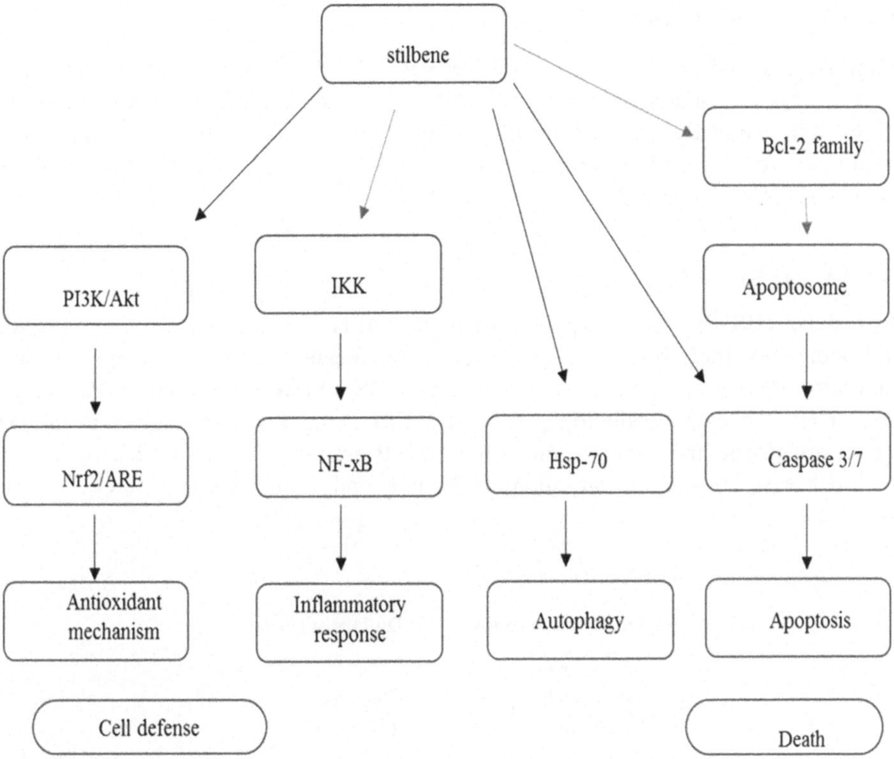

FIGURE 4.3 Anticarcinogenic mechanisms induced by major stilbenes.

upregulation of p53 and p21, suppression of growth factor receptors and trophic effectors (Hewlings and Kalman 2017).

4.4.8 Terpenoids

Terpenoids are secondary metabolites, primarily produced by plants. Terpenoids are classified as carotenoids, phytosterols, and β-sitosterol (Kamran et al. 2022). The most common plant source for terpene is cannabis and other sources include tea, thyme, Spanish sage, citrus fruits and mandarins (Georgian et al. 2019).

4.4.9 Carotenoids

Carotenoids are tetraterpenes that are responsible for the yellow, orange, and red colour pigments in many fruits, flowers, and plants without chlorophyll. Carotenoids are divided into apocarotenoids, carotenes, xanthophylls, and derivative chemicals that have anticancer efficacy through controlling pro-apoptotic signalling. Bell peppers, broccoli, carrot, mango, orange, papaya and spinach have rich concentrations of carotenoids (Koklesova et al. 2020; Olatunde et al. 2020).

4.4.10 Phytosterols

Plant sterols and their saturated derivatives, are referred to as "phytosterols." Phytosterols are bioactive substances with a structure that resembles cholesterol, which are naturally present in plant-origin foods. Vegetable oils like corn, sunflower, soybean, olive, orange, and cauliflower are sources of phytosterols in food (Cabral and Klein 2017).

4.4.11 β-sitosterol

β-sitosterol (BS) is a subcomponent of phytosterols. BS is found in various foods and botanicals, including rice bran, wheat germ, peanuts, soybeans, corn oils, saw palmetto, rye grass pollen, and stinging nettles. BS inhibits the growth of Pancreatic Cancer (PC) cells by reducing proliferation, inducing cell cycle arrest at G0/G1 phase, apoptosis, and suppression of the NF-kB activity (Cao et al. 2019).

Functional groups of various polyphenols and their dietary sources are as follows:

Functional groups	Dietary sources
Caffeic acid	Coffee
Gallic acid	Green tea
Rosmarinic acid	Rosemary
Anacardic acid	Cashew
Chlorogenic acid	Coffee
Ellagic acid	Pomegranate

Functional groups of various stilbenes, curcuminoids and their dietary sources are as follows:

Functional groups	Dietary sources
Piceatannol	Grapes
Pterostilbene	Blueberries
Resveratrol	Red grapes, berries
Curcuminoids	
Bisdemethoxycurcumin	
Curcumin	Turmeric
Desmethoxycurcumin	
Phytosterols	
β-Sitosterol	Nuts, grains

Functional groups of various carotenoids and non-carotenoids and their dietary sources are as follows:

Functional groups	**Dietary sources**
Carotenoids	
Lycopene	Tomato, watermelon
β-carotene	Carrots
Crocetin	Saffron
Lutein	Spinach
Non- carotenoids	
Limonene	Citrus fruits, cherries
Anethole	Sweet fennel
Ginsenoside Rg3	Ginseng
Ursolic acid	Rosemary, basil
Carnosol	Rosemary
Bisacurone	Turmeric
Lupeol	Mango, strawberry

Flavonoids have very good antioxidant activity. Functional groups of flavonoids and their dietary sources are as follows:

Functional groups	**Dietary sources**
Apigenin	Parsley, celery, pepper
Luteolin	dandelions
Fisetin	Strawberry, apples
Kaempferol	Tea, broccoli,
Quercetin	grapes, onion, apple
Catechin gallate	Green tea
Epicatechin gallate	
(-)-Epigallocatechin-3-gallate	
Myricetin	Grapes, onions, tea
Naringenin	
Tangeretin	
Daidzein	
Genistein	Soybeans
Delphinidin	Cranberry, strawberry, pomegranates
Licochalcone-A	Licorice (*Glycyrrhiza glabra*)
Isoliquiritigenin	
Silibinin	Milk thistle (*Silybum marianum*)
Xanthohumol	Beer (from *Humulus lupulus*)
Cyanidin	Wild blueberry (*Vaccinium myrtillus*)
Butein	Indian cashew

4.5 VITAMINS AND MINERALS

Vitamins and minerals are crucial in cancer prevention and management, with patients often using nutritional supplements as potent chemo-preventive agents, typically in adequate amounts.

4.5.1 Vitamins

Vitamin A, vitamin B complex, vitamin C, vitamin D, vitamin E, and vitamin K have major contributions in cancer treatment.

4.5.1.1 Vitamin A

Vitamin A is a natural fat-soluble vitamin that is present in many foods. A gene associated with more aggressive kinds of breast cancer, cerbB, is expressed less when retinoic acid is present. Retinoic acid, on the other hand, also prevents proliferation in human mammary epithelial cells that have had the tumour suppressor p53 inactivated (Mamede et al. 2011).

4.5.1.2 Vitamin B

The vitamin B complex is made up of water-soluble vitamins. Brewer's yeast, liver, whole-grain cereals, grains, nuts, milk, eggs, meat, fish, fruits, leafy green vegetables, and a variety of other foods contain these vitamins (Mamede et al. 2011). Lack of vitamin B causes DNA damage, oxidative stress, and a chronic inflammatory state that shows in epigenetic changes and subsequent cancer. Vitamin B6 has antioxidant nutrients and a dominant protective role against inflammation and cancer progression (Mikkelsen et al. 2019).

4.5.1.3 Vitamin C

Vitamin C is water-soluble and exists in two chemical forms: the reduced form, ascorbic acid (AA), and the oxidized form, dehydroascorbic acid (DHA). AA is a potent antioxidant that efficiently smoothers potentially damaging free radicals produced through biological processes (Mamede et al. 2011). Vitamin C is abundant in citrus fruits, green and red peppers, strawberries, tomatoes, broccoli, turnips, Indian gooseberries, and other leafy vegetables (Khanna et al. 2014).

4.5.1.4 Vitamin D

Vitamin D is a fat-soluble compound which has antiproliferative effects involved in bone development and the immune system. Calcitriol causes cell cycle arrest in the G0/G1 phase of the cell cycle, which prevents the proliferation of many malignant cells by upregulation of the expression of the cyclin-dependent kinase inhibitors and downregulation of the activity of cyclin-dependent kinase 2 (CDK2) in PC cells (Kim et al. 2012).

4.5.1.5 Vitamin E

Vitamin E is a fat-soluble antioxidant nutrient from the Tocols family that includes four tocopherols and four tocotrienols. These are the different forms of vitamin E.

All tocopherols and tocotrienols block oxidative stress-induced DNA damage. Tocopherol-rich dietary oils like corn, soybean, sesame, cottonseed, and nut are abundant, while tocotrienols are abundant in palm oil and low in wheat and corn bran oils (Jiang 2017).

4.5.1.6 Vitamin K

Vitamin K (VK) is an essential lipid-soluble nutrient that exists in natural and synthetic forms. It suppresses the proliferation of cancer cells by cell cycle arrest. In cancer cells, VK2 downregulates the expression of cyclin D1. Green leafy vegetables like kale, romaine lettuce, broccoli, cabbage, and spinach are major sources of vitamin K (Simes et al. 2020).

4.5.2 Minerals

4.5.2.1 Selenium

Selenium (Se), is an essential mineral which is a prominent protective agent against cancer. It controls cancers by antioxidant protection through selenoenzymes, activation of DNA repair, and apoptosis. Se is primarily sourced from cereals, grains, and animal foods like fish, meat, dairy products, milk, and eggs (Yang et al. 2012).

4.5.2.2 Zinc

Zinc is a key element in cell metabolism. Particularly in malignant cells, it controls oxidative stress response, DNA replication, and apoptosis, and is responsible for the activation of the tumour suppressor p53 protein. Zn primarily exists in meat, fish, legumes, nuts, and other dietary sources, but the absorption varies based on food sources (Vinceti et al. 2018).

4.5.2.3 Molybdenum (Mo)

Molybdenum (Mo), is an essential trace metal. Earlier investigational study indirectly implicates that molybdenum deficiency is the etiology of cancer (Dhawan and Chadha 2010). Mo involves a generation of free radicals and plays a pivotal role in the functioning of antioxidant enzymes and targeting radiation towards the cancer cells (Costello and Franklin 2012). Molybdenum-rich plants produce cereal grains, cheese, green vegetables, legumes, milk, nuts, and organ meats (Indrakumar and Korrapati 2020).

4.6 CONCLUSION

The scientific world has been interested in nutraceutical-based cancer therapy in recent years, and it is obvious that it is essential to understand the etiology of many diseases, particularly cancer. Nutraceuticals, such as phytoconstituents, vitamins, minerals, and other micronutrients, offer a fantastic supply of chemicals with cancer-preventing properties. Additionally, they are affordable, and the majority of them show no signs of toxicity or pain. With respect to cancer, the results obtained by this strategy prove that nutraceutical-based cancer therapy could be a promising way to treat cancer.

REFERENCES

Aggarwal, B.B., Van Kuiken, M.E., Iyer, L.H., Harikumar, K.B., & Sung, B. (2009). Molecular targets of nutraceuticals derived from dietary spices: potential role in suppression of inflammation and tumorigenesis. *Experimental Biology and Medicine*, 234(8), 825–849.

Alharbi, K.S., Almalki, W.H., Makeen, H.A., Albratty, M., Meraya, A.M., Nagraik, R., et al. (2022). Role of medicinal plant-derived nutraceuticals as a potential target for the treatment of breast cancer. *Journal of Food Biochemistry*, 46(12), e14387.

Amalraj, A., Pius, A., & Gopi, S. (2017). Biological activities of curcuminoids, other biomolecules from turmeric and their derivatives - A review. *Journal of Traditional Complementary Medicine*, 7(2), 205–233.

Bagchi, D., Preuss, H.G., & Swaroop, A. (2015). *Nutraceuticals and Functional Foods in Human Health and Disease Prevention*. CRC Press.

Boots, A., Haenen, G., & Bast, A. (2008). Health effects of quercetin: From antioxidant to nutraceutical. *European Journal of Pharmacology*, 585, 325–337.

Cabral, C.E., & Klein, M.R.S.T (2017). Phytosterols in the treatment of hypercholesterolemia and prevention of cardiovascular diseases. *Arquivos Brasileiros de Cardiologia*, 109(5), 475–482.

Calvani, M., Pasha, A., & Favre, C. (2020). Nutraceutical boom in cancer: Inside the labyrinth of reactive oxygen species. *International Journal of Molecular Sciences*, 21(6), 1936.

Cao, Z.Q., Wang, X.X., Lu, L., Xu, J.W., Li, X.B., Zhang, G.R. et al. (2019). "β-sitosterol and gemcitabine exhibit synergistic anti-pancreatic cancer activity by modulating apoptosis and inhibiting epithelial–mesenchymal transition by deactivating Akt/GSK 3β signaling. *Frontiers in Pharmacology*, 9, 1525.

Costello, L.C., & Franklin, R.B. (2012). Cytotoxic/tumor suppressor role of zinc for the treatment of cancer: an enigma and an opportunity. *Expert Review of Anticancer Therapy*, 12(1), 121–128.

Dhawan, D.K., & Chadha, V.D. (2010). Zinc: a promising agent in dietary chemoprevention of cancer. *Indian Journal of Medical Research*, 132(6), 676–682.

Georgian, D., Ramadoss, N., Dona, C., & Basu, C. (2019). Therapeutic and medicinal uses of terpenes. *Medicinal Plants: From Farm to Pharmacy*, 333–359. https://doi.org/10.1007/978-3-030-31269-5_15

Gonzalez-Vallinas, M., González-Castejon, M., Rodríguez-Casado, A., & de Molina, A.R. (2013). Dietary phytochemicals in cancer prevention and therapy: a complementary approach with promising perspectives. *Nutrition Reviews*, 71(9), 585–599.

Goradel, N.H., Najafi, M., Salehi, E., Farhood, B., & Mortezaee, K. (2019). Cyclooxygenase-2 in cancer: A review. *Journal of Cellular Physiology*, 234(5), 5683–5699.

Hewlings, S.J., & Kalman, D.S. (2017). Curcumin: A review of its effects on human health. *Foods*, 6(10), 92.

Huang, Y., Cai, Y.C., & Zhang, Y. (2010). Natural phenolic compounds from medicinal herbs and dietary plants: potential use for cancer prevention. *Nutrition and Cancer*, 62(1), 1–20.

Ibrahim, S.A.E.F., Abudu, A., Johnson, E., Aftab, N., Conrad, S., & Fluck, M. (2018). The role of AP-1 in self-sufficient proliferation and migration of cancer cells and its potential impact on an autocrine/paracrine loop. *Oncotarget*, 9, 34259–34278.

Indrakumar J., & Korrapati, P.S. (2020). Steering efficacy of nano molybdenum towards cancer: Mechanism of action. *Biological Trace Element Research*, 194, 121–134.

Jiang, Q. (2017). Natural forms of vitamin E as effective agents for cancer prevention and therapy. *Advances in Nutrition*, 8(6), 850–867.

Kamran, S., Sinniah, A., Abdulghani, M.A.M., & Alshawsh, M.A. (2022). Therapeutic potential of certain terpenoids as anticancer agents: A scoping review. *Cancers (Basel)*, 14, 5.

Kelley, G.M. (2016). The importance of the Ras-Raf pathway in cancer development. *Inquiries Journal*, 8(6), 1.

Khanna, S., Karki, R.D., Pande, K., & Negi, D. (2014). Inflammation, free radical damage, oxidative stress and cancer. *International Journal of Inflammation, Cancer and Integrative Therapy*, 1(1), 109.

Kim, J.E., Kang, J.S., & Lee, W.J. (2012). Vitamin C induces apoptosis in human colon cancer cell line, HCT-8 Via the modulation of calcium influx in endoplasmic reticulum and the dissociation of bad from 14-3-3β. *Immune Network*, 12(5), 189–195.

Ko, J.H., Sethi, G., Um, J.Y., Shanmugam, M.K., Arfuso, F., Kumar, A.P., et al. (2017). The role of resveratrol in cancer therapy. *International Journal of Molecular Sciences*, 18(12), 2589.

Koklesova, L., Liskova, A., Samec, M., Buhrmann, C., Samuel, S.M., Varghese, E. et al. (2020). Carotenoids in cancer apoptosis — The road from bench to bedside and back. *Cancers (Basel)*, 12(9), 2425.

Li, W., Saud, S.M., Young, M.R., Chen, G., & Hua, B. (2015). Targeting AMPK for cancer prevention and treatment. *Oncotarget*, 6(10), 7365–7378.

Li, Y.L., Zhao, H., & Ren, X.B. (2016). Relationship of VEGF/VEGFR with immune and cancer cells: staggering or forward? *Cancer Biology Medicine*, 13(2), 206–214.

Maiuolo, J., Gliozzi, M., Carresi, C., Musolino, V., Oppedisano, F., & Scarano, F. (2021). Nutraceuticals and cancer: Potential for natural polyphenols *Nutrients*, 13, 11.

Mamede, A.C., Tavares, S.D., Abrantes, A.M., Trindade, J., Maia, J.M., & Botelho, M.F. (2011). The role of vitamins in cancer: A review. *Nutritional Cancer*, 63(4), 479–494.

Mikkelsen, K., Prakash, M.D., Kuol, N., Nurgali, K., Stojanovska, L., & Apostolopoulos, V. (2019). AntiTumor effects of vitamin B2, B6 and B9 in promonocytic lymphoma cells. *International Journal of Molecular Sciences*, 20(15), E3763.

Olatunde, A., Tijjani, H., Ishola, A., Egbuna, C., Hassan, S., & Akram, M. (2020). Carotenoids as functional bioactive compounds. *Functional Foods and Nutraceuticals*, 415–444. https://doi.org/10.1007/978-3-030-42319-3_20

Ranzato, E., Martinotti, S., Calabrese, C., & Giorgio, C. (2014). Role of nutraceuticals in cancer therapy *Journal of Food Research*, 3(4), 18–25.

Rascio, F., Spadaccino, F., Rocchetti, M.T., Castellano, G., Stallon, G., Netti, G.S. et al. (2021). The pathogenic role of PI3K/AKT pathway in cancer onset and drug resistance: An updated review. *Cancers (Basel)*, 13(16), 3949.

Santini, A., Tenore, G.C., & Novellino, E. (2017). Nutraceuticals: A paradigm of proactive medicine. *European Journal of Pharmaceutical Sciences*, 96, 53–61.

Sever, R., & Brugge, J.S. (2015). Signal transduction in cancer. *Cold Spring Harbor Perspectives in Medicine*, 5(4), a006098.

Shanmugalingam, T., Bosco, C., Ridley, A.J., & Van Hemelrijck, M. (2016). Is there a role for IGF-1 in the development of second primary cancers? *Cancer Medicine*, 5(11), 3353–3367.

Sherman, R., Firth, R., Charlton, M., De, P., Green, D., Hofer, B., Hofferkamp, J., Hsieh, M., Johnson, C., Kohler, B., Morawski, B., Nash, S., Qiao, B., & Wie, H. (2020). *Cancer in North America: 2013–2017. Volume Two: Registry-specific Cancer Incidence in the United States and Canada*. North American Association of Central Cancer Registries.

Simes, D.C., Viegas, C.S.B., Araújo, N., & Marreiros, C. (2020). Vitamin K as a diet supplement with impact in human health: Current evidence in age-related diseases. *Nutrients*, 12(1), 138.

Sirerol, J.A., Rodríguez, M.L., Mena, S., Asensi, M.A., Estrela, J.M., & Ortega, A.L. (2016). Role of natural stilbenes in the prevention of cancer. *Oxidative Medicine and Cellular Longevity*, 3128951. 10.1155/2016/3128951

Sung, B., Prasad, S., Yadav, V.R., & Aggarwal, B.B. (2012). Cancer cell signaling pathways targeted by spice-derived nutraceuticals. *Nutrition and Cancer*, 64(2), 173–197.

Tian, T., Li, X., & Zhang, J. (2019). mTOR signaling in cancer and mTOR inhibitors in solid tumor targeting therapy. *International Journal of Molecular Sciences*, 20(3), 755.

Vinceti, M., Filippini, T., Del Giovane, C., Dennert, G., Zwahlen, M., Brinkman, M., Zeegers, M.P., Horneber, M., D′Amico, R., & Crespi, C.M. (2018). Selenium for preventing cancer. *Cochrane Database Systematic Review*, 1(1), CD005195.

Wang, X., & Lin, Y. (2008). Tumor necrosis factor and cancer, buddies or foes? *Acta Pharmacologica Sinica*, 29(11), 1275–1288.

Xia, L., Tan, S., Zhou, Y., Lin, J., Wang, H., Oyang, L., et al. (2018). Role of the NFκB-signaling pathway in cancer. *OncoTargets and Therapy*, 11, 2063–2073.

Yang, C.S., Suh, N., & Kong, A.N.T. (2012). Does vitamin E prevent or promote cancer? *Cancer Prevention Research*, 5(5), 701–705.

Yousuf, M., Shamsi, A., Khan, P., Shahbaaz, N., AlAjmi, M.F., Hussain, A., et al. (2020). Ellagic acid controls cell proliferation and induces apoptosis in breast cancer cells via inhibition of cyclin-dependent kinase 6. *International Journal of Molecular Sciences*, 21(10), 3526.

Yuan, J., Yin, Z., Tao, K., Wang, G., & Gao, J. (2018). Function of insulin-like growth factor 1 receptor in cancer resistance to chemotherapy. *Oncology Letters*, 15(1), 41–47.

Zhou, G.X., Ding, X.L., Wu, S.B., Zhang, H.F., Cao, W., Qu, L.S. et al. (2015). Inhibition of 5lipoxygenase triggers apoptosis in pancreatic cancer cells. *Oncology Reports*, 33(2), 661–668.

Zou, Z., Tao, T., Li, H., & Zhu, X. (2020). MTOR signaling pathway and mTOR inhibitors in cancer: Progress and challenges. *Cell & Bioscience*, 10, 31.

5 Insight into the Role of Prebiotics in Diabetes Therapy

Akash Kumar, Jhilam Pramanik, Swati Joia, Dimple Chauhan, Rajju Priya Soni, and Bhupendra G Prajapati

5.1 INTRODUCTION

Diabetes, characterized by insufficient insulin production or utilization, has subtypes like type 1, gestational, and type 2 diabetes. It ranks fifth in global causes of death, with 1.6 million deaths attributed (Roglic et al. 2005). Type 1 and type 2 diabetes reduce life expectancy by 10–20 years (Tancredi et al. 2015). Globally, 8.8% of 20–79-year-olds have diabetes, and projections suggest 693 million cases by 2045 (IDF 2017).

5.2 RELATIONSHIPS BETWEEN THE GUT MICROBIOTA AND DIABETES MELLITUS

Research in both humans and animals highlights dysbiosis in type 2 diabetes (T2D) and its connection to non-communicable diseases. In T2D, the microbiome shows lower levels of specific microorganisms. Initial studies using gene-targeted methods and qPCR revealed reduced Firmicutes, Clostridia, Betaproteobacteria, and a positive link with fasting glucose. The Bacteroidetes/Firmig3cutes ratio was also lower (Larsen et al. 2010). Genome-wide association studies indicated higher levels of bacteria like *Bacteroides intestinalis, Clostridium hathewayi*, etc., in diabetes (Wang et al. 2012). However, inconsistencies exist; for example, the *Firmicutes/Bacteroidetes* ratio changes due to diabetes are debated (Sircana et al. 2018), requiring more investigation. Diabetes progression and complications like retinopathy affect the microbiome profile (Das et al. 2021). Figure 5.1 depicts the mechanism that relates diabetes and intestinal flora (Gurung et al. 2020). Diabetes correlates with elevated inflammatory proteins, chemokines, and pro-inflammatory cytokines. Lipopolysaccharides (LPS), produced by certain gut microbes, trigger low-grade inflammation and metabolic endotoxemia, while others stimulate chemokines and anti-inflammatory cytokines (Plovier et al. 2016).

DOI: 10.1201/9781003392934-5

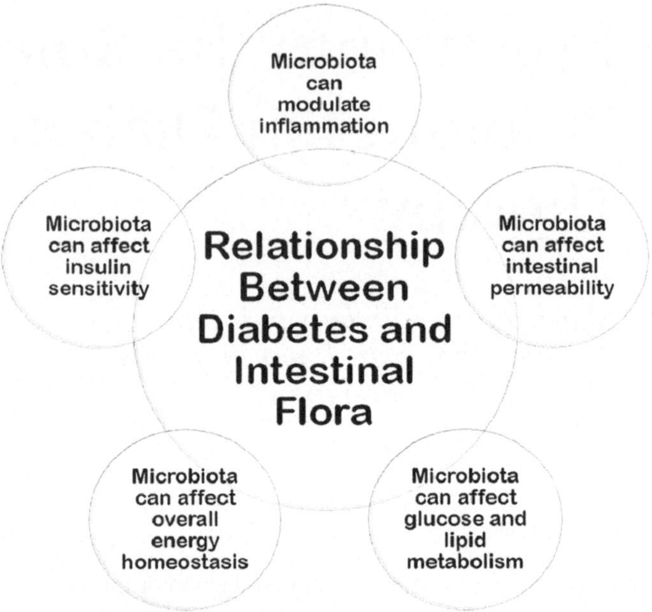

FIGURE 5.1 Mechanism that relates diabetes and intestinal flora (Gurung et al. 2020).

5.3 OVERVIEW OF PREBIOTICS

In the 1990s, Gibson and Roberfroid coined prebiotics as "a non-digestible food ingredient that beneficially affects the host by selectively stimulating the growth and/or activity of one or a limited number of bacteria in the colon, and thus improves host health" (Gibson & Roberfroid 1995). A newer definition from the International Scientific Association of Probiotics and Prebiotics states prebiotics are "substrates selectively used by host microorganisms for health benefits a substrate that is selectively utilized by host microorganisms conferring a health benefit" (ISAPP). This update considers impact, selectivity, substrates, host utilization, and health benefits, encompassing non-carbohydrate compounds like polyunsaturated fatty acids, polyphenols, and minerals. Notably, inulin, xylooligosaccharides (XOS), fructooligosaccharides (FOS), and galactooligosaccharides (GOS) are carbohydrate-based prebiotics (Gibson et al. 2017). The term "prebiotic" extends beyond the gut, covering other sites like the skin and vaginal tract. Specific microbial-mediated mechanisms determine their action. This definition acknowledges diverse microbial taxa like *Eubacterium, Roseburia*, and *Faecalibacterium* spp. alongside *Bifidobacteria* and *Lactobacilli* for conferring health benefits (Gibson et al. 2017).

5.4 RELATIONSHIPS BETWEEN THE GUT MICROBIOTA AND PREBIOTICS

Prebiotic treatments induce specific changes in gut microbiota composition. Different types of prebiotics stimulate the growth of various beneficial bacteria in the gastrointestinal tract, particularly *Lactobacilli*, and *Bifidobacteria*, and maintain intestinal health (Kumar et al. 2022; Kumar et al. 2023). They could offer beneficial effects for gastrointestinal conditions like ulcerative colitis, Crohn's disease, and irritable bowel syndrome (Akutko & Stawarski 2021).

FOS reduced *Fusobacterium*, *Bacteroides*, and *Clostridium* while promoting *Bifidobacteria* growth (Gibson & Roberfroid 1995). GOS ferments gut microbiota to produce SCFAs and lower pH (Tran et al. 2020). PDX alters gut flora, improves bowel movements, lowers pH, and reduces glucose absorption (Toporovski et al. 2021). Lactulose selectively increases *Bifidobacterium, Lactobacillus*, and *Streptococcus*. Lactosucrose boosts *Bifidobacteria* population (Li et al. 2015), fermenting to SCFAs and pH reduction (Nath et al. 2018). XOS improves fecal weight and moisture, bone characteristics, and quantity of Bifidobacteria in various animal and human studies (Berger et al. 2021). Prebiotic fermentation products, like SCFAs, alter gut pH and microbial populations, demonstrating prebiotics' potential to modulate gut microbiota composition.

5.5 MECHANISM OF DIABETES REGULATION BY THE INTESTINAL FLORA

Several studies suggest that intestinal flora may impact the onset of diabetes by modulating bile acid metabolism, improving SCFA production, and modifying intestinal permeability.

5.5.1 Effect of Intestinal Flora on the Development of Diabetes via Bile Acid Metabolism

Intestinal flora affects insulin resistance through bile acid metabolism, where the liver converts cholesterol into bile acids. Liver and intestinal flora cooperation is crucial for this process (Zaborska & Cummings 2018). Intestinal bacteria's enzymes convert primary to secondary bile acids in the liver (Ma et al. 2019). The farnesoid X receptor (FXR) controls bile acid, lipid, glucose, and energy metabolism. FXR deficiency in obesity enhances glucose and energy homeostasis (Prawitt et al. 2011). Intestinal endocrine cells release glucagon-like peptide-1 (GLP-1) via bile acid-triggered TGR-5 signaling. GLP-1 boosts insulin production by islet beta cells for improved glucose response (Lee et al. 2019). Diabetes involves changes in these bile acid metabolisms and signaling mechanisms.

5.5.2 Effect of Intestinal Flora on the Development of Diabetes via Alterations of Short-Chain Fatty Acids (SCFAs)

Bacteria ferment dietary fiber in the colon, producing short-chain fatty acids (SCFAs) like butyrate, acetate, and propionate, which enter the bloodstream from the colon. SCFAs activate G protein-coupled receptors 41 (GPR41) and 43 (GPR43) receptors, promoting hormone release and insulin control and impacting gut immunity, hunger, and energy balance. Research highlights SCFAs' potential to alleviate diabetes symptoms; dietary SCFA supplementation may increase peptide

YY (PYY) and GLP-1 levels (Byrne et al. 2015). These findings suggest SCFAs influence host metabolism and have complex effects on conditions like obesity, diabetes, and hypertension. Further understanding of SCFAs' role in diabetes pathophysiology is crucial.

5.5.3 Intestinal Flora Affects Diabetes Development by Changing Intestinal Permeability

The intestinal mucosa barrier shields against harmful substances entering the bloodstream. Pathological conditions can compromise this barrier, raising intestinal permeability and allowing elements like endotoxins to cause endotoxemia and inflammation. Impaired barrier function disrupts homeostasis, leading to systemic infection, inflammation, and metabolic disorders like diabetes. In a mouse model, *Bacteroides vulgatus* and *dorei* improved intestinal integrity, reducing endotoxemia by enhancing tight junction genes in the colon (Yoshida et al. 2018). *Akkermansia muciniphila* activated AMPK, bolstering tight junctions (Chelakkot et al. 2018).

5.6 RELATIONSHIP BETWEEN PREBIOTICS AND TYPE I DIABETES

Various studies demonstrate the positive impact of dietary fibers on gut permeability and microbiota balance, contributing to delaying T1DM development, as shown in Table 5.1. For example, administering long-chain fructans to NOD mice regulates gut-barrier function, microbiota, and pancreatic immunity, delaying T1DM progression and cytokine production (Chen et al. 2017). Human milk oligosaccharides (HMOs) promote the growth of beneficial gut microbes and aid in preventing T1DM by modulating immune response through SCFA production. Dietary resistant starch (RS) delays diabetic neuropathy progression by maintaining vitamin-D balance in STZ-induced T1DM rats (Koh et al. 2016). Extracted caffeic acid fractions from *Prunella vulgaris* L. exhibit potential as a therapeutic agent for T1DM treatment in alloxan-induced diabetic mice (Raafat et al. 2016).

Prebiotics positively impact gut microbiota in school-age children (8–17 years), elevating *Bacteroidetes* and lactic acid bacteria, thereby improving intestinal permeability, reducing inflammation, enhancing glycemic control, and lowering T1D risk (Ho et al. 2016). Increased dietary fiber intake (>30 g/day) by T1D patients reduces coronary heart disease risk and inflammation (Bernaud et al. 2014). Breastfeeding lowers autoimmune risk, possibly due to long-chain polyunsaturated fatty acids (PUFA) in human milk that mitigate primary islet autoimmunity and immune antigens (Niinistö et al. 2017). Human milk, likely due to its oligo- and polysaccharides, reduces autoimmunity and improves T1D outcomes (Mishra et al. 2019). Table 5.2 represents human studies of prebiotic interventions and T1DM.

5.7 RELATIONSHIP BETWEEN PREBIOTICS AND TYPE II DIABETES

Male rats with induced T2DM were orally given different doses of feruloylated oligosaccharides for eight weeks. 600 mg/kg/day of feruloylated oligosaccharides

TABLE 5.1
Characteristics of Some Animal Studies of Prebiotic Interventions and T1DM

Intervention/ Source	Design/Model Type	Dose/Duration	Mechanism of Action	Outcomes	Reference
Inulin-type fructan	NOD mice	24 weeks	Changes in cytokines production. Increased (CD4+ CD25+ Treg+ Foxp3) cells, SCFA, tight junction proteins, and alleviate dysbiosis	Modulates gut-pancreatic immunity and T-cell response which delays T1DM development	(Chen et al. 2017)
β-glucan	TIDM animal model	2 consecutive weeks	Reduced *Firmicutes* and increased *Verrucomicrobia,* and *Bacteroidetes*	Suppressed insulitis, improved carbohydrate metabolism, and immune function	(Gudi et al. 2019)
HMOs	NOD mice	6 weeks	Regulated the immune system and reduced the destruction of pancreatic islets	Increased SCFAs, improved intestinal barrier, increased Treg cells, altered microbial diversity	(Xiao et al. 2018)
XOS	NOD mice	13 weeks	Decreased $CD8^+$ T-cells, $CD11c^+$ M1 macrophages and increased regulatory T-cells	Reduction in the incidence of T1DM and reduction in insulitis	(Hansen et al. 2019)

TABLE 5.2
Characteristics of Some Human Studies of Prebiotic Interventions and T1DM

Type of Study	Interventions	Results/Findings	References
Controlled trial	OF – enriched inulin	Potentially novel, cheap, and low-risk treatment for T1DM	(Ho et al. 2016)
Controlled trial	Galacto-oligosaccharide	Hemoglobin level not decreased and no effect on BMI	(Gonai et al. 2017)
Controlled trial	Galacto-oligosaccharide	FBG and TG significantly reduced and HDL-C levels increased	(Pedersen et al. 2016)
Controlled trial	Breast milk	Inversely increased the abundance of Bifidobacterium correlated with T1DM risk	(Insel & Knip 2018)

notably reduced plasma glucose, LDL, aspartate transaminase, fasting insulin, and creatine kinase levels (Huang et al. 2018). Rats given guava juice enriched with quercetin and trehalose for four weeks exhibited improved insulin, OGTT, HOMA-β, and HOMA-IR, protecting the kidney and pancreas (Lin et al. 2016). Administration of 0.5 g/kg of *Trigonella foenum graecum* soluble dietary fiber (Tf-sdf) orally twice daily for 28 days lowered serum fructosamine and atherogenic lipids (Hannan et al. 2003). Table 5.3 represents the impact of prebiotics on T2DM animal models.

FOS supplementation led to lower glucose and insulin levels while increasing PYY compared to the placebo (Parnell & Reimer 2009). Resistant starch consumption improved insulin sensitivity in healthy subjects (Bodinham et al. 2014). Consumption of barley kernel-based bread increased short-chain fatty acid (SCFA) levels, and improved insulin sensitivity (Nilsson et al. 2015). In T2DM patients, FOS-enriched inulin improved inflammatory markers, reduced fasting blood sugar, and decreased glycosylated hemoglobin when compared to a placebo (Dehghan et al. 2014). Table 5.4 provides a summary of the impact of prebiotics on T2DM in human models.

5.8 RELATIONSHIP BETWEEN PREBIOTICS AND GESTATIONAL DIABETES

Chinese women face a high risk of gestational diabetes mellitus (GDM). Meta-analysis reveals that adopting low-glycemic load (GL) diets, low-glycemic index (GI) diets, and high fiber diets during pregnancy leads to improved glycemic control and pregnancy outcomes (Wan et al. 2019). Dietary patterns rich in grains, vegetables, and beans, and low in full-fat dairy, sweets, and cookies, along with high fiber content, are inversely associated with GDM and thrombosis risk (Sartorelli et al. 2019). During pregnancy, dietary changes positively impact maternal gestational weight gain, nutritional intake, and glycemic control, with increased fiber intake reducing neonatal birth weight and preventing excessive maternal weight gain (McGowan et al. 2013). Poor dietary habits, such as high

TABLE 5.3
Characteristics of Some Animal Studies of Prebiotic Interventions and T2DM

Intervention/Source	Design/Model Type	Dose/Duration	Mechanism of Action	Outcomes	Reference
Feruloylated oligosaccharides	STZ-induced T2DM male rats	600 mg/kg/day for 8 weeks	Inhibition of NF-κB pathway	Drastically reduced the levels of fasting insulin, TG, FPG, and LDL-c	(Huang et al. 2018)
Quercetin-rich guava juice in combination with trehalose	STZ, nicotinamide, and combination with HFD-induced T2DM Wistar rats	Different levels 2.5 μg/kg BW to 12.6 μg/kg BW per day 4 weeks	ROS, 4-hydroxynonenal, IL-1β/pyroptosis, caspase-3/apoptosis, and LC3-B/autophagy and were drastically reduced	Protects the pancreas and kidney against T2DM-induced injury	(Lin et al. 2016)
XOS and FOS	STZ-induced diabetic rats	10% in the diet for 6 weeks	significantly increased the population of *bifidobacteria* and *lactobacilli*	The level of plasma glucose was decreased significantly	(Gobinath et al. 2010)
Trigonella foenum graecum soluble dietary fiber	T2DM rats	0.5 g/kg for 28 days	NA	No significant change in the level of insulin while the beneficial effect on dyslipidemia	(Hannan et al. 2003)

TABLE 5.4
Characteristics of Some Human Studies of Prebiotic Interventions and T2DM

Interventions	Results/Findings	References
NBS	Reduced fasting blood glucose	(Arias-Córdova et al. 2021)
GOS syrup	Improved *Bifidobacteriaceae*	(Gonai et al. 2017)
Acarbose	Improved glycemic control, and increased *Bifidobacterium longum*	(Gu et al. 2017)
High fiber diet	Improved HbA1c	(Zhao et al. 2018)

sugar intake and fast-food consumption, increase the risk of preterm delivery (Alves-Santos et al. 2019). Evidence also suggests that higher dietary fiber intake is associated with a reduced risk of gestational diabetes (Zhang et al. 2006). While there is limited human research on the effects of resistant starch (RS) on maternal hyperglycemia, studies in pregnant GK diabetic rats have shown improved glycemic control with RS consumption (Shen et al. 2011).

5.9 CONCLUSIONS

According to our analysis, Prebiotics and compounds with prebiotic characteristics may enhance metabolic and inflammatory indicators linked to diabetes. According to the abundance of articles and quality assessments, the interventions using resistant starch, resistant dextrin, and oligofructose-enriched inulin showed the greatest evidence to ameliorate diabetes. Even though there was insufficient research, several prebiotics and compounds with prebiotic characteristics also exhibit a positive impact on diabetic models.

REFERENCES

Akutko, K., & Stawarski, A. (2021). Probiotics, prebiotics and synbiotics in inflammatory bowel diseases. *Journal of Clinical Medicine*, 10(11), 2466.

Alves-Santos, N.H., Cocate, P.G., Benaim, C., Farias, D.R., Emmett, P.M., & Kac, G. (2019). Prepregnancy dietary patterns and their association with perinatal outcomes: A prospective cohort study. *Journal of the Academy of Nutrition and Dietetics*, 119(9), 1439–1451.

Arias-Córdova, Y., Ble-Castillo, J.L., García-Vázquez, C., Olvera-Hernández, V., Ramos-García, M., Navarrete-Cortes, A., Jiménez-Domínguez, G., Juárez-Rojop, I.E., Tovilla-Zárate, C.A., Martínez-López, M.C., & Méndez, J.D. (2021). Resistant starch consumption effects on glycemic control and glycemic variability in patients with type 2 diabetes: A randomized crossover study. *Nutrients*, 13(11), 4052.

Berger, K., Burleigh, S., Lindahl, M., Bhattacharya, A., Patil, P., Stålbrand, H., Nordberg Karlsson, E., Hållenius, F., Nyman, M., & Adlercreutz, P. (2021). Xylooligosaccharides increase Bifidobacteria and Lachnospiraceae in mice on a high-fat diet, with a concomitant increase in short-chain fatty acids, especially butyric acid. *Journal of Agricultural and Food Chemistry*, 69(12), 3617–3625.

Bernaud, F.S.R., Beretta, M.V., do Nascimento, C., Escobar, F., Gross, J.L., Azevedo, M.J., & Rodrigues, T.C. (2014). Fiber intake and inflammation in type 1 diabetes. *Diabetology and Metabolic Syndrome*, 6(1), 1–10.

Bodinham, C.L., Smith, L., Thomas, E.L., Bell, J.D., Swann, J.R., Costabile, A., Russell-Jones, D., Umpleby, A.M., & Robertson, M.D. (2014). Efficacy of increased resistant starch consumption in human type 2 diabetes. *Endocrine Connections*, 3(2), 75–84.

Byrne, C.S., Chambers, E.S., Morrison, D.J., & Frost, G. (2015). The role of short chain fatty acids in appetite regulation and energy homeostasis. *International Journal of Obesity*, 39(9), 1331–1338.

Chelakkot, C., Choi, Y., Kim, D.K., Park, H.T., Ghim, J., Kwon, Y., Jeon, J., Kim, M.S., Jee, Y.K., Gho, Y.S., Park, H.S., Kim, Y.K., & Ryu, S.H. (2018). Akkermansia muciniphila-derived extracellular vesicles influence gut permeability through the regulation of tight junctions. *Experimental & Molecular Medicine*, 50(2), e450–e450.

Chen, K., Chen, H., Faas, M.M., de Haan, B.J., Li, J., Xiao, P., Zhang, H., Diana, J., de Vos, P., & Sun, J. (2017). Specific inulin-type fructan fibers protect against autoimmune diabetes by modulating gut immunity, barrier function, and microbiota homeostasis. *Molecular Nutrition & Food Research*, 61(8). 10.1002/mnfr.201601006

Das, T., Jayasudha, R., Chakravarthy, S.K., Prashanthi, G.S., Bhargava, A., Tyagi, M., Rani, P.K., Pappuru, R.R., Sharma, S., & Shivaji, S. (2021). Alterations in the gut bacterial microbiome in people with type 2 diabetes mellitus and diabetic retinopathy. *Scientific Reports*, 11(1), 1–15.

Dehghan, P., Pourghassem Gargari, B., & Asghari Jafar-abadi, M. (2014). Oligofructose-enriched inulin improves some inflammatory markers and metabolic endotoxemia in women with type 2 diabetes mellitus: A randomized controlled clinical trial. *Nutrition*, 30(4), 418–423.

Gibson, G.R., Hutkins, R., Sanders, M.E., Prescott, S.L., Reimer, R.A., Salminen, S.J., Scott, K., Stanton, C., Swanson, K.S., Cani, P.D., Verbeke, K., & Reid, G. (2017). Expert consensus document: The International Scientific Association for Probiotics and Prebiotics (ISAPP) consensus statement on the definition and scope of prebiotics. *Nature Reviews Gastroenterology & Hepatology*, 14(8), 491–502.

Gibson, G.R., & Roberfroid, M.B. (1995). Dietary modulation of the human colonic microbiota: Introducing the concept of prebiotics. *The Journal of Nutrition*, 125(6), 1401–1412.

Gobinath, D., Madhu, A.N., Prashant, G., Srinivasan, K., & Prapulla, S.G. (2010). Beneficial effect of xylo-oligosaccharides and fructo-oligosaccharides in streptozotocin-induced diabetic rats. *British Journal of Nutrition*, 104(1), 40–47.

Gonai, M., Shigehisa, A., Kigawa, I., Kurasaki, K., Chonan, O., Matsuki, T., Yoshida, Y., Aida, M., Hamano, K., & Terauchi, Y. (2017). Galacto-oligosaccharides ameliorate dysbiotic Bifidobacteriaceae decline in Japanese patients with type 2 diabetes. *Beneficial Microbes*, 8(5), 705–716.

Gu, Y., Wang, X., Li, J., Zhang, Y., Zhong, H., Liu, R., Zhang, D., Feng, Q., Xie, X., Hong, J., Ren, H., Liu, W., Ma, J., Su, Q., Zhang, H., Yang, J., Wang, X., Zhao, X., Gu, W., … Wang, W. (2017). Analyses of gut microbiota and plasma bile acids enable stratification of patients for antidiabetic treatment. *Nature Communications*, 8(1), 1–12.

Gudi, R., Perez, N., Johnson, B.M., Sofi, M.H., Brown, R., Quan, S., Karumuthil-Melethil, S., & Vasu, C. (2019). Complex dietary polysaccharide modulates gut immune function and microbiota, and promotes protection from autoimmune diabetes. *Immunology*, 157(1), 70–85.

Gurung, M., Li, Z., You, H., Rodrigues, R., Jump, D.B., Morgun, A., & Shulzhenko, N. (2020). Role of gut microbiota in type 2 diabetes pathophysiology. *EBioMedicine*, 51, 102590.

Hannan, J.M.A., Rokeya, B., Faruque, O., Nahar, N., Mosihuzzaman, M., Azad Khan, A.K., & Ali, L. (2003). Effect of soluble dietary fibre fraction of Trigonella foenum graecum on glycemic, insulinemic, lipidemic and platelet aggregation status of Type 2 diabetic model rats. *Journal of Ethnopharmacology*, 88(1), 73–77. 10.1016/S0378-8741(03)00190-9

Hansen, C.H.F., Larsen, C.S., Petersson, H.O., Zachariassen, L.F., Vegge, A., Lauridsen, C., Kot, W., Krych, Ł., Nielsen, D.S., & Hansen, A.K. (2019). Targeting gut microbiota and barrier function with prebiotics to alleviate autoimmune manifestations in NOD mice. *Diabetologia*, 62(9), 1689–1700.

Ho, J., Reimer, R.A., Doulla, M., & Huang, C. (2016). Effect of prebiotic intake on gut microbiota, intestinal permeability and glycemic control in children with type 1 diabetes: Study protocol for a randomized controlled trial. *Trials*, 17(1), 1–8. 10.1186/S13063-016-1486-Y/TABLES/2

Huang, J., Wang, X., Tao, G., Song, Y., Ho, C., Zheng, J., & Ou, S. (2018). Feruloylated oligosaccharides from maize bran alleviate the symptoms of diabetes in streptozotocin-induced type 2 diabetic rats. *Food & Function*, 9(3), 1779–1789.

Insel, R., & Knip, M. (2018). Prospects for primary prevention of type 1 diabetes by restoring a disappearing microbe. *Pediatric Diabetes*, 19(8), 1400–1406.

International Diabetes Federation. (2017). *IDF Diabetes Atlas*, 8th ed. Brussels, Belgium: International Diabetes Federation. 9–44.

Koh, G.Y., Rowling, M.J., Schalinske, K.L., Grapentine, K., & Loo, Y.T. (2016). Consumption of dietary resistant starch partially corrected the growth pattern despite hyperglycemia and compromised kidney function in streptozotocin-induced diabetic rats. *Journal of Agricultural and Food Chemistry*, 64(40), 7540–7545.

Kumar, A., Prajapati, B.*, & Pramanik, J.(2022). Prebiotics as adjunctive therapy in diabetes: A review of prebiotics in diabetes. *Current Nutraceuticals*, 3(3), e180822207618.

Kumar, A., Pramanik, J., Goyal, N., Chauhan, D., Sivamaruthi, B.S., Prajapati, B.G., & Chaiyasut, C. (2023). Gut microbiota in anxiety and depression: Unveiling the relationships and management options. *Pharmaceuticals*, 16(4), 565.

Larsen, N., Vogensen, F.K., van den Berg, F.W.J., Nielsen, D.S., Andreasen, A.S., Pedersen, B.K., Al-Soud, W.A., Sørensen, S.J., Hansen, L.H., & Jakobsen, M. (2010). Gut microbiota in human adults with type 2 diabetes differs from non-diabetic adults. *PLoS One*, 5(2), e9085.

Lee, S.G., Lee, Y.H., Choi, E., Cho, Y., & Kim, J.H. (2019). Fasting serum bile acids concentration is associated with insulin resistance independently of diabetes status. *Clinical Chemistry and Laboratory Medicine*, 57(8), 1218–1228.

Li, W., Yu, S., Zhang, T., Jiang, B., Stressler, T., Fischer, L., & Mu, W. (2015). Efficient biosynthesis of lactosucrose from sucrose and lactose by the purified recombinant levansucrase from leuconostoc mesenteroides B-512 FMC. *Journal of Agricultural and Food Chemistry*, 63(44), 9755–9763.

Lin, C.F., Kuo, Y.T., Chen, T.Y., & Chien, C.T. (2016). Quercetin-rich guava (Psidium guajava) juice in combination with trehalose reduces autophagy, apoptosis and pyroptosis formation in the kidney and pancreas of type II diabetic rats. *Molecules*, 21(3), 334.

Ma, Q., Li, Y., Li, P., Wang, M., Wang, J., Tang, Z., Wang, T., Luo, L., Wang, C., & Zhao, B. (2019). Research progress in the relationship between type 2 diabetes mellitus and intestinal flora. *Biomedicine & Pharmacotherapy*, 117. 10.1016/j.biopha.2019.109138

McGowan, C.A., Walsh, J.M., Byrne, J., Curran, S., & McAuliffe, F.M. (2013). The influence of a low glycemic index dietary intervention on maternal dietary intake, glycemic index and gestational weight gain during pregnancy: A randomized controlled trial. *Nutrition Journal*, 12(1), 1–9.

Mishra, S., Wang, S., Nagpal, R., Miller, B., Singh, R., Taraphder, S., & Yadav, H. (2019). Probiotics and prebiotics for the amelioration of type 1 diabetes: Present and future perspectives. *Microorganisms*, 7(3), 67.

Nath, A., Haktanirlar, G., Varga, Á., Molnár, M.A., Albert, K., Galambos, I., Koris, A., & Vatai, G. (2018). Biological activities of lactose-derived prebiotics and symbiotic with probiotics on gastrointestinal system. *Medicina*, 54(2), 18.

Niinistö, S., Takkinen, H.M., Erlund, I., Ahonen, S., Toppari, J., Ilonen, J., Veijola, R., Knip, M., Vaarala, O., & Virtanen, S.M. (2017). Fatty acid status in infancy is associated with the risk of type 1 diabetes-associated autoimmunity. *Diabetologia*, 60(7), 1223–1233.

Nilsson, A.C., Johansson-Boll, E.V., & Björck, I.M.E. (2015). Increased gut hormones and insulin sensitivity index following a 3-d intervention with a barley kernel-based product: a randomised cross-over study in healthy middle-aged subjects. *British Journal of Nutrition*, 114(6), 899–907.

Parnell, J.A., & Reimer, R.A. (2009). Weight loss during oligofructose supplementation is associated with decreased ghrelin and increased peptide YY in overweight and obese adults. *The American Journal of Clinical Nutrition*, 89(6), 1751–1759.

Pedersen, C., Gallagher, E., Horton, F., Ellis, R.J., Ijaz, U.Z., Wu, H., Jaiyeola, E., Diribe, O., Duparc, T., Cani, P.D., Gibson, G.R., Hinton, P., Wright, J., la Ragione, R., & Robertson, M.D. (2016). Host–microbiome interactions in human type 2 diabetes following prebiotic fibre (galacto-oligosaccharide) intake. *British Journal of Nutrition*, 116(11), 1869–1877.

Plovier, H., Everard, A., Druart, C., Depommier, C., van Hul, M., Geurts, L., Chilloux, J., Ottman, N., Duparc, T., Lichtenstein, L., Myridakis, A., Delzenne, N.M., Klievink, J., Bhattacharjee, A., van der Ark, K.C.H., Aalvink, S., Martinez, L.O., Dumas, M.E., Maiter, D., … Cani, P.D. (2016). A purified membrane protein from Akkermansia muciniphila or the pasteurized bacterium improves metabolism in obese and diabetic mice. *Nature Medicine*, 23(1), 107–113.

Prawitt, J., Abdelkarim, M., Stroeve, J.H.M., Popescu, I., Duez, H., Velagapudi, V.R., Dumont, J., Bouchaert, E., van Dijk, T.H., Lucas, A., Dorchies, E., Daoudi, M., Lestavel, S., Gonzalez, F.J., Oresic, M., Cariou, B., Kuipers, F., Caron, S., & Staels, B. (2011). Farnesoid X receptor deficiency improves glucose homeostasis in mouse models of obesity. *Diabetes*, 60(7), 1861–1871.

Raafat, K., Wurglics, M., & Schubert-Zsilavecz, M. (2016). Prunella vulgaris L. active components and their hypoglycemic and antinociceptive effects in alloxan-induced diabetic mice. *Biomedicine & Pharmacotherapy*, 84, 1008–1018.

Roglic, G., Unwin, N., Bennett, P.H., Mathers, C., Tuomilehto, J., Nag, S., Connolly, V., & King, H. (2005). The burden of mortality attributable to diabetes realistic estimates for the year 2000. *Diabetes Care*, 28(9), 2130–2135.

Sartorelli, D.S., Zuccolotto, D.C.C., Crivellenti, L.C., & Franco, L.J. (2019). Dietary patterns during pregnancy derived by reduced-rank regression and their association with gestational diabetes mellitus. *Nutrition*, 60, 191–196.

Shen, L., Keenan, M.J., Raggio, A., Williams, C., & Martin, R.J. (2011). Dietary-resistant starch improves maternal glycemic control in Goto-Kakizaki rat. *Molecular Nutrition & Food Research*, 55(10), 1499–1508.

Sircana, A., Framarin, L., Leone, N., Berrutti, M., Castellino, F., Parente, R., de Michieli, F., Paschetta, E., & Musso, G. (2018). Altered gut microbiota in type 2 diabetes: Just a coincidence? *Current Diabetes Reports*, 18(10), 1–11.

Tancredi, M., Rosengren, A., Svensson, A.-M., Kosiborod, M., Pivodic, A., Gudbjörnsdottir, S., Wedel, H., Clements, M., Dahlqvist, S., & Lind, M. (2015). Excess mortality among persons with type 2 diabetes. *New England Journal of Medicine*, 373(18), 1720–1732.

Toporovski, M.S., de Morais, M.B., Abuhab, A., & Crippa Júnior, M.A. (2021). Effect of polydextrose/fructooligosaccharide mixture on constipation symptoms in children aged 4 to 8 years. *Nutrients*, 13(5), 1634.

Tran, N.T., Tang, Y., Li, Z., Zhang, M., Wen, X., Ma, H., & Li, S. (2020). Galactooligosaccharides and resistant starch altered microbiota and short-chain fatty acids in an in vitro fermentation study using gut contents of mud crab (Scylla paramamosain). *Frontiers in Microbiology*, 11, 1352.

Wan, C.S., Nankervis, A., Teede, H., & Aroni, R. (2019). Dietary intervention strategies for ethnic Chinese women with gestational diabetes mellitus: A systematic review and meta-analysis. *Nutrition & Dietetics*, 76(2), 211–232.

Wang, J., Qin, J., Li, Y., Cai, Z., Li, S., Zhu, J., Zhang, F., Liang, S., Zhang, W., Guan, Y., Shen, D., Peng, Y., Zhang, D., Jie, Z., Wu, W., Qin, Y., Xue, W., Li, J., Han, L., & Wang, J. (2012). A metagenome-wide association study of gut microbiota in type 2 diabetes. *Nature*, 490(7418), 55–60.

Xiao, L., Van't Land, B., Engen, P.A., Naqib, A., Green, S.J., Nato, A., Leusink-Muis, T., Garssen, J., Keshavarzian, A., Stahl, B., & Folkerts, G. (2018). Human milk oligosaccharides protect against the development of autoimmune diabetes in NOD-mice. *Scientific Reports*, 8(1). 10.1038/s41598-018-22052-y

Yoshida, N., Emoto, T., Yamashita, T., Watanabe, H., Hayashi, T., Tabata, T., Hoshi, N., Hatano, N., Ozawa, G., Sasaki, N., Mizoguchi, T., Amin, H.Z., Hirota, Y., Ogawa, W., Yamada, T., & Hirata, K.I. (2018). Bacteroides vulgatus and bacteroides dorei reduce gut microbial lipopolysaccharide production and inhibit atherosclerosis. *Circulation*, 138(22), 2486–2498.

Zaborska, K.E., & Cummings, B.P. (2018). Rethinking bile acid metabolism and signaling for type 2 diabetes treatment. *Current Diabetes Reports*, 18(11), 1–10.

Zhang, C., Liu, S., Solomon, C.G., & Hu, F.B. (2006). Dietary fiber intake, dietary glycemic load, and the risk for gestational diabetes mellitus. *Diabetes Care*, 29(10), 2223–2230.

Zhao, L., Zhang, F., Ding, X., Wu, G., Lam, Y.Y., Wang, X., Fu, H., Xue, X., Lu, C., Ma, J., Yu, L., Xu, C., Ren, Z., Xu, Y., Xu, S., Shen, H., Zhu, X., Shi, Y., Shen, Q., … Zhang, C. (2018). Gut bacteria selectively promoted by dietary fibers alleviate type 2 diabetes. *Science*, 359(6380), 1151–1156.

6 Nutraceuticals for Hormonal Imbalance Management

Sheetal Sonawdekar, Mala M. Parab, Amit Kumar Shrivastava, and Pramodkumar P. Gupta

6.1 INTRODUCTION

6.1.1 Hormones-Biochemical Emissaries

Hormones, biochemical emissaries, or stimulants, play a pivotal role in various metabolic processes in all living organisms. In the absence of these emissaries, a child's growth can get stunted, fertility can be abridged, sleep circadian cycles may get arrhythmic, and metabolic disorders may ensue. In the human body, the maximum genres of molecules are defined under the catalog of hormones. Many metabolites including the prostaglandins and thromboxanes belong to the eicosanoids group, brassinosteroid and estrogen from the group of steroids, ethylene and nitric oxide as gases, auxins, and epinephrine are well-known amino acid derivatives and from the clusters of protein and peptides are insulin and CLE peptides are well-defined hormones (Hiller-Sturmhöfel and Bartke 1998).

The hormones are well known to activate or deactivate the biological mechanism within the organism, they affect the distant cells by interacting and binding to their specific indigenous receptor/target protein within the target cells elucidating the change in function of the cell. It has been observed and well-studied that hormone binding to its indigenous receptor results in the stimulation and activation of the biochemical signal transduction pathway, typically actuating the transcription process and increasing the expression of target proteins. They also play a vital role in non-genomic pathways that synergize with the genomic effects. Peptides and amines-based hormones are hydrophilic in nature and generally are water-soluble hormones, and via second messengers they mostly act on the surface of the target cells. Steroid hormones are mostly hydrophobic in nature and are lipid-soluble hormones. Eventually, they pass through the plasma membranes (cytoplasmic and nuclear) of the target cells to act within their nuclei.

Polyhydroxy-type steroids like Brassinosteroids are known as the sixth class of plant hormones and are vital in the development and growth of the plant. This hormone may be advantageous as an anticancer drug by encouraging apoptosis in

DOI: 10.1201/9781003392934-6

the cancer cells for endocrine-responsive tumors. Though the brassinosteroids are lipid soluble, they are never attached to their receptor at the cell surface (Giorgio et al. 1974).

6.1.2 Hormonal Imbalance

A hormonal imbalance is an upshot from the inappropriate functioning of the endocrine system. The system includes the glands that are composed of the secreted hormones, the indigenous receptors that specifically respond to their indigenous hormones, and the associated organs that are undeviatingly influenced by the hormones. An imbalance may be represented as an excess of the particular hormone in certain cases, while in others there may be a scarcity. Depending on the type of hormone that is gone off the balance; a momentous impact on the signs and symptoms and associated risks shall be observed. A hormone flux may be thus contemplated as a hushed executioner and is impending as a legitimate epidemic not only to a specific nation but to the entire globe. At present, with a rapidly mounting society, privatization, transformation, globalization, and rigorous progression in agriculture, the lifestyle and food habits of humankind have become more susceptible to irritability, anxiety, edginess, mood fluctuations, vexation, and depression. All these factors have been observed to affect the metabolic activities of life forms grossly (Epel 2009). These effects usually occur with age and lead to comorbid disorders in many. A few studies on rats and humans have shown that environmental pollution has also contributed to the worsening of the individual's health at almost all ages by instigating the change and disruption of hormones. Furthermore, medications and therapeutics taken to treat a disease or disorder may instigate disturbance in bio-metabolic processes and intervene in the secretion and production of hormones (Ye et al. 2020).

Several studies have reported that, in comparison to male counterparts, the hormonal balance/flux frequency is more observed in females. Alterations in hormone secretion become more noticeable during menstruation, pregnancy, and menopause duration. In females, there are multifarious risk factors and symptoms of hormone imbalance, including an increase in the levels of free estrogen (hyperestrogenism) leading to early menarche, disorders of eating, endometriosis, premenstrual syndrome, uterine fibroids, muscular cramps, heavy bleeding and pain, infertility, and various cancers (Moridi et al. 2019).

6.2 ROLE OF DIET ON HORMONAL IMBALANCE AND RELATED METABOLIC DISORDERS

Hyperestrogenism can be attributed to lifestyle and dietary habits that may include a high intake of fatty foods, which are principally involved in causing obesity, along with an augmented translation of testosterone, the primary male hormone, to estrogens associated with the female reproductive organ in the existence of enzyme aromatase. It may also be accredited to hyperinsulinism, a condition with unregulated insulin secretion, and may result from mild to severe hypoglycemia (Collison et al. 2011).

It also intensifies the synthesis of testosterone in the ovary and lowers sex hormone-binding globulins, giving an upsurge in the level of free estrogen within the human blood. Thus, the appropriate diet significantly regulates the synthesis of estrogen, its metabolism, and its receptor activity (Malik 2021). Alcohol consumption obstructs the detoxification process of estrogen within the liver, increasing the levels of estradiol levels within the blood, which may lead to breast cancer in a human (Deshpande 1976). The estrogenic substances that are present in dairy products and food are also a foremost health concern for many. Studies supporting the causal agents such as hormones present in dairy products, estrogens, and insulin-like growth factor-1, cause a plausible impact on human health as they are triggering factors to breast, endometrial, and prostate tumors (Malekinejad and Rezabakhsh 2015).

The xenoestrogenic compounds used as herbicides and pesticides are now moved into our food chain causing multiple ill-health effects. Hormones that are causatively used to increase livestock and milk production have now been known to be effective agents that increase human susceptibility to environmental estrogens. These exogenous estrogens mimic endogenous hormones or interfere with endocrine processes, thereby ensuing disruption of routine cellular functions, development, and regulation of hemostasis in the nervous system and urogenital tract (Singleton and Khan 2003). Antibiotics, preservatives, and food coloring agents may also be a causative agent or a triggering factor in the high threat of breast cancer by varying gut flora involved in the enterohepatic circulation of estrogens (Dey and Nagababu 2022). Furthermore, the deficiencies of Vit A, Vit B6, Vit C, VitD3, Zinc, and overconsumption of sugar and saturated fats are directly correlated with the reduction levels of progesterone, which may eventually lead to an imbalance between progesterone and estrogen. As a consequence, a woman may undergo joint pain, weight gain, vaginal dryness, and urinary infection (Harmon et al. 2020). Likewise, prolonged and chronic stress mechanisms raise the levels of cortisol and adrenaline from the adrenal gland, which may prime suppression of the immune system and other opportunistic metabolic disorders. This process intensifies the blood flow and supply of glucose and oxygen to the neurons.

Diet constitution has also been insinuated to positively oscillate pancreatic beta cell responsiveness and subsequent insulin sensitivity. Insulin being a primary regulator of carbohydrate, fat, and protein metabolism, is a pivotal hormone in living forms. The deposited fat within the adipose tissues gets lipolysed, and in the liver, gluconeogenesis takes place, which accelerates the translocation of the GLUT-4 protein to push the glucose into muscle cells, besides the gene expression of proteins that are essential for the growth, cellular repair, and cellular function, and here it designates the metabolic availability of several fuels to the brain (Sears and Perry 2015).

The consumption of excess processed foods, saturated and trans fats, aerated drinks, canned juices, vitamin water, and artificial energy boosters all limit the complete functions of the hormone insulin and eventually lead to metabolic disorders like Diabetes Mellitus and inflammation-induced oxidative stress. Insulin resistance may also upsurge the quantity of androgens, and it may be the prime cause of acne, the occurrence of dark patches of skin on the neck region, or skin tags, facial hair growth, loss of head hair, or infertility (Ryan and Seeley 2013).

The basal metabolic rate of the human body is controlled by the thyroid hormones that act as a rheostat. A little decline in the secretion level of thyroid hormone, i.e., hypothyroidism, to an upsurge in level, i.e., hyperthyroidism, may result in various physiological changes. Hypothyroidism leads to cold intolerance, constipation, depression, dry skin, hair loss, and much more. Whereas, hyperthyroidism causes high energy and diarrhea, weight loss, and a warm body with increased metabolism all the time.

Cortisol has been reported to control glucose and insulin levels, inflammation, bone matrix deposition, muscle building, mood and mental focus, stamina, sex drive, and sleep cycles. Whereas, when stress increases, the levels of cortisol fluctuate and trigger blood sugar and imbalances in insulin, food cravings, and inhibition of thyroid function. A prolonged increase in glucocorticoids (cortisol) that transpire in times of stress, aging, and other traumatic conditions has also been associated with impaired metabolic functions of insulin and other hormones in the body (John E. Hall 2010). Across the globe, around 5–10% of women of reproductive age are affected by a multifaceted endocrine disorder known as polycystic ovary syndrome (PCOS).

It generally co-exists with oligo and/or anovulatory cycles, hirsutism, and polycystic ovaries, together with an extensive pervasiveness of insulin resistance. Through the productive period, it may cause anovulatory infertility and could be related to amplified prevalence of gestational tribulations, such as gestational diabetes, preeclampsia, and miscarriage. The condition may worsen and the patient may be exposed to a high risk of cardiovascular disease, diabetes, hypertension, and other types of numerous metabolic complications, especially after menopause. Most often, diets high in trans-fat, high sugar intake, Iodine and Zinc deficiency, smoking, and pollution are related to the onset of PCOS in the early age of females. Birth control pills and overdoses of some classes of antibiotics have also been found to escalate poly-ovulation and infertility in women (Szczuko et al. 2021). With an imbalance in insulin levels, the ovaries try to reimburse by producing more ovarian hormones, which eventually primes for disturbance in several metabolic processes of the body (Szczuko et al. 2021).

Few researchers have indicated that fluxes in the estrogen and progesterone levels may lead to intensification in abdominal painful and non-painful indications throughout the menstrual cycle and during the early menopause (perimenopause) transition in women with or without irritable bowel syndrome. Hormonal imbalance is well associated with pain in the head and back, bloating, obesity, cramping from mild to severe, hunger for sweet or salty food, sensitivity to allergic reactions, and temperature (Roop 2018). Administration of estrogen is well known to increase serotonin levels by declining the breakdown of serotonin and varying the mRNA and protein levels of numerous types of serotonin markers.

These changes may have a straight inference on female mood disorders, like during the menopausal transition, premenstrual disorders, and depression during pregnancy and postpartum (Epperson et al. 2012). If your diet consists of Xenoestrogens, then it may lead to the dominance of estrogen in the body, and that's a major cause for endometriosis, fibroids, hyperthyroidism, and eventually may lead to breast cancer too. The dominance of estrogen and unhealthy body conditions may cause hysterectomy – surgical removal of uterus or ovariectomy – surgical removal of ovaries or both, which might cause a sudden drop in the levels of estrogen, progesterone, and testosterone. Such conditions may mainly exhibit a decrease in bone density, causing osteoporosis, muscle mass, heart palpitations, stress, and depression (Szczuko et al. 2021).

Thus, augmented intake of simple sugars and high-fat content conveyed by a Western-style diet, followed by physical inactivity, are major reasons for the rising obesity epidemic in modern society. The postponement of the human lifespan and its natural effects far ahead of the reproductive age augmented the numerous burdens of metabolic disorders that are commonly associated with over-nutrition and age-related hypogonadism. Whereas considering sex steroids, which are essential regulators in both energy metabolism and reproductive function, an imbalance widely causes abnormality and disease in the human body, including dyslipidemia, glucose intolerance, increase in appetite, infertility, and, finally, obesity.

6.3 NEED FOR NUTRACEUTICALS

The standard treatment for curing or ameliorating the symptoms of hormonal imbalances includes mainly synthetic Hormone replacement therapy (HRT), especially if there is deficiency, hypo-synthesis, expression, or hormone activity. If the hormone levels are high in an individual, the different therapy alternatives include medication, surgery, radiotherapy, or combination therapy. However, the latest Hormone replacement therapy is an alternative, but it has a risk of an increased chance of heart disease, stroke, and it may cause a condition or blood clots to form, problems with gallbladder, and breast issues. Other risks, such as bloating in the stomach, pain in the head, and hot flashes, are few. Oral contraceptive pills may upsurge the resistance to insulin and may lead to an abnormal intolerance to glucose. However, all these factors may also put an individual at high risk of mounting Type-2 diabetes, high blood pressure, and cardiovascular disorders. Synthetic hormones may cause positive and negative side effects, including: breast sensitivity – inflamed or painful – stomach bloating, nausea, acne changes, variations in bleeding pattern, fluctuations in cholesterol levels, and alterations in risk to some cancers ("Diagnostic tests for metastatic breast cancer," n.d.).

Clinical and translational studies have thus suggested that dietary restriction along with complementary and alternative practices as adjuncts, can progress the metabolic and reproductive results of hormone-related pathologies, comprising the deficiency of testosterone in male and natural menopause and hyperandrogenemia in female insulin, thyroid, growth hormone, etc. Minimizing metabolic and reproductive decline through rationally designed therapeutics with natural bioactive compounds or nutraceuticals (as they are known) can help extend human reproductive age and promote a healthy lifestyle (Sharokhyan et al. 2022). In the current era, the incipient class of natural products are nutraceuticals that mark the fading contour between food and drugs. They have been used positively in therapeutic areas such as anti-arthritic, blood pressure, cold and cough, cancer, diabetes, digestion problems, osteoporosis, cholesterol control, painkillers, depression, and sleep disorders.

6.4 DISEASE ASSOCIATED WITH HORMONAL IMBALANCE

6.4.1 PCOS and Infertility

Among the various endocrine disorders identified in women, Polycystic ovarian syndrome is the most common occurring in one out of seven during the reproductive age. Nearly two-thirds of the women will not ovulate steadily and will seek treatment (Hart 2008). In common diagnosis, infertility was not identified as a root cause for the increased risk of cardiovascular disease or metabolic dysfunction disorder. But it was specific that women with infertility linked with polycystic ovarian syndrome (PCOS), do seem more likely to develop a high risk of cardiovascular or metabolic dysfunction disorders such as diabetes (Hanson et al. 2017).

For this current generation, the most common and well-known abnormal endocrine condition for women is (PCOS) polycystic ovarian syndrome. Indications of hyperandrogenism (a condition of the presence of a high proportion of male sex hormones androsterone, androstenedione, and testosterone in women and the consequences that they have on the female body (Ashraf et al. 2019; "Hyperandrogenism," n.d.)), irregular menstrual periods, and insulin resistance are all traits associated with PCOS (Zehravi et al. 2021). Studies reported that PCOS patients treated with insulin sensitizers, metformin, or thiazolidinediones, have implicated a positive outcome where an increase in ovulation rates is reported, followed by a number of successful pregnancies (Froment and Touraine 2006). The study also mentioned that the inhibition of hepatic gluconeogenesis is carried by metformin and thus the decrease in the insulin level (Lauretta et al. 2016; Shaw et al. 2005). Hence it is noted that metformin-based treatment for PCOS women helps in overcoming reproductive-based abnormalities, restoration of ovulation, and positive regulation of fertility (Dronavalli and Ehrmann 2007; Lauretta et al. 2016; Talaulikar et al. 2016).

6.4.2 Diabetes

Diabetes mellitus, or diabetes, is a group of heterogeneous disorders in which there is an increase in blood glucose concentration (Roden 2016; Taylor 2021). Today, Diabetes mellitus (DM) and diabetes-associated impediments are amidst the foremost reasons for fatality across the globe. As per the International Diabetes Federation (IDF), by 2035 there will be an estimated 592 million people who will suffer from diabetes mellitus (Patel et al. 2022). There are four types of diabetes: prediabetes, type 1 diabetes, type 2 diabetes, and gestational diabetes. Insulin, a peptide hormone, is produced by the pancreatic β-cells and has a major role in maintaining the homeostasis of glucose in humans. Studies have reported that deficiency in β-cell insulin production leads to a disturbance in the maintenance of blood glucose levels and the onset of type 1 diabetes and type 2 diabetes, including multiple metabolic disorders associated with high or abnormal levels of blood glucose (Rachdaoui 2020).

Prediabetes, or intermediate hyperglycemia, is a condition where the glycaemic variables are above standard but lesser than diabetes edge. The condition intensifies the high-risk state for an individual to become diabetic in the near future. Experts predicted that by the year 2030, there will be around 470 million people suffering from prediabetes (Tabák et al. 2012; Taylor 2021). The prediabetes condition estimates a high risk for type 2 diabetes, heart disease, and stroke (Taylor 2021). Type 1 diabetes is a prolonged autoimmune disease considered by insulin deficit that is subsequent to the hyperglycemia condition (DiMeglio et al. 2018).

Type 1 diabetes damages the tiny blood vessels in the eyes – diabetic retinopathy damages the nerves – diabetic neuropathy damages the kidneys – and diabetic nephropathy is followed by a high risk of heart disease and stroke (Taylor 2021). Type 2 diabetes is a disease condition where the levels of sugar in the blood are very high or in a hyperglycemic condition. Usually, the peptide hormone "Insulin," produced by the beta cells of the pancreatic islets encoded by the INS gene in humans, controls the level of glucose (sugar) in the human bloodstream and helps the glucose get into the cell to give them energy ("MedlinePlus," n.d.). Incidents with a change in lifestyle and obesity have increased the incidence of gestational diabetes mellitus (GDM) including perinatal complications (Lende and Rijhsinghani 2020). The diabetes diagnosed foremost during pregnancy (gestation) is known as gestational pregnancy. Like the pre- Type 1- and Type 2 diabetes, gestational diabetes also affects the glucose (sugar) metabolism in an individual, which leads to high blood sugar, and may affect the mother's and fetus' health and cause many complications ("Gestational Diabetes," n.d.). The common symptoms of diabetes are often urination (mostly in night), feeling very thirsty, loss of weight, feeling hungry most of the time, numb or tingling of hands or feet, feeling tired mostly, dry skin, slowly healing soares, more infection episodes ("Diabetes Symptoms," 2022; Lal 2016) and many of which that are not yet identified or classified in detail.

6.4.3 Obesity

Over or excess body weight is one of the major risk factors for the onset of many diseases among populations worldwide. Due to obesity, numerous adverse consequences exist for human health diseases including cardiovascular disease, type 2 diabetes, and several cancers. The diseases are due to complex pathological processes imitating environmental and genetic interactions, too. It is also aggravated by age-related factors, reduction in physical activity and mobility, dietary changes, and overconsumption of food (Haslam and James 2005). It is well-defined that the causal agent for obesity is the difference between energy intake and energy expenditure. Worldwide, the prevalence of obesity is more severe in females compared to males, and obesity-related disease risk factors are more diverse in women than with respect to men. Pre-clinical and clinical studies suggest the role of ovarian hormone might play a major role in the obesity of female counterparts (Leeners et al. 2017). Numerous studies reported the change in the hormonal milieu during the menopause transition is widely associated with the upsurge in total body fat and rise in abdominal fat. In the midlife age of an individual, an increase in body weight raises the menace of cardiovascular disease, metabolic disease, including impacts on the quality of life and sexual function. The overall impact of weight gain sometimes leads to additional psychological and physical morbidity. However, studies suggest that the overall body fat mass can be reduced with the help of estrogen-progestin therapy, which enhances insulin sensitivity in the individual and may lower the rate of development of type 2 diabetes (Davis et al. 2012).

6.4.4 Hair Loss

Alopecia or Hair loss marks both men and women of all ages and considerably disturbs social and psychological comfort (Springer et al. 2003). Numerous reasons are known for hair loss such as hereditary (family history), hormonal changes, and medical conditions, side effects of medication and supplements, radiation therapy, stress, hairstyles, and treatment ("Hair loss," 2022). In women, hair loss is a clinical grievance as it is associated with severe emotional distress (Tosti et al. 2009). The most common form of hair loss is Androgenetic alopecia, with a specific pattern in men where temporal-frontal loss of hair is identified, and in women, central thinning (Springer et al. 2003). It has been reported that deficiency of proteins, minerals, essential fatty acids, and vitamins, due to inborn errors or a decrease in intake may lead to various structural abnormalities in an individual including loss of hair (Finner 2013).

6.5 WHAT ARE NUTRACEUTICALS?

For ages, humans have recognized the healing potential of the foods and food products that are naturally available. They have tested many foods and herbal extracts that have been known to be a classical modus operandi to achieving complete wellbeing, especially in the primitive ayurvedic system in India, as also in the case of traditional Chinese, Roman, and Greek medicines. Since then, scientists have tried to explore food's hidden potential to benefit our health. And, with this exploration today we have a category of food which is called Nutraceuticals. The term Nutraceutical was coined by DeFelice in 1939. The word, Nutraceutical has two parts: nutrition and pharmaceutical (Chaudhari 2017). One can say that a nutraceutical is a nutritional food or a food product that plays a key role in maintaining a healthy body and acts as a necessary supplement required for various metabolic activities regulating body functions and preventing infections or diseases (Chanda et al. 2019). Nutraceuticals are known to provide extra health benefits, other than the basic nutritional value found in foods. Nowadays, nutraceuticals are gaining considerable interest not only due to their potential nutritional effects but also due to their safety, and therapeutic effects. As side effects and antimicrobial resistance can be associated with some pharmaceutical drugs, the emergence of nutraceutical compounds has gained attention as precautionary measures as well as an alternative therapy alongside their supremacy in affordability and easy availability (AlAli et al. 2021). Several studies have significantly shown the beneficial effects of nutraceutical ingredients in curing several diseases including the ones related to hormonal imbalances. Recent studies have shown promising results for many such compounds in treating various complications.

The main aim of this chapter is to give an overview of several types of nutraceuticals and highlight their properties along with their potential therapeutic activities in treating hormonal imbalances. Additionally, the safety of nutraceuticals will also be discussed.

6.6 TYPES OF NUTRACEUTICALS

There are different ways in which nutraceuticals can be classified. They can be clustered based on their natural resources, chemical composition, along with pharmacological conditions and composition, Figure 6.1. Quite often they are relegated as dietary supplements, functional food, medicinal food, and pharmaceuticals.

In this chapter, we will be focusing more on nutraceuticals as dietary supplements or the ones with medicinal value, especially in curing hormonal imbalance. The PCOS, PMS, and menopausal transition are part of almost every woman's life and directly affect the reproductive hormones. Similarly, with lifestyle changes many times hormonal imbalance is caused resulting in Type 2 Diabetes and other diseases. Hormone replacement therapy (HRT) is the first choice in the treatment of such hormonal imbalances, but the several side effects associated with the therapy and the high cost of the treatment make patients look for natural, alternative treatments.

As mentioned above, several types of nutraceuticals can be used to treat different diseases related to hormonal imbalance, here we will consider them based on their natural sources.

6.6.1 NUTRACEUTICALS FROM PLANTS

Phytochemicals are plant-derived biomolecules that are majorly classified into categories like Phytoestrogens, fatty acids, polyphenols, catechins, flavonoids, phytosterols, dietary fibers, etc. Phytoestrogens are presently the most popular form

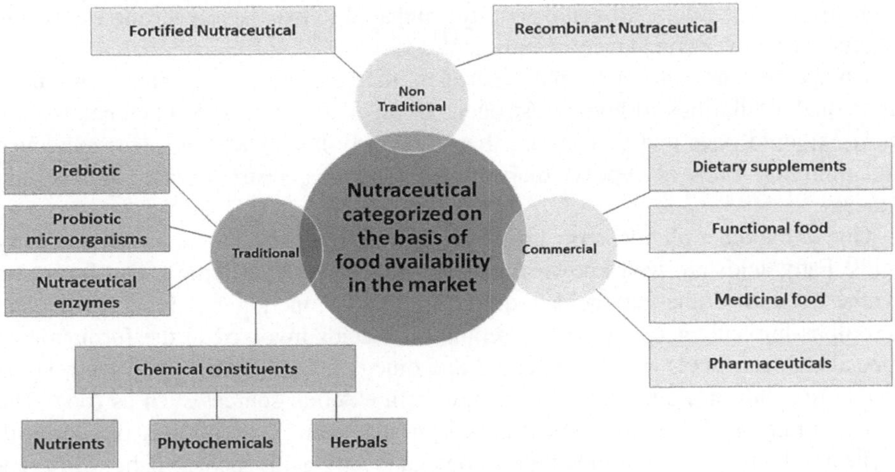

FIGURE 6.1 Nutraceutical category (Chaudhari 2017).

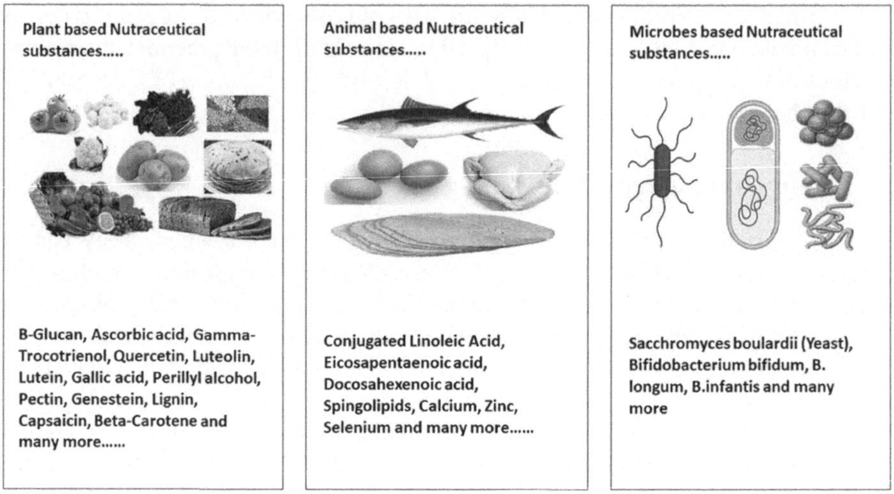

FIGURE 6.2 Nutraceutical substance from different sources.

of alternative therapy used for PMS and PCOS-related problems. The main classes are isoflavones, lignans, cumestan, and lactones. The commonly explored food sources include soy flour, legumes, fruits and vegetables, cereals, olive oil, wheat, etc., Figure 6.2.

Phytoestrogens can cause estrogenic or/and anti-estrogenic effects because of their structural similarity with estradiol (17-β-estradiol). They compete with more potent estrogens for "receptor binding sites" on cells. When the hormone comes in contact with the "receptor binding site," they exert their cellular effect. If the body has low levels of estrogen, then receptor binding sites can be occupied by phytoestrogen to gently mimic the role of estrogens. On the contrary, if the estrogen level in the body is too high, phytoestrogen competes with estrogen to access receptor sites. They try to exert their own milder estrogenic activity compared to excessively strong estrogenic effects due to over-abundance of estrogen.

Isoflavones are one such phytoestrogen that are known to have structural/functional similarities to human estrogen. In this category Soy isoflavones are the most explored ones and consuming them regularly has exhibited lower incidence and mortality rates of type II diabetes, osteoporosis, heart disease, and certain cancers.

One of the other phytochemicals used to treat different hormonal balances is fatty acids. Fatty acids are well known for their role in body functioning. Our body can synthesize most of the fatty acids required for proper functioning. However, linoleic and alpha-linolenic acids are two essential fatty acids involved in the formation of specialized fatty acids such as omega-3 and omega-6 fatty acids, which the body is unable to synthesize and needs to procure from external sources such as food. The omega-6 fatty acid, Linoleic acid is present in abundance in sunflower oil, corn oil, soybean oil, etc whereas, foods high in omega-3 fatty acids include fishes, different nuts and seeds, spinach, flaxseed oil, canola oil, etc. Dietary fatty acids have a significant impact on hormone, and neuropeptide concentrations as well as their receptors. Polyunsaturated fatty acids (PUFA) increase plasma insulin concentration and decrease insulin resistance. Hence, supplementing the daily diet with PUFAs can lead to the betterment of the symptoms associated with diabetes and obesity. In patients diagnosed with diabetes, Omega-3 fatty acids have been proposed to reduce glucose tolerance. Ethyl esters of n–3 fatty acids also are under exploration for their beneficial effects in diabetic patients.

6.6.2 Nutraceuticals from Animals

Molecules obtained from animal sources also referred to as zoo chemicals, have been explored extensively by nutritionists. One of the common nutraceuticals obtained from animal sources is Fatty acids. As mentioned above our body cannot synthesize two essential fatty acids, linoleic and alpha-linolenic, that are responsible for building omega-3 and omega-6 fatty acids, and need to be obtained externally via food. The omega-6 fatty acid, Linoleic acid is present in abundance in animal meat whereas, Omega 3 fatty acids are commonly found in different fishes such as salmon, halibut, sardines, albacore, trout, herring, shrimp, clams, light chunk tuna, catfish, cod, etc., Figure 6.2. The normal functioning of the endocrine system is also found to be strongly associated with fatty acids. They direct the secretion of endocrine hormones to their target cells. They are responsible for the production and synthesis of hormone-like substances known as prostaglandins, steroids, and other fatty acids that are needed for many physiologic processes. Prostaglandins play a very critical role in normal physiological processes such as homeostatic regulation, synovial pressure regulation, the body's response to pain, immune responses, regulating bodily secretions, and maintenance of viscosity.

6.6.3 Nutraceuticals from Microorganisms

Most of the hormonal imbalances are associated with diet as mentioned earlier. Along with that, having the proper digestive system is equally important. Our gut is colonized by unicellular eukaryotes, and Bacteria, including Bacteroidetes, Firmicutes, and Actinobacteria. These organisms not only aid in maintaining a healthy gut but also play a key role in the endocrine and reproductive system. Fortunately, any dysbiosis associated with these systems can be treated with probiotics, especially Lactobacilli and Bifidobacteria. Many times, in relieving pre and post-menopausal symptoms microbiotas can be really useful. Few works have reported that maintaining adequate estrogen before the onset of menopause can act as an antioxidant to substantially balance oxidative stress (Chen et al. 2022).

During the course of menopause, estrogen synthesis is found to be inconsistent and leads to an increase in oxidative stress which is a key contributor to the aging process as well as exacerbation of menopausal symptoms. With the help of different studies conducted it can be said that LAB can act as a good antioxidant and can prevent stress due to different oxidative mechanisms. In vitro studies, quite a few LAB strains and their metabolites have exhibited resistance against oxidative stress either by scavenging molecules such as 1,1-diphenyl-2-picrylhydrazyl, O_2^-, and H_2O_2 (Leeners et al. 2017) or by chelation of metal ions like Fe2+ and Cu2+. From studies, scientists have also proposed that the antioxidant capacity of LAB is possibly due to the chelation of metal ions (Davis et al. 2012). Also, LAB has enzymatic regulation as another mode of action, including regulation of certain ROS-producing enzymes, induction of the activity of host antioxidative enzymes, and regulation of the auto-secretion of antioxidant enzymes. In addition to this, LAB helps phytoestrogens to bind to estrogen receptors more efficiently and convert them into their active biomolecular form which has stronger estrogenic and anti-estrogenic properties. Furthermore, LAB supplements may also influence estrogen metabolism by regulating the estrobolome. Several studies have shown that LAB is directly or indirectly involved in regulating hypothalamic-pituitary hormones (Erdman and Poutahidis 2014) Figure 6.2.

6.7 CONCLUSION

Over time, scientists have been working on Nutraceuticals and have collected substantial evidence for their health benefits and disease prevention capability. They provide all the essential substances that should be present in a healthy diet for humans. In the present scenario where people prefer self-medication before approaching the experts, nutraceuticals are surely playing a major role in therapeutic development. Also, in comparison to pharmaceuticals, there are very few side effects associated with Nutraceuticals. But without any doubt, their success depends on how well their quality, purity, safety, and efficacy are maintained.

REFERENCES

AlAli, M., Alqubaisy, M., Aljaafari, M.N., AlAli, A.O., Baqais, L., Molouki, A., … Lim, S.-H. E. (2021). Nutraceuticals: Transformation of conventional foods into health promoters/disease preventers and safety considerations. *Molecules*, *26*(9), 2540. 10.3390/molecules26092540

Ashraf, S., Nabi, M., Rasool, S. ul A., Rashid, F., & Amin, S. (2019). Hyperandrogenism in polycystic ovarian syndrome and role of CYP gene variants: a review. *Egyptian Journal of Medical Human Genetics*, *20*(1), 25. 10.1186/s43042-019-0031-4

Chanda, S., Tiwari, R.K., Kumar, A., & Singh, K. (2019). Nutraceuticals inspiring the current therapy for lifestyle diseases. *Advances in Pharmacological Sciences*, *2019*, 1–5. 10.1155/2019/6908716

Chaudhari, S.P. (2017). Nutraceuticals: A review. *World Journal of Pharmacy and Pharmaceutical Sciences*, *6*(8), 681–739. 10.20959/wjpps20178-9825

Chen, Q., Wang, H., Wang, G., Zhao, J., Chen, H., Lu, X., & Chen, W. (2022). Lactic acid bacteria: A promising tool for menopausal health management in women. *Nutrients*, *14*(21), 4466. 10.3390/nu14214466

Collison, K.S., Zaidi, M.Z., Saleh, S.M., Inglis, A., Mondreal, R., Makhoul, N.J., … Al-Mohanna, F.A. (2011). Effect of trans-fat, fructose and monosodium glutamate feeding on feline weight gain, adiposity, insulin sensitivity, adipokine and lipid profile. *British Journal of Nutrition*, *106*(2), 218–226. 10.1017/S000711451000588X

Davis, S.R., Castelo-Branco, C., Chedraui, P., Lumsden, M.A., Nappi, R.E., Shah, D., … Writing Group of the International Menopause Society for World Menopause Day 2012. (2012). Understanding weight gain at menopause. *Climacteric: The Journal of the International Menopause Society*, *15*(5), 419–429. 10.3109/13697137.2012.707385

Deshpande, N. (1976). Hormonal imbalance in breast cancer. In *Proceedings of the fourth international congress on hormonal steroids* (pp. 735–741). Elsevier. 10.1016/B978-0-08-019682-4.50096-2

Dey, S., & Nagababu, B.H. (2022). Applications of food color and bio-preservatives in the food and its effect on the human health. *Food Chemistry Advances*, *1*, 100019. 10.1016/j.focha.2022.100019

Diabetes Symptoms. (2022). Retrieved from https://www.cdc.gov/diabetes/basics/symptoms.html

Diagnostic tests for metastatic breast cancer. (n.d.). Retrieved from https://www.ncbi.nlm.nih.gov/books/NBK361015/

DiMeglio, L.A., Evans-Molina, C., & Oram, R.A. (2018). Type 1 diabetes. *Lancet (London, England)*, *391*(10138), 2449–2462. 10.1016/S0140-6736(18)31320-5

Dronavalli, S., & Ehrmann, D.A. (2007). Pharmacologic therapy of polycystic ovary syndrome. *Clinical Obstetrics and Gynecology*, *50*(1), 244–254. 10.1097/GRF.0b013e31802f35a0

Epel, E. (2009). Psychological and metabolic stress: A recipe for accelerated cellular aging? *Hormones*, *8*(1), 7–22. 10.14310/horm.2002.1217

Epperson, C.N., Amin, Z., Ruparel, K., Gur, R., & Loughead, J. (2012). Interactive effects of estrogen and serotonin on brain activation during working memory and affective processing in menopausal women. *Psychoneuroendocrinology*, *37*(3), 372–382. 10.1016/j.psyneuen.2011.07.007

Erdman, S.E., & Poutahidis, T. (2014). Probiotic "glow of health": it's more than skin deep. *Beneficial Microbes*, *5*(2), 109–119. 10.3920/BM2013.0042

Finner, A.M. (2013). Nutrition and hair: deficiencies and supplements. *Dermatologic Clinics*, *31*(1), 167–172. 10.1016/j.det.2012.08.015

Froment, P., & Touraine, P. (2006). Thiazolidinediones and fertility in polycystic ovary syndrome (PCOS). *PPAR Research*, *2006*, 73986. 10.1155/PPAR/2006/73986

Gestational Diabetes. (n.d.). Retrieved February 13, 2023, from https://www.mayoclinic.org/diseases-conditions/gestational-diabetes/symptoms-causes/syc-20355339

Giorgio, N.A., Johnson, C.B., & Blecher, M. (1974). Hormone receptors. *Journal of Biological Chemistry*, *249*(2), 428–437. 10.1016/S0021-9258(19)43048-2

Hair loss. (2022). Retrieved February 13, 2023, from https://www.mayoclinic.org/diseases-conditions/hair-loss/symptoms-causes/syc-20372926

Hanson, B., Johnstone, E., Dorais, J., Silver, B., Peterson, C.M., & Hotaling, J. (2017). Female infertility, infertility-associated diagnoses, and comorbidities: a review. *Journal of Assisted Reproduction and Genetics*, *34*(2), 167–177. 10.1007/s10815-016-0836-8

Harmon, Q.E., Kissell, K., Jukic, A.M.Z., Kim, K., Sjaarda, L., Perkins, N.J., … Mumford, S.L. (2020). Vitamin D and reproductive hormones across the menstrual cycle. *Human Reproduction*, *35*(2), 413–423. 10.1093/humrep/dez283

Hart, R. (2008). PCOS and infertility. *Panminerva Medica*, *50*(4), 305–314. Retrieved from http://www.ncbi.nlm.nih.gov/pubmed/19078871

Haslam, D.W., & James, W.P.T. (2005). Obesity. *Lancet (London, England)*, *366*(9492), 1197–1209. 10.1016/S0140-6736(05)67483-1

Hiller-Sturmhöfel, S., & Bartke, A. (1998). The endocrine system: an overview. *Alcohol Health and Research World*, *22*(3), 153–164. Retrieved from http://www.ncbi.nlm.nih.gov/pubmed/15706790

Hyperandrogenism. (n.d.). Retrieved February 15, 2023, from https://www.topdoctors.co.uk/medical-dictionary/hyperandrogenism#

John E. Hall, J.E.H. (2010). *Guyton and Hall Textbook of Medical Physiology* (12th ed.). Retrieved from https://www.uk.elsevierhealth.com/guyton-and-hall-textbook-of-medical-physiology-e-book-9781437726749.html

Lal, B.S. (2016). Diabetes: Causes, symptoms and treatments. In B.S. Lal (Ed.) *Public health environment and social issues in India* (1st ed., pp. 55–67). Serials Publications.

Lauretta, R., Lanzolla, G., Vici, P., Mariani, L., Moretti, C., & Appetecchia, M. (2016). Insulin-sensitizers, polycystic ovary syndrome and gynaecological cancer risk. *International Journal of Endocrinology, 2016*, 8671762. 10.1155/2016/8671762

Leeners, B., Geary, N., Tobler, P.N., & Asarian, L. (2017). Ovarian hormones and obesity. *Human Reproduction Update, 23*(3), 300–321. 10.1093/humupd/dmw045

Lende, M., & Rijhsinghani, A. (2020). Gestational diabetes: Overview with emphasis on medical management. *International Journal of Environmental Research and Public Health, 17*(24). 10.3390/ijerph17249573

Malekinejad, H., & Rezabakhsh, A. (2015). Hormones in dairy foods and their impact on public health - A narrative review article. *Iranian Journal of Public Health, 44*(6), 742–758. Retrieved from http://www.ncbi.nlm.nih.gov/pubmed/26258087

Malik Aubead, N. (2021). Role of sex hormones in human body. In C. Marsh (Ed.) *Reproductive hormones*. IntechOpen. 10.5772/intechopen.95778

MedlinePlus. (n.d.). Retrieved February 16, 2022, from https://medlineplus.gov/diabetestype2.html

Moridi, A., Roozbeh, N., Yaghoobi, H., Soltani, S., Dashti, S., Shahrahmani, N., & Banaei, M. (2019). Etiology and risk factors associated with infertility. *International Journal of Women's Health and Reproduction Sciences, 7*(3), 346–353. 10.15296/ijwhr.2019.57

Patel, R., Parmar, N., Pramanik Palit, S., Rathwa, N., Ramachandran, A.V., & Begum, R. (2022). Diabetes mellitus and melatonin: Where are we? *Biochimie, 202*, 2–14. 10.1016/j.biochi.2022.01.001

Rachdaoui, N. (2020). Insulin: The friend and the foe in the development of type 2 diabetes mellitus. *International Journal of Molecular Sciences, 21*(5). 10.3390/ijms21051770

Roden, M. (2016). [Diabetes mellitus: definition, classification and diagnosis]. *Wiener Klinische Wochenschrift, 128 Suppl*, S, 37–40. 10.1007/s00508-015-0931-3

Roop, J.K. (2018). Hormone imbalance—A cause for concern in women. *RJLBPCS, 4*(2), 23–251. 10.26479/2018.0402.18

Ryan, K.K., & Seeley, R.J. (2013). Food as a hormone. *Science, 339*(6122), 918–919. 10.1126/science.1234062

Sears, B., & Perry, M. (2015). The role of fatty acids in insulin resistance. *Lipids in Health and Disease, 14*(1), 121. 10.1186/s12944-015-0123-1

Sharokhyan Rezaee, M., Farzinpour, A., Farshad, A., & Hatfaludi, T. (2022). The regulative effect of Urtica dioica on sex hormones imbalance: elevated follicle-stimulating hormone/luteinizing hormone ratio ≥4.5 is associated with low performance in aged breeder quails. *Italian Journal of Animal Science, 21*(1), 142–152. 10.1080/1828051X.2021.2007801

Shaw, R.J., Lamia, K.A., Vasquez, D., Koo, S.-H., Bardeesy, N., Depinho, R.A., … Cantley, L.C. (2005). The kinase LKB1 mediates glucose homeostasis in liver and therapeutic effects of metformin. *Science (New York, N.Y.), 310*(5754), 1642–1646. 10.1126/science.1120781

Sinai Talaulikar, V., Tang, T., & Yasmin, E. (2016). Role of metformin in women's health: Review of its current place in clinical practice and emerging indications for future. *Obstetrical & Gynecological Survey, 71*(5), 307–317. 10.1097/OGX.0000000000000312

Singleton, D.W., & Khan, S.A. (2003). Xenoestrogen exposure and mechanisms of endocrine disruption. *Frontiers in Bioscience: A Journal and Virtual Library, 8*, s110–s118. 10.2741/1010

Springer, K., Brown, M., & Stulberg, D.L. (2003). Common hair loss disorders. *American Family Physician, 68*(1), 93–102. Retrieved from http://www.ncbi.nlm.nih.gov/pubmed/12887115

Szczuko, M., Kikut, J., Szczuko, U., Szydłowska, I., Nawrocka-Rutkowska, J., Ziętek, M., ... Saso, L. (2021). Nutrition strategy and life style in polycystic ovary syndrome—Narrative review. *Nutrients*, *13*(7), 2452. 10.3390/nu13072452

Tabák, A.G., Herder, C., Rathmann, W., Brunner, E.J., & Kivimäki, M. (2012). Prediabetes: a high-risk state for diabetes development. *Lancet (London, England)*, *379*(9833), 2279–2290. 10.1016/S0140-6736(12)60283-9

Taylor, R.B. (2021). Types of Diabetes Mellitus. Retrieved February 15, 2023, from https://www.webmd.com/diabetes/guide/types-of-diabetes-mellitus

Tosti, A., Piraccini, B.M., Sisti, A., & Duque-Estrada, B. (2009). Hair loss in women. *Minerva Ginecologica*, *61*(5), 445–452. Retrieved from http://www.ncbi.nlm.nih.gov/pubmed/19749676

Ye, X., Pan, W., Li, C., Ma, X., Yin, S., Zhou, J., & Liu, J. (2020). Exposure to polycyclic aromatic hydrocarbons and risk for premature ovarian failure and reproductive hormones imbalance. *Journal of Environmental Sciences*, *91*, 1–9. 10.1016/j.jes.2019.12.015

Zehravi, M., Maqbool, M., & Ara, I. (2021). Polycystic ovary syndrome and infertility: an update. *International Journal of Adolescent Medicine and Health*, *34*(2), 1–9. 10.1515/ijamh-2021-0073

7 Nutraceuticals for Hypertension Management

A. Prabitha Priyadharshini, M. Dhivya Sree, S. Lakshmana Prabu, and M. Vijayalakshmi

7.1 INTRODUCTION

Nutraceuticals are the products developed from food or part of food, isolated nutrients, or any dietary supplements that are intended for any physiological benefit or therapeutic advantage. These act in diversified ways based on the functional compounds present in them by exhibiting preventative or remedial effects. Hypertension (HTN) is a chronic disease condition marked by persistent high blood pressure in arteries. Its etiology is multifactorial involving multiple pathophysiological, environmental, genetic factors where many are complexly interplayed. Various functional compounds have been characterized to study their anti-hypertensive effects and confirmed to possess the potential to regulate the disturbances occurring in physiological systems. Hence, understanding their mechanism of action can play a key role in treating the disease condition better based on its etiological origin. HTN is both preventable and treatable. Utilization of nutraceuticals accordingly can have a significant contribution to better prevention and management of HTN. This chapter deals with the pathophysiology of HTN and the clinical aspects which can be targeted with nutraceuticals possessing anti-hypertensive potential.

7.2 HYPERTENSION – PATHOPHYSIOLOGY

Blood pressure (BP) in the human physiological system is denoted by systolic (the pressure exerted by blood on the blood vessels during heart contraction) to the diastolic (pressure exerted during heart relaxation) ratio. Normal blood pressure lies below the range of 120 mmHg /80 mmHg. The risk of hypertension increases with an increase in the above value. The condition can be classified into two types based on the origin of cause, essential, idiopathic, or primary hypertension and secondary hypertension. High BP having no known cause or not due to any other medical condition defines the former one. The majority (90–95%) of the cases fall into this category (Oparil et al. 2018). Risk factors contributing may include smoking, alcohol consumption, family history, lifestyle modifications, obesity, improper diet, stress, etc. The same with known causes occurring due to underlying medical

 DOI: 10.1201/9781003392934-7

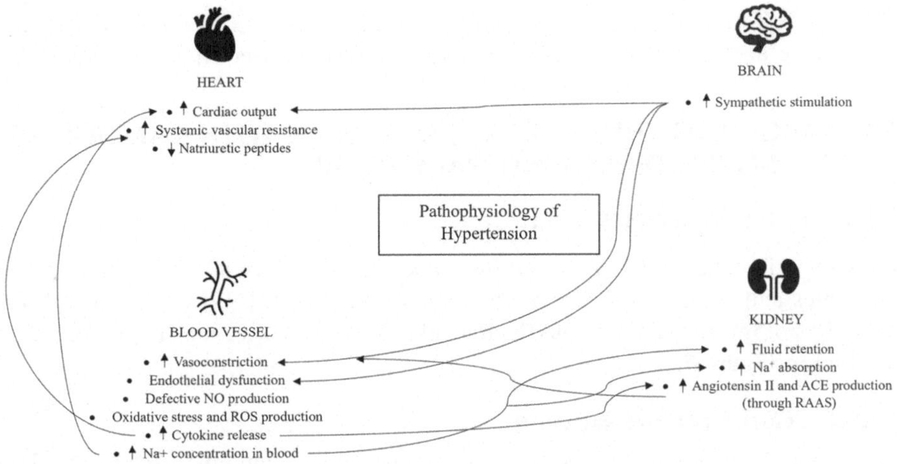

FIGURE 7.1 Pathophysiology of hypertension.

conditions like stroke, CVDs, kidney disease, adrenal and thyroid dysfunctions, sleep apnea, etc. defines the latter one. This is a rare phenomenon appearing in only about 10–5% cases of all. The pathophysiology of Hypertension is depicted in Figure 7.1.

The blood pressure homeostasis is regulated by various components of the physiological system. Each of the factors discussed below can interplay and act in a complex manner to maintain the BP. Sympathetic stimulation may lead to increased cardiac output in some patients which causes an increase in vascular resistance leading to high blood pressure (Beevers and O'Brien 2001). An increase in the sodium ion (Na^+) concentration in the blood causes fluid retention in the kidney raising the blood volume and cardiac output. This is regulated by nitric oxide (NO), a gaseous compound produced in the endothelium which shows vasodilating effect. Any dysfunction in the endothelium affects the NO production and can disturb sodium ion regulation. Renin is a hormone secreted from the kidney when low BP is sensed. It acts on angiotensinogen to form angiotensin I and II. The latter is a potent vasoconstrictor. It acts on endothelium causing blood vessel constriction and an increase in the BP. It also acts on adrenal glands to release aldosterone. Aldosterone raises BP by regulating the Na^+ ions and water retention. Both angiotensin-II and aldosterone elevate NADPH oxidase causing excessive oxidative stress due to increased reactive oxygen species (ROS) production inciting hypertension (Oparil et al. 2018; Beevers and O'Brien 2001). Endothelium lines the entire vascular system and controls functions like vasoconstriction and vasodilation. It produces Nitric oxide (NO). It acts on the smooth muscle and reduces its contraction, leading to vasodilation and reduction in blood pressure (Spieker et al. 2006). Notably, its production is severed or severely imbalanced in HTN. Oxidative stress produces ROS such as hydrogen peroxide (H_2O_2) and superoxide (O_2^-) ions. This binds to NO and decreases its bioavailability. These are mediated by various enzyme systems like NADPH oxidase and cyclooxygenase (Dharmashankar and Widlansky 2010). Other factors which exhibit vasodilatory effects include bradykinin, prostacyclin, and substance P. Substances such as angiotensin-II, endothelin 1 (ET-1), thromboxane, and prostaglandins act as potent vasoconstrictors (Oparil et al. 2018).

7.3 TARGETING THE CLINICAL CONDITION WITH VARIOUS ANTI-HYPERTENSIVE NUTRACEUTICALS

7.3.1 Green Vegetables, Fruits

Many experimental studies revealed the advantageous effect of the intake of green vegetables and fruits in the diet for the management of HTN. Correction of HTN pathophysiology through various Nutraceuticals and its Mechanism of Action is depicted in Figure 7.2.

7.3.1.1 Garlic (Allium sativum)

Garlic is rich in flavonoids, polyphenols, anthocyanins, tannins, ascorbic acid. It possesses high anti-oxidant properties and helps in reducing plasma cholesterol level, blood pressure, and in prevention of heart disease (Gorinstein et al. 2007). The anti-hypertensive activity of aged garlic extract was significantly higher as it is rich in S-allylcysteine, an organosulfur compound responsible for anti-hypertensive activity (Ali et al. 2000). It exhibits anti-hypertensive effect by inhibiting angiotensin-converting enzyme (ACE) production, reducing the production of thromboxane and prostaglandin, production of NO due to its active compound allicin, peroxynitrite scavenging activity (Chen et al. 2009).

7.3.1.2 Onion (Allium cepa)

Onions are rich in thiosulfinates, sulfur-containing, and phenolic compounds. Dried onions, green leafy, and raw welsh onion types are reported to possess significant BP-lowering activity rather than cooked ones. It increases the bioavailability of NO,

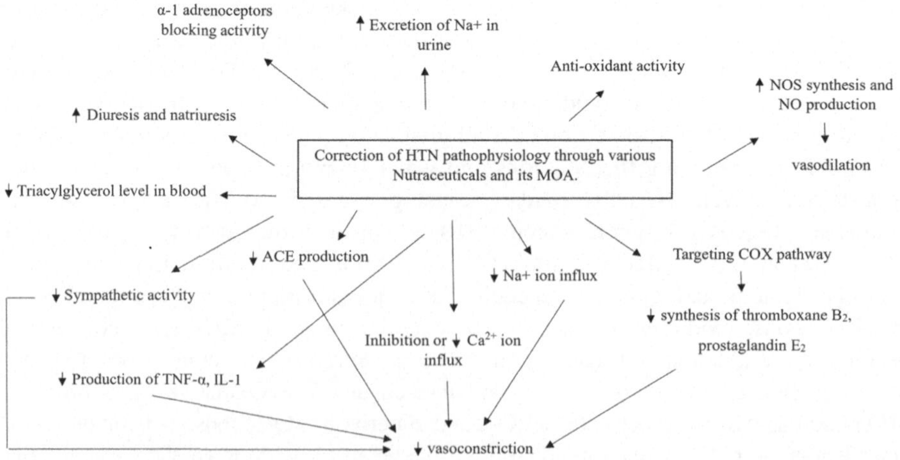

FIGURE 7.2 Correction of HTN pathophysiology through various nutraceuticals and its mechanism of action.

inhibits the angiotensin-II production, inhibits calcium ion influx into the cell, and 3-mercapto-2-methylpentan-1-ol (3-MP) present in it acts as a peroxynitrite radical scavenger (Sakai et al. 2003; Rose et al. 2003).

7.3.1.3 Tea

Green tea contains catechins which show BP-lowering activity. Cell culture and animal studies showed inhibition of ACE production, promotion of NO production, α-1 adrenoceptors blockage activity (Lorenz et al. 2009). Its composition of GMA and theanine has been observed to elicit anti-hypertensive activity even though its mechanism is not fully understood (Chen et al. 2009).

7.3.1.4 Soybean Protein

Soy protein is rich in proteins and lowers the ACE activity. Investigation of soy nuts showed blood pressure lowering potential. However, another clinical study found that it increased systolic blood pressure indicating its contradicting potential (Harrison et al. 2004). Its ACE inhibitory potential is due to the short peptides obtained during enzymatic hydrolysis in the gastrointestinal tract. The presence of phytoestrogens is also observed to possess anti-hypertensive activity (Chen et al. 2009; Fang et al. 2001).

7.3.1.5 Pomegranate Juice (Punica granatum L.)

Pomegranate juice is rich in polyphenols and contains ellagitannins and anthocyanins which are considered high anti-oxidants. A clinical study conducted with supplementation of pomegranate juice indicated a significant reduction in systolic BP and a minimal reduction in diastolic BP (Sahebkar et al. 2017).

7.3.1.6 Beetroot Juice (Beta vulgaris)

Beetroot juice is rich in Nitrate (NO_3^-) which helps in nitric oxide (NO) production. Consumption of 250 mL/day led to a reduction in BP (Kapil et al. 2015). Another study also showed a reduction in systolic BP upon daily intake (Borghi et al. 2020).

7.3.2 Spices

7.3.2.1 Ginger (Zingiber officinale)

Ginger contains zingerone, shogaols, gingerols, and volatile oils which exhibit anti-hyperglycemic activity. Its active compounds (6)-shogaol and (6)-gingerol reduced the BP at lower doses. It blocks the Ca^{2+} channel activity and increases the NO availability by scavenging peroxynitrite (Chen et al. 2009). Other spices like cinnamon, turmeric, curcumin, paprika, saffron, black, white, and red peppers are also established to exhibit BP modulatory activity (Lampe et al. 2003).

7.3.2.2 Turmeric (Curcuma longa)

Turmeric rhizomes and roots are rich in phenolic and terpenoid compounds which exhibit anti-oxidant activity. Clinical studies conducted signified that curcumin is shown to have BP-lowering potential (Alwi et al. 2008). It increases the endothelial nitric oxide synthase (eNOS) in the vasculature (Ghaffari and Roshanravan 2020).

7.3.2.3 Cinnamon (Cinnamomum verum)

Cinnamon possesses anti-oxidant properties. In animal studies, it has been proven to reduce systolic BP (Preuss et al. 2006). A clinical study conducted with 500 mg/day of cinnamon extract showed systolic BP fall (Ziegenfuss et al. 2006). The polyphenolic polymers present in cinnamon are shown to exhibit an anti-oxidant effect by reducing ROS levels (Ghaffari and Roshanravan 2020).

7.3.2.4 Saffron (Crocus sativus L.)

Saffron has strong anti-oxidant and radical scavenging potential. It inhibits cyclooxygenase 1 and 2 enzymes and prostaglandin E2 productions, blocks the inflammatory mediators such as TNF-α, blocks the calcium channel transport, exerts smooth muscle relaxation effect, reduces ACE activity, promotes eNOS production and NO bioavailability (Poma et al. 2012). An investigational study on the aqueous extract of saffron stigma in an animal study is shown to reduce BP (Ghaffari and Roshanravan 2020; Imenshahidi et al. 2010).

7.3.3 Dietary Fibers

Soluble fiber, guar gum, guava, psyllium, and oat bran all have been shown to lower BP and reduce the intake of anti-hypertensive medications in hypertensive individuals. Administration of 50 g/day of mixed fiber exhibited a reduction in BP level. It increases endothelial function, reduces sympathetic activity, or increases the excretion of sodium (Houston 2013).

7.3.4 Nutrients (Minerals)

7.3.4.1 Sodium

Sodium is a major mineral required for maintaining systemic homeostasis. However, its increased intake can increase blood pressure. Reduced intake of Na^+ has led to a reduction in BP in hypertensive patients. A minimum of 500 mg/day is an optimal requirement for sodium (Kotchen et al. 1998).

7.3.4.2 Calcium

Regular intake of calcium more than 1 g/day showed a significant reduction of BP. Maternal supplementation of calcium during pregnancy may contribute a significant effect on HTN development in an offspring's later life (Borghi et al. 2020). However, prolonged intake of calcium has also been shown to develop adverse effects such as the risk of Myocardial infarction (MI).

7.3.4.3 Magnesium

A study on the role of magnesium revealed a fall in both systolic and diastolic BP (Jee et al. 2002). A similar study showed Mg supplementation at 300 mg/day for a period of one month sufficiently contributed to the reduction in BP. It promotes prostacyclin and Nitric oxide formation and has anti-oxidant and anti-inflammatory properties. It is also a calcium antagonist (Borghi et al. 2020; Houston 2011).

7.3.4.4 Potassium

Low dietary intake of potassium has been reported to elevate the BP. It also leads to increased retention of sodium and reduced excretion of it. A study was conducted where 90–120 mEq/day of potassium supplementation reduced the BP in hypertensive patients (Aburto et al. 2013). Potassium can be supplemented as citrate, bicarbonate, and chloride salts for treating BP. The recommended intake of potassium for healthy individuals would be 650 mEq/day.

7.3.4.5 Zinc

Optimal zinc levels in serum are required for healthy well-being, and a low level has been attributed to HTN. An experimental study demonstrated the inverse correlation between serum Zinc level and BP. It affects the membrane ion exchange, influences the RAAS system, or shows an effect on the sympathetic nervous system.

7.3.5 Nutrients (Vitamins)

Vitamin C influences the BP through many mechanisms. It increases NO and PGI_2 release, promotes diuresis and natriuresis, increases cGMP production, activates potassium channel, reduces intracellular calcium level, and inhibits the activity of angiotensin-II. Experimental studies on Vit. C as a supplement at 500 mg/day showed a reduction in systolic BP (Juraschek et al. 2012). Vitamin E and Vitamin B have been documented to promote endothelial function in hypertensive patients (Turner et al. 2016). 1, 25-dihydroxycholecalciferol (1,25 $[OH]_2$ D3), the active form of Vitamin D, has a significant effect on lowering the BP. It is known to modulate BP by exerting effects on Ca^{2+}-phosphate metabolism, RAAS system, immune system, endocrine system, and endothelium. Importantly Vitamin D3 has been reported to directly suppress the renin transcription through Vitamin D receptors (VDR) mediated mechanism (Li et al. 2002).

7.3.6 Bioactive Compounds

7.3.6.1 Flavonoids

Flavonoids are rich in fruits, vegetables, red wine, tea, soy, etc. They act as free-radical scavengers and exert effects like vascular relaxation. Resveratrol is a flavonoid found in red wine and red grapes which possesses high anti-oxidant effect. Its administration in a clinical study showed a reduction in arterial BP (Karatzi et al. 2005).

7.3.6.2 Lycopene

Lycopene is abundant in tomatoes, guava, pink grapefruit, watermelon, apricots, and papaya. A clinical study data reported significant Systolic BP reduction upon 10–50 mg/day consumption. A synergic effect was documented when lycopene was administered along with anti-hypertensive drugs (Borghi et al. 2020).

7.3.6.3 Quercetin

Quercetin is found in apples, berries, and onions with anti-oxidant potential and helps reduce BP. Various experimental studies confirmed its anti-hypertensive potential (Larson et al. 2012). The recommended dose of 500 mg twice a day of quercetin may show a significant effect in the prevention and management of HTN (Houston 2013).

7.3.6.4 Pycnogenol

Pycnogenol extracted from the bark of *Pinus pinaster* is considered a natural ACE inhibitor. At 100 mg daily along with anti-hypertensive drugs showed synergistic potential in the reduction of HTN (Zibadi et al. 2008).

7.3.6.5 Alpha Lipoic Acid

Alpha lipoic acid exhibits natural scavenging activity against ROS. Upon aging, its production is reduced and can lead to endothelial dysfunction. Daily intake of 600 mg as a supplement showed a significant reduction in both Systolic and diastolic BP (Mohammadi et al. 2018).

7.3.6.6 L-arginine

L-arginine is the primary precursor of NO and is given as a dietary supplement. An experimental study conducted with 10 g/day of L-arginine administration exhibited a fall in BP (Siani et al. 2000). It is considered one of the major constituents of the DASH (Dietary Approaches to Stop Hypertension) diet.

7.3.7 Other Functional Compounds

7.3.7.1 Fish Oil and Omega-3, Omega-6 Polyunsaturated Fatty Acid (PUFA)

Animal studies conducted with fish oil showed a reduction in BP (Bond et al. 1989). Studies with dietary supplementation of fish oil or omega-3 PUFA indicated a significant reduction in BP at higher doses (>3 g/ day) (Russo et al. 1995). The activity is due to eicosapentaenoic acid (EPA) and docosahexaenoic acid (DHA) (Kasuya et al. 1986; Engler et al. 2003). It influences the eNOS production, increases the synthesis of vasodilatory prostacyclins, decreases thromboxane (TX A_2) level, decreases the production and action of TNF-α and Interleukin-1 (IL-1) and simultaneous production of acetylcholine (ACH) exhibiting relaxation of smooth muscle, reduces the triacylglycerol levels in blood, reduces the sodium ion influx and promotes NO bioavailability (Nyby et al. 2005, Chen et al. 2009). The omega-6 fatty acid which includes linolenic acid (LA), dihomo-gamma-linolenic acid (DGLA), gamma-linolenic acid (GLA), and arachidonic acid does not decrease BP however may help in preventing the rise in BP induced by saturated fats (Morris 1994).

7.3.7.2 Olive Oil

Olive oil is rich in monounsaturated fatty acid (MUFA), Omega-9 FA, and oleic acid, and all possess BP and lipid-lowering potential. In a comparative study conducted between MUFA and PUFA-treated subjects, a reduction in Systolic and Diastolic BP was observed in the former one. Also, the requirement of anti-hypertensive drugs was reduced to 48% in subjects treated with MUFA, whereas it was only 4% in PUFA (omega-6 FA).

7.3.7.3 Co-enzyme q10

It is an anti-oxidant, free-radical scavenger which reduces systemic vascular resistance and BP. In an experimental study, it showed a significant decrease in Systolic BP (Borghi et al. 2020). In another study conducted, intake of 100–225 mg/day led to a fall in BP (Rosenfeldt et al. 2007).

7.3.7.4 Seaweed

Wakame (*Undaria pinnatifida*) is the most popular seaweed and has the potential to treat HTN. A clinical study outlined a reduction in both Systolic and Diastolic BP with 3.3 g of dried wakame intake daily for four weeks. It inhibits ACE activity through its di, tri, and tetrapeptides, especially those containing amino acid sequences with Tyr-Lys. Other seaweeds are also reported to exhibit BP-lowering activity through reduced intestinal Na^+ absorption and increased intestinal K^+ absorption.

7.3.7.5 Cocoa

Cocoa is rich in flavanols and increases NO bioavailability. Dark chocolates are one such source which elicits a significant effect in both normal and hypertensive individuals. A study at 5 g/day with regular increased intake showed a reduction in BP (Zhang et al. 2013). Another study showed a reduction in both Systolic and Diastolic BP (Borghi et al. 2020).

7.4 CONCLUSION

Most of the nutraceuticals studied possessed strong anti-oxidant and anti-inflammatory potential that showed a direct effect on reducing blood pressure. Thus, these can be used either as a single treatment for initial treatment stages such as in mild hypertension, or in combination with other pharmacological drugs in order to improve the efficacy of the treatment outcome. When used in combination, duration and dose of drug therapies can be shortened and side effects can be prevented or reduced. However, many clinical studies are required in this approach to confirm their potential and efficacy. Proper understanding of their mechanism of action would once again help in treating the HTN condition based on the etiology of its origin. This can lead to the development of better HTN treatment strategies. Besides that, the safety aspect is also of major concern. Any product developed as a nutraceutical should be sufficiently bioavailable, acceptable to patients, and inexpensive. The health benefit of nutraceuticals to prevent and manage the disease condition is immense, and appropriate considerations would help in better development of nutraceutical products in the prevention and management of HTN.

REFERENCES

Aburto, N.J., Hanson, S., Gutierrez, H., Hooper, L., Elliott, P., & Cappuccio, F.P. (2013). Effect of increased potassium intake on cardiovascular risk factors and disease: Systematic review and meta-analyses. *BMJ (Online)*, *346*(7903). 10.1136/bmj.f1378

Ali, M., Al-Qattan, K.K., Al-Enezi, F., Khanafer, R.M.A., & Mustafa, T. (2000). Effect of allicin from garlic powder on serum lipids and blood pressure in rats fed with a high cholesterol diet. *Prostaglandins Leukotrienes and Essential Fatty Acids*, *62*(4), 253–259. 10.1054/plef.2000.0152

Alwi, I., Santoso, T., Suyono, S., Sutrisna, B., Suyatna, F.D., Kresno, S.B., & Ernie, S. (2008). The effect of curcumin on lipid level in patients with acute coronary syndrome. *Acta Medica Indonesiana*, *40*(4), 201–210.

Beevers, G., Lip, G.Y., & O'Brien, E. (2001). ABC of hypertension: The pathophysiology of hypertension. *BMJ (Clinical research ed.)*, *322*(7291), 912–916. 10.1136/bmj.322.7291.912

Bond, V., Ordor, O., Bruckner, G., Webb, P., Kotchen, T., Tearney, R.J., & Adams, R.G. (1989). Effects of dietary fish oil or pectin on blood pressure and lipid metabolism in the DOCA-salt hypertensive rat. *Journal of Nutrition*, *119*(5), 813–817. 10.1093/jn/119.5.813

Borghi, C., Tsioufis, K., Agabiti-Rosei, E., Burnier, M., Cicero, A.F.G., Clement, D., & Mancia, G. (2020). Nutraceuticals and blood pressure control: A European Society of Hypertension position document. *Journal of Hypertension*. 10.1097/HJH.0000000000002353

Chen, Z.Y., Peng, C., Jiao, R., Wong, Y.M., Yang, N., & Huang, Y. (2009). Anti-hypertensive nutraceuticals and functional foods. *Journal of Agricultural and Food Chemistry*, *57*(11), 4485–4499. 10.1021/jf900803r

Dharmashankar, K., & Widlansky, M.E. (2010, December). Vascular endothelial function and hypertension: Insights and directions. *Current Hypertension Reports*. 10.1007/s11906-010-0150-2

Engler, M.M., Engler, M.B., Pierson, D.M., Molteni, L.B., & Molteni, A. (2003). Effects of docosahexaenoic acid on vascular pathology and reactivity in hypertension. *Experimental Biology and Medicine*, *228*(3), 299–307. 10.1177/153537020322800309

Fang, Z., Carlson, S.H., Chen, Y.F., Oparil, S., & Wyss, J.M. (2001). Estrogen depletion induces NaCl-sensitive hypertension in female spontaneously hypertensive rats. *American Journal of Physiology - Regulatory Integrative and Comparative Physiology*, *281*(6). 10.1152/ajpregu.2001.281.6.r1934

Ghaffari, S., & Roshanravan, N. (2020). The role of nutraceuticals in prevention and treatment of hypertension: An updated review of the literature. *Food Research International*. 10.1016/j.foodres.2019.108749

Gorinstein, S., Jastrzebski, Z., Namiesnik, J., Leontowicz, H., Leontowicz, M., & Trakhtenberg, S. (2007). The atherosclerotic heart disease and protecting properties of garlic: Contemporary data. *Molecular Nutrition and Food Research*. 10.1002/mnfr.200700064

Harrison, R.A., Sagara, M., Rajpura, A., Armitage, L., Birt, N., Birt, C.A., & Yamori, Y. (2004). Can foods with added soya-protein or fish-oil reduce risk factors for coronary disease? A factorial randomised controlled trial. *Nutrition, Metabolism, and Cardiovascular Diseases: NMCD*, *14*(6), 344–350. 10.1016/s0939-4753(04)80024-3

Houston, M. (2011). The role of magnesium in hypertension and cardiovascular disease. *Journal of Clinical Hypertension*. 10.1111/j.1751-7176.2011.00538.x

Houston, M. (2013). Nutrition and nutraceutical supplements for the treatment of hypertension: Part II. *Journal of Clinical Hypertension*, *15*(11), 845–851. 10.1111/jch.12212

Imenshahidi, M., Hosseinzadeh, H., & Javadpour, Y. (2010). Hypotensive effect of aqueous saffron extract (Crocus sativus L.) and its constituents, safranal and crocin, in normotensive and hypertensive rats. *Phytotherapy Research*, *24*(7), 990–994. 10.1002/ptr.3044

Jee, S.H., Miller, E.R., Guallar, E., Singh, V.K., Appel, L.J., & Klag, M.J. (2002). The effect of magnesium supplementation on blood pressure: a meta-analysis of randomized clinical trials. *American Journal of Hypertension*, *15*(8), 691–696. 10.1016/s0895-7061(02)02964-3

Juraschek, S.P., Guallar, E., Appel, L.J., & Miller, E.R. (2012). Effects of vitamin C supplementation on blood pressure: A meta-analysis of randomized controlled trials. *American Journal of Clinical Nutrition*, *95*(5), 1079–1088. 10.3945/ajcn.111.027995

Kapil, V., Khambata, R.S., Robertson, A., Caulfield, M.J., & Ahluwalia. (2015). Dietary nitrate provides sustained blood pressure lowering in hypertensive patients: A randomized, phase 2, double-blind, placebo-controlled study. *Hypertension*, *65*(2), 320–327. 10.1161/HYPERTENSIONAHA.114.04675

Karatzi, K.N., Papamichael, C.M., Karatzis, E.N., Papaioannou, T.G., Aznaouridis, K.A., Katsichti, P.P., & Mavrikakis, M.E. (2005). Red wine acutely induces favorable effects on wave reflections and central pressures in coronary artery disease patients. *American Journal of Hypertension*, *18*(9), 1161–1167. 10.1016/j.amjhyper.2005.03.744

Kasuya, Y., Utsunomiya, N., & Matsuki, N. (1986). Attenuation of the development of hypertension in spontaneously hypertensive rats by chronic oral administration of eicosapentaenoic acid. *Journal of Pharmacobio-Dynamics*, *9*(3), 239–243. 10.1248/bpb1978.9.239

Kotchen, T.A., & McCarron, D.A. (1998). Dietary electrolytes and blood pressure. *Circulation*, *98*(6), 613–617. 10.1161/01.cir.98.6.613

Lampe, J.W. (2003). Spicing up a vegetarian diet: Chemopreventive effects of phytochemicals. *American Journal of Clinical Nutrition*, *78*. 10.1093/ajcn/78.3.579s

Larson, A., Witman, M.A.H., Guo, Y., Ives, S., Richardson, R.S., Bruno, R.S., & Symons, J.D. (2012). Acute, quercetin-induced reductions in blood pressure in hypertensive individuals are not secondary to lower plasma angiotensin-converting enzyme activity or endothelin-1: Nitric oxide. *Nutrition Research*, *32*(8), 557–564. 10.1016/j.nutres.2012.06.018

Li, Y.C., Kong, J., Wei, M., Chen, Z., Liu, S.Q., & Cao, L. (2002). Commentary - 2002 - 1, 25-Dihydroxyvitamin D 3 is a negative endocrine regulator of the renin-angiotensin system - Li et al.pdf. *Commentary*, *110*(2), 229–238.

Lorenz, M., Urban, J., Engelhardt, U., Baumann, G., Stangl, K., & Stangl, V. (2009). Green and black tea are equally potent stimuli of NO production and vasodilation: New insights into tea ingredients involved. *Basic Research in Cardiology*, *104*(1), 100–110. 10.1007/s00395-008-0759-3

Mohammadi, V., Khorvash, F., Feizi, A., & Askari, G. (2018). Does alpha-lipoic acid supplementation modulate cardiovascular risk factors in patients with stroke? A randomized, double-blind clinical trial. *International Journal of Preventive Medicine*, *9*. 10.4103/ijpvm.IJPVM_32_17

Morris M.C. (1994). Dietary fats and blood pressure. *Journal of Cardiovascular Risk*, *1*(1), 21–30.

Nyby, M.D., Matsumoto, K., Yamamoto, K., Abedi, K., Eslami, P., Hernandez, G., Smutko, V., Berger, M.E., & Tuck, M.L. (2005). Dietary fish oil prevents vascular dysfunction and oxidative stress in hyperinsulinemic rats. *American Journal of Hypertension*, *18*(2 Pt 1), 213–219. 10.1016/j.amjhyper.2004.08.030

Oparil, S., Acelajado, M.C., Bakris, G.L., Berlowitz, D.R., Cífková, R., Dominiczak, A.F., Grassi, G., Jordan, J., Poulter, N.R., Rodgers, A., & Whelton, P.K. (2018). Hypertension. *Nature Reviews. Disease Primers*, *4*, 18014. 10.1038/nrdp.2018.14

Poma, A., Fontecchio, G., Carlucci, G., & Chichiriccò, G. (2012). Anti-inflammatory properties of drugs from saffron crocus. *Anti-inflammatory & Anti-allergy Agents in Medicinal Chemistry*, *11*(1), 37–51. 10.2174/187152312803476282

Preuss, H.G., Echard, B., Polansky, M.M., & Anderson, R. (2006). Whole cinnamon and aqueous extracts ameliorate sucrose-induced blood pressure elevations in spontaneously hypertensive rats. *Journal of the American College of Nutrition*, *25*(2), 144–150. 10.1080/07315724.2006.10719525

Rose, P., Widder, S., Looft, J., Pickenhagen, W., Ong, C.N., & Whiteman, M. (2003). Inhibition of peroxynitrite-mediated cellular toxicity, tyrosine nitration, and alpha1-antiproteinase inactivation by 3-mercapto-2-methylpentan-1-ol, a novel compound isolated from Allium cepa. *Biochemical and Biophysical Research Communications*, *302*(2), 397–402. 10.1016/s0006-291x(03)00193-1

Rosenfeldt, F.L., Haas, S.J., Krum, H., Hadj, A., Ng, K., Leong, J.Y., & Watts, G.F. (2007). Coenzyme Q10 in the treatment of hypertension: a meta-analysis of the clinical trials. *Journal of Human Hypertension*, *21*(4), 297–306. 10.1038/sj.jhh.1002138

Russo, C., Olivieri, O., Girelli, D., Azzini, M., Stanzial, A.M., Guarini, P., Friso, S., De Franceschi, L., & Corrocher, R. (1995). Omega-3 polyunsaturated fatty acid supplements and ambulatory blood pressure monitoring parameters in patients with mild essential hypertension. *Journal of Hypertension*, *13*(12 Pt 2), 1823–1826.

Sahebkar, A., Ferri, C., Giorgini, P., Bo, S., Nachtigal, P., & Grassi, D. (2017). Effects of pomegranate juice on blood pressure: A systematic review and meta-analysis of randomized controlled trials. *Pharmacological Research*, *115*, 149–161. 10.1016/j.phrs.2016.11.018

Sakai, Y., Murakami, T., & Yamamoto, Y. (2003). Antihypertensive effects of onion on NO synthase inhibitor-induced hypertensive rats and spontaneously hypertensive rats. *Bioscience, Biotechnology, and Biochemistry*, *67*(6), 1305–1311. 10.1271/bbb.67.1305

Siani, A., Pagano, E., Iacone, R., Iacoviello, L., Scopacasa, F., & Strazzullo, P. (2000). Blood pressure and metabolic changes during dietary L-arginine supplementation in humans. *American Journal of Hypertension*, *13*(5 Pt 1), 547–551. 10.1016/s0895-7061(99)00233-2

Spieker, L.E., Flammer, A.J., & Lüscher, T.F. (2006). The vascular endothelium in hypertension. *Handbook of Experimental Pharmacology*, (176 Pt 2), 249–283. 10.1007/3-540-36028-x_8

Turner, J.M., & Spatz, E.S. (2016). Nutritional supplements for the treatment of hypertension: A practical guide for clinicians. *Current Cardiology Reports* *18*(12), 126. 10.1007/s11886-016-0806-x

Zhang, Z., Xu, G., & Liu, X. (2013). Chocolate intake reduces risk of cardiovascular disease: evidence from 10 observational studies. *International Journal of Cardiology*, *168*(6), 5448–5450. 10.1016/j.ijcard.2012.12.036

Zibadi, S., Rohdewald, P.J., Park, D., & Watson, R.R. (2008). Reduction of cardiovascular risk factors in subjects with type 2 diabetes by Pycnogenol supplementation. *Nutrition Research*, *28*(5), 315–320. 10.1016/j.nutres.2008.03.003

Ziegenfuss, T.N., Hofheins, J.E., Mendel, R.W., Landis, J., & Anderson, R.A. (2006). Effects of a water-soluble cinnamon extract on body composition and features of the metabolic syndrome in pre-diabetic men and women. *Journal of the International Society of Sports Nutrition*, *3*(2), 45–53. 10.1186/1550-2783-3-2-45

8 Nutraceuticals for Respiratory Disease Management

S. Diksha, S. Meganathan, N. Tamilselvan, M. Vijayalakshmi, and M. Dhivya Sree

8.1 INTRODUCTION

In recent years, chronic respiratory disorders (CRD) have been the leading cause of morbidity and mortality worldwide. CRDs are disorders which cause damage and deterioration of the lungs. CRDs generally consist of diseases like chronic obstructive pulmonary disease (COPD), Asthma, Pulmonary Fibrosis, Pneumonia, Lung Cancer, Tuberculosis, and Pulmonary Sarcoidosis. Numerous studies validate that the influence of the surrounding environment, genetic factors, and exposure to fine particles play a major role in the prevalence of CRDs. As per the National Health Policy of India 2017, premature mortality due to non-communicable diseases including CRDs should be reduced by 2025. The leading causes of CRDs are smoking, exposure to air pollution indoors and outside, allergies, occupational exposure, poor diet, obesity, inactivity, and other factors (Soriano et al. 2020).

For the management of Respiratory diseases, Nutraceuticals play a vital role in diversified ways by promoting the health of CRD patients. Recently, medicinal plant extracts and their important phytoconstituents like quercetin, a common flavonoid, polyphenol, iridoids, and terpenes have been used for the management of several respiratory diseases in the conventional and modern systems of medicine. Furthermore, quite a lot of scientific investigations demonstrated that nutraceutical products are considered to be a major alternative source of treatment for several human disorders, including respiratory diseases like Asthma, COPD, Pulmonary Fibrosis, Pneumonia, and Lung cancer (Vestbo et al. 2013).

8.2 ROLE OF NUTRACEUTICALS IN THERAPEUTICS

Regarding potential growth and expansion for improved health, the term "Nutraceuticals" has a lot of potential. It has shown subsequent benefits in minimising the need for traditional medications and has lessened the possibility of adverse effects, depending on the type and alternative usage as a contemporary medicine. They are currently utilised across all medical specialties in the world (Ahmad et al. 2013).

DOI: 10.1201/9781003392934-8

The vital role of nutraceuticals in the prevention and treatment of various diseases has been amply supported by studies in many different ways. The majority of people prefer a natural cure for any illness. Nutraceuticals have been found to be the only solution, replacing chemotherapy with a new method called phytotherapy, which is also known as using extracts from natural sources for treatment. Due to its numerous health advantages and apparent absence of toxicity and side effects, natural products have attracted a lot of interest recently for the purpose of illness prevention. It is less expensive than other therapies, which is another benefit (Saikia and Deka 2011).

8.3 RESPIRATORY DISEASES

8.3.1 Asthma

Asthma is referred to as chronic inflammation of the airway epithelial cells caused by eosinophilia, mast cells, and activated T helper lymphocytes. An asthma exacerbation goes through two stages: the early stage and the late stage. Plasma cells sensitise and release IgE antibodies, which start the early phase. When a pollutant or risk factor is inhaled, the mast cells will degranulate and produce cytokines. Upon inhalation of an irritant, the mast cell Eosinophil counts often rise, and the lamina reticularis thickens, among other typical changes in the airways. T lymphocytes particularly Th2 lymphocytes play a crucial role in the inflammation by generating different interleukins (IL-4, IL-5, IL-13) (Sinyor and Concepcion Perez 2023; Subbarao et al. 2009). The pathogenesis of asthma is shown in Figure 8.1a.

8.3.2 Chronic Obstructive Pulmonary Disorder (COPD)

COPD is a significant respiratory disorder which causes airway obstruction. Chronic inflammation causes structural modification to the airways that may lead to alveolar attachment to small airways and suppression of lung elastic recoil. In addition to inflammation, an imbalance between proteases and anti-proteases, and oxidative stress (an imbalance between oxidants and antioxidants) inside the lungs are the two other most important mechanisms that greatly influence the pathogenesis of COPD (Alfahad et al. 2021; MacNee 2006) which was depicted in Figure 8.1b.

8.3.3 Pulmonary Fibrosis

Idiopathic Pulmonary Fibrosis (IPF) results in the disruption of homoeostasis between alveolar and epithelial cells that activate the alveolar epithelium. Abnormal activation of alveolar epithelial cells starts the migration, proliferation, and activation of lung fibroblastic foci are produced as a result of mesenchymal cells. Other than the cytokines and growth factors, other proteinoids, like PGE2, are also produced which ultimately cause IPF (Dua et al. 2021).

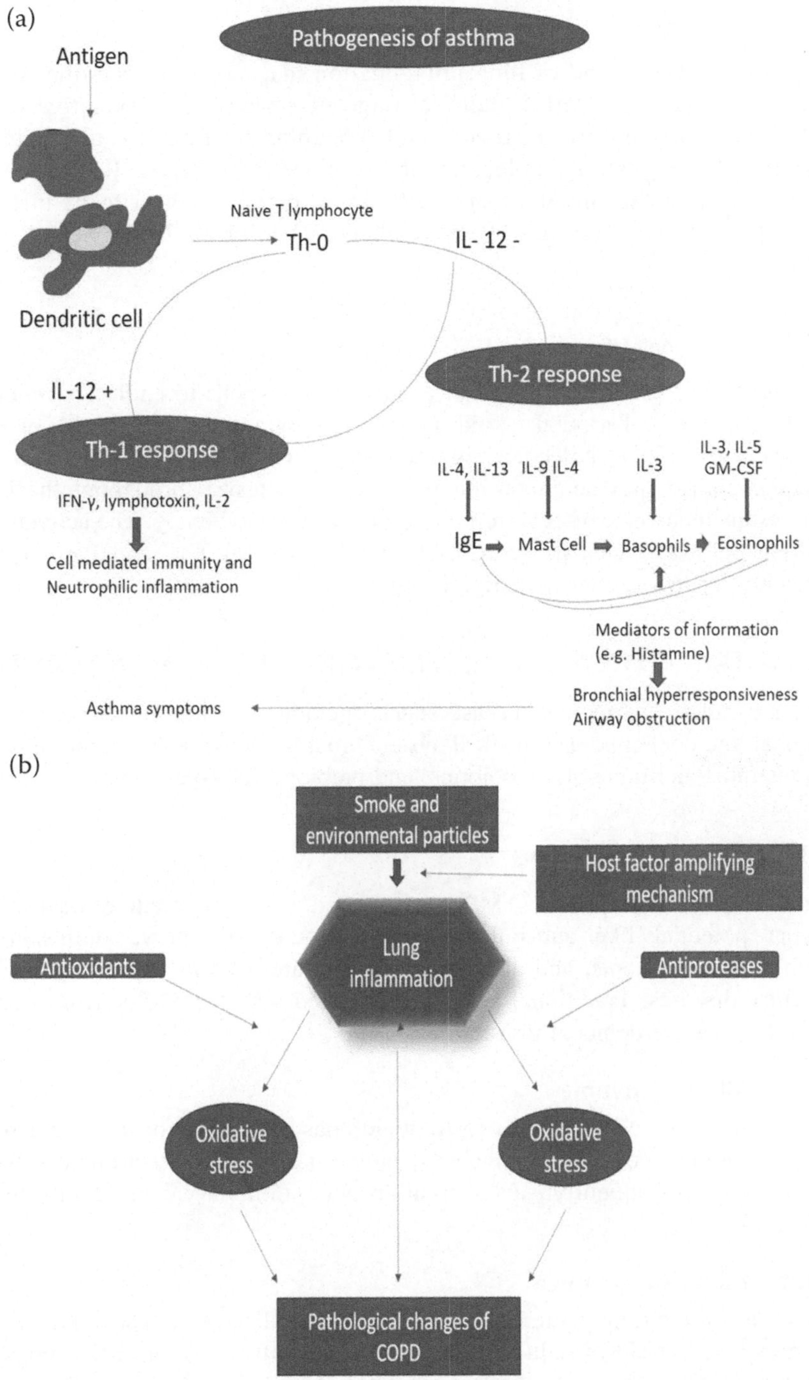

FIGURE 8.1 Pathogenesis of prevalent respiratory disease (a) Asthma (b) COPD.

8.3.4 Pneumonia

Pneumonia is also a kind of lung inflammation that mostly affects the tiny air sacs known as alveoli with a definite range of severity. A productive or dry cough, chest discomfort, a fever, and breathing difficulties are common symptoms. The signalling molecules or cytokines like TNF-α, IL-8, and IL-1 are released, and the inflammatory cells are attracted to the site of infection when pathogens are engulfed by macrophages (Jain et al. 2023; Nelson et al. 1995).

8.3.5 Lung Cancer

In lung cancer, a molecular mutation enables tumour cells to endlessly replicate, promote blood vessel growth, avoid apoptosis (programmed cell death), produce pro-growth signalling molecules, ignore anti-growth signalling molecules, and eventually spread into neighbouring tissue or metastasize throughout the body, which results in adverse effects from radiation and chemotherapy. The activation of signalling pathways such as Akt/GSK3Beta, MEK-ERK, Fas, and Par6 may be responsible for this (Potter and Higginson 2004).

8.4 NUTRACEUTICALS IN RESPIRATORY DISEASE MANAGEMENT

In order to treat a variety of disease states, including respiratory disorders, both traditional and contemporary medical systems make extensive use of nutrients and food, vitamins and minerals, probiotics, and prebiotics (Kasper et al. 2015).

8.4.1 Nutraceutical Herbs

Traditional medicinal plants (TMPs) have been used as herbal remedies with excellent potential like anti-inflammatory, immunomodulatory, antihistaminic, smooth-muscle relaxants, and allergic action that are used in the management of respiratory diseases. Traditional benefits associated with the TMPs against Lung-related diseases are depicted in Table 8.1.

8.4.1.1 Allium sativum

Allium sativum is well known as garlic which has been used for treating asthma, whooping cough, cold, flu, bronchitis, and other respiratory ailments. As an expectorant, it is frequently used to treat bronchopulmonary disorders (Taur and Patil 2011).

8.4.1.2 Tamarindus indica

Tamarindus indica is also referred to as tamarind and has strong anti-inflammatory properties that can aid in reducing discomfort and inflammation in the lungs and respiratory system. This tree's bark is extremely beneficial for treating asthma and eye problems (Rivers and Mark 2017).

TABLE 8.1
Traditional Benefits of TMPs against Respiratory Diseases

S.No	Scientific Name	Family	Parts Used	Traditional Use	References
1	*Acacia Jacquemontii*	Myrsinacae	Flower, seed, Leaves, Stem	Asthma	(Ahmad et al. 2014)
2	*Achyranthes Aspera Linn*	Amaranthacae	Leaves	Pneumonia, Asthma	(Qureshi et al. 2009)
3	*Apium Graveocens L*	Pinaceae	Seed, Root	Bronchitis, Asthma	(Bibi et al. 2014)
4	*Astragulus Tragacantha*	Asteraceae	Leaves	Respiratory infections	(Murad et al. 2013)
5	*Bergenia Stracheyi*	Saxifragaceae	Leaves, Root	Cough, Asthma, Lung Cancer, Respiratory problems	(Abbas et al. 2014)
6	*Datura Metal Linn*	Solanaceae	Whole Plant	Asthma	(Ishtiaq et al. 2015)
7	*Ephedra Gerardiana*	Ephedraceae	Stem	COPD, Asthma, Breathing problems	(Bibi et al. 2014)
8	*Foeniculum Vulgare Miller*	Papilionaceae	Seed and Leaves	Cough, Pneumonia	(Ullah et al. 2014)
9	*Helianthus Annuus*	Papilionaceae	Flower, Root, Seed, Leaves	Asthma, Bronchial	(Khan et al. 2007)
10	*Iris Hookeriana*	Iriddaceae	Flower	Asthma, Cough, Bronchitis	(Hussain et al. 2008)
11	*Lanata Camara*	Amaranthaceae	Leaves, Root and Flowers	Respiratory diseases	(Jabeen et al. 2009)
12	*Medicago Denticulate*	Podceae	Seeds	Respiratory diseases	(Ibrar et al. 2007)
13	*Onosma Hispida*	Boraginaceae	Leaves, flower	Cough and others	(Khan et al. 2007)
14	*Oxalis Carniculata L*	Ranunculaceae	Leaves	Bronchitis, Asthma	(Shaheen et al. 2014)
15	*Polygonum Affine*	Polygonaceae	Root	Lung disorder	(Bano et al. 2014)
16	*Salvia Nubicola*	Labiateae	Leaves	Cough, Asthma, and Others	(Khan et al. 2007)
17	*Zinger officinalis*	Asclepiadaceae	Stem, Leaves	Asthma, Flu	(Ishtiaq et al. 2015)

8.4.1.3 Zingiber officinale

It is found on Southern islands and is commonly known as ginger. It is effective in treating bronchitis, coughs, and colds. It has antiviral, anti-inflammatory, and anti-asthmatic properties; it contains some essential oils, gingerols, and sesquiterpene hydrocarbon (Yusuf et al. 2018).

8.4.1.4 Boswellia serrata Roxb

Numerous Unani and Ayurvedic preparations use the oleo gum resin of *Boswellia serrata*. According to reports, it can help with bronchitis, asthma, cough, sore throat, and a variety of digestive issues. Boswellic acid, 3′ hydroxyl urs-9, -amyrins, 11-keto-a-boswellic acid, 3′-acetoxy urs-9, 11-dien-24-oic acid, and other important terpenoids are present in the plant's gum resin (Upaganlawar and Ghule 2009).

8.4.1.5 Curcuma Longa L

Curcumin is a potential phytoconstituent widely present in *Curcuma Longa* L which has anti-inflammatory activity by inhibiting cyclooxygenase-2, 5-lipoxygenase, and nitric oxide synthase. Other mechanisms involved in its anti-inflammatory activities are inhibiting prostaglandin synthesis, arachidonic acid metabolism, and inhibiting the activation of proinflammatory transcription factors including NF-B and c-Jun/AP-1 (Venkatesan et al. 2007).

8.4.2 Phytoconstituents as Nutraceuticals

Most of the existing phytochemicals play several vital roles as nutraceutical supplements with potential pharmacological activity. Various phytoconstituents used as nutraceutical structures are depicted in Table 8.2.

8.4.2.1 Flavonoids

Flavonoids are the most significant single group of polyphenols which are secondary plant metabolites having antioxidant properties. Based on its chemical structure, they fall into the categories of flavans, flavanones, isoflavanones, flavones, isoflavones, anthocyanidins, and flavonolignans. These polyphenols are abundantly present in vegetables, fruits, tea, coffee, wine, nuts, and different parts of plants such as seeds, flowers, stems, and roots. Phytoconstituents such as chrysin and luteolin have anti-asthmatic activity (Kawai et al. 2007; Kumar and Pandey 2013).

8.4.2.2 Resveratrol

Resveratrol is trans-3,5,4′-trihydroxy stilbene and has potent antioxidative, potent metabolic regulator, antiasthma, anticancer, and anti-inflammatory properties. This resveratrol can be obtained from the bark of red fruits. Its antioxidative potential is in neutralising intracellular ROS by stimulating and stabilising antioxidants. Also has anti-inflammatory activity by inhibiting prostaglandin synthesis. By preventing the production of co-stimulatory molecules, resveratrol can also influence innate immune response. Administration of resveratrol through oral has been considered a powerful natural remedy for asthma sufferers (Akgedik et al. 2012).

8.4.2.3 Quercetin

Quercetin (3,30,40,5,7-pentahydroxy flavone) is a phenolic compound belonging to the flavonoid family. It is present in food products such as onions, apples, and broccoli. In addition to protecting against oxidative stress and lung inflammation, it

TABLE 8.2
Structure of Important Phytoconstituents as Nutraceuticals

Name	Structure
Resveratrol	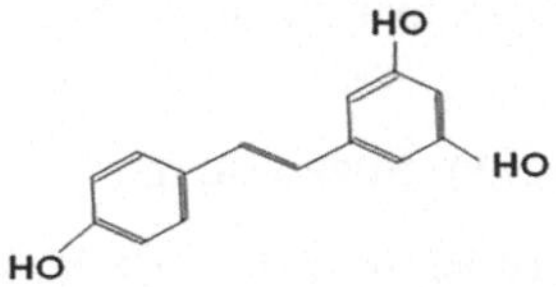
Quercetin	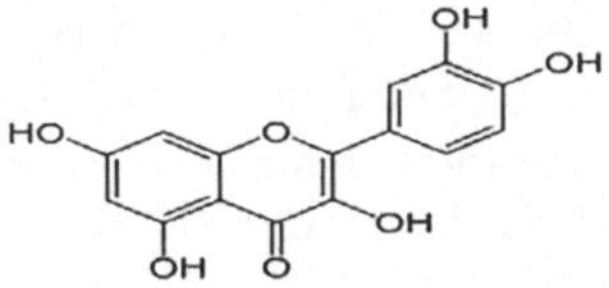
Silymarin	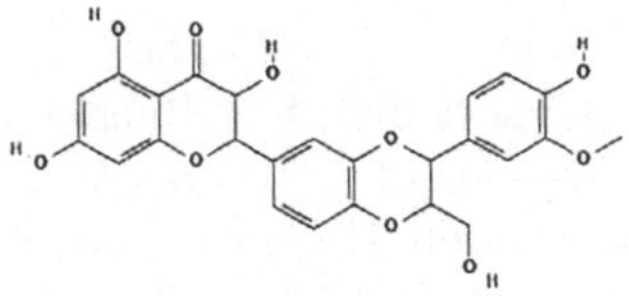
Berberine	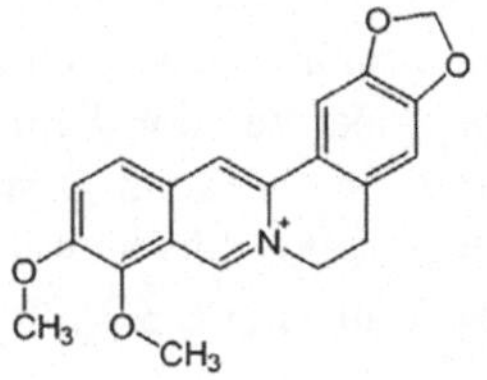
Baicalein	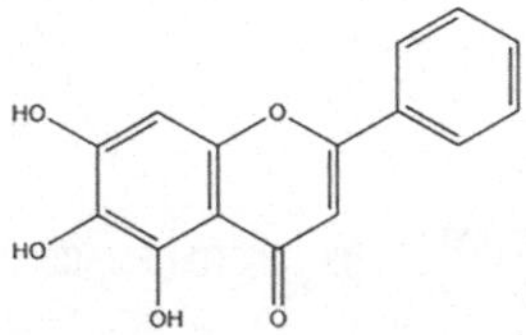

significantly improves antioxidant levels and pulmonary function in the COPD murine model. In pulmonary disease, it works by activating antioxidant enzymes and inhibiting the NF-κB pathway. Quercetin reduces both lung injury and lung inflammation caused by cigarette smoking. It reduces the release of inflammatory mediators and oxidative mediators thereby acting as anti-inflammatory and antioxidative agents (Araújo et al. 2022).

8.4.2.4 Silymarin

Silymarin is a natural flavonoid ligand compound obtained from the dried fruits of milk plants and weeds as a natural active substance. Silymarin reduces oxidative stress and increases ROS production by preventing the phosphorylation of the peripheral blood neutrophil membrane protein, NADPH oxidase, and p47phox factor (Xu et al. 2021).

8.4.2.5 Berberine

Rather like other polyphenols, berberine does not induce apoptosis, it shows anticancer activity by inhibiting the DNA repair and replication. Berberine works by inhibiting the proliferation of NSCLC cells by inducing the G1/S phase of cell cycle arrest. It down-regulates the RRM1, RRM2, POLE2 and LIG1 expressions in A549, H1299, H1975 cells that suppress DNA repair and replication (Ni et al. 2022).

8.4.3 Role of Dietary Supplements

The current age of consuming lots of junk and the decline in the intake of nutrients and vitamins has led to all these complications in respiratory illness. Based on the critical condition of the disease, regular intake of fruits and vegetables may reduce the worst rate. Rich sources of antioxidants like fruits and vegetables, vitamin E, vitamin C, flavonoids, which can be used regularly (Mercader-Barcelo et al. 2020).

Furthermore, Vitamin C is found to be more potent, especially for the treatment of asthma and other respiratory disorders. Vitamin E and Vitamin C both show synergistic activity. Vitamin E consists of 4 tocopherols and 4 tocotrienols. α-tocopherol reduces allergic airway inflammation. Due to its capacity to oxidise reactive nitrogen species, γ-tocopherol may aid in the resolution of inflammation brought on by ozone exposure and endotoxin-induced neutrophilic airway inflammation. Vitamin D is essential for the growth of lungs and its proper function. Through the lack of the vitamin D receptor and parenchyma degradation, low vitamin D status may also have an impact on the progression of COPD. The relationship between obstructive pulmonary disease and dietary supplements is shown in Figure 8.2.

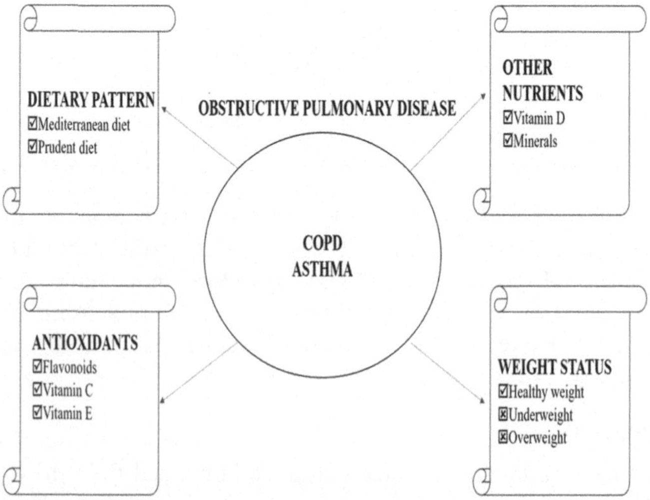

FIGURE 8.2 Relationship between obstructive pulmonary disease and nutrients. ☑ represents positive effect, ☑ represents positive effect, ☒ represents negative effect, ☒ represents negative effect.

8.4.4 Prebiotics and Probiotics

8.4.4.1 Probiotics

Probiotics are living organisms, and when given to patients in large doses can produce favourable effects on their health. When these probiotics are given in sufficient quantities in several pathologic illness conditions, showed some positive physiological impact on the host. Certain lactic acid bacteria that are present in a variety of fermented foods, including yoghurt, cheese, and pickles, are widely accepted under probiotics. In order to maximise the effectiveness of probiotics, it is crucial to combine them with other supplements, such as postbiotics, prebiotics, minerals, vitamins, lactoferrin, and nutraceuticals. Numerous supplements claim to improve both the probiotics' effectiveness and their processes. Probiotics are advised to be ingested every day in order to promote human health (Anwar et al. 2021). The recognised health advantages include improving lactose digestion to lessen lactose intolerance symptoms, preventing allergic disease onset, preventing ischemic heart syndromes, maintaining intestinal pH, lowering blood cholesterol levels, increasing dietary calcium's bioavailability, producing vitamin B, and enhancing immune function. Probiotics have been demonstrated to provide therapeutic management of several disorders like HIV, rotavirus, hemagglutinin, neuraminidase type 1 (H1N1) influenza virus, and gastric coronavirus. A significant COVID-19 consequence called ARDS may be less severe because of their usage (Darbandi et al. 2021). Numerous studies have documented the impact of probiotics against different coronavirus species. It has been demonstrated that probiotic bacteria have a lot of positive immunological and health impacts. They have a role in controlling the bacterial environment and modulating immune cells in addition to improving the bioavailability of nutrients and maintaining general health. Based on prior research on various infectious diseases, it is clear that we can avoid infectious diseases by enhancing and stimulating immune activity in human beings through the ingesting of a nutritious and healthy diet, supplements like probiotics, vitamins, minerals, and fibre (Infusino et al. 2020).

8.4.4.2 Prebiotics

Prebiotics are first described as "non-digestible" dietary supplements that benefit the host by specifically promoting the development of one or a restricted number of bacteria already present in the colon. Like probiotics, prebiotics can be administered orally to reach the intestines or directly to the vaginal canal and skin to reach microbially colonised bodily areas. Compounds such as resistant starch, lactosucrose, lactobionic acid, galactomannan, psyllium, polyphenols, polyunsaturated fatty acids, fructans, oligosaccharides, arabino oligosaccharides, sialyloligosaccharides, and xylooligosaccharides are categorised under prebiotics. Probiotics have the activity of destruction of infections and activation of the immune system, which accounts for their health benefits to the GI tract. Although an indirect impact may be speculated, there is currently no information explicitly connecting prebiotics to respiratory infections in any way (Infusino et al. 2020).

8.5 CONCLUSION

Chronic Respiratory Disorders (CRD) have been considered more widespread than ever and can cause grave health problems. Recent investigational studies have shown that different mechanisms are highlighted for this pulmonary ailment. Nutraceuticals have shown subsequent benefits in minimising the need for traditional medications and lessening the possibility of adverse effects. The progression of nutraceuticals has greatly increased the importance of pursuing the maximum degree of wellness. Phytotherapy is an alternative therapy that uses extracts from natural sources as medications or health-improving substances. Probiotics have been suggested as antimicrobial agents against viruses that cause respiratory tract infections. Nutraceuticals are considered to be the major source as an alternative for several human disorders, including respiratory diseases like lung cancer, asthma, COPD, pneumonia, and pulmonary fibrosis. This chapter explained the efficacy of nutraceuticals as a remedy for the management of respiratory diseases. When compared to the traditional treatment methodologies for treating respiratory diseases, nutraceuticals with certain nutritional and pharmacological activity have shown a drastic effect in treating the disease. However, these nutraceuticals-based investigations in this present era will make a new approach, especially in the therapeutic ability for pulmonary diseases in the near future.

REFERENCES

Abbas, Q., Khan, S.W., Khatoon, S., Hussain, S.A., Hassan, S.N., Hussain, A., … & Hussain, I. (2014). Floristic biodiversity and traditional uses of medicinal plants of Haramosh valley Central Karakoram National Park of Gilgit district, Gilgit-Baltistan. *Pakistan Journal of Biological Sciences*, *5*, 75–86.

Ahmad, M.F., Ahmad, F.A., Azad, Z.A., Alam, M.S., & Ashraf, S.A. (2013). Nutraceutical is the need of hour. *World Journal of Pharmaceutical Sciences*, *2*, 2516–2525.

Ahmad, M., Sultana, S., Fazl-i-Hadi, S., Ben Hadda, T., Rashid, S., Zafar, M., … & Yaseen, G. (2014). An ethnobotanical study of medicinal plants in high mountainous region of Chail valley (District Swat-Pakistan). *Journal of Ethnobiology and Ethnomedicine*, *10*, 1–18.

Akgedik, R., Akgedik, S., Karamanli, H., Uysal, S., Bozkurt, B., Ozol, D., & Yildirim, Z. (2012). Effect of resveratrol on treatment of bleomycin-induced pulmonary fibrosis in rats. *Inflammation*, *35*, 1732–1741.

Alfahad, A.J., Alzaydi, M.M., Aldossary, A.M., Alshehri, A.A., Almughem, F.A., Zaidan, N.M., & Tawfik, E.A. (2021). Current views in chronic obstructive pulmonary disease pathogenesis and management. *Saudi Pharmaceutical Journal: SPJ: The Official Publication of the Saudi Pharmaceutical Society*, *29*(12), 1361–1373.

Anwar, F., Altayb, H.N., Al-Abbasi, F.A., Al-Malki, A.L., Kamal, M.A., & Kumar, V. (2021). Antiviral effects of probiotic metabolites on COVID-19. *Journal of Biomolecular Structure and Dynamics*, *39*(11), 4175–4184.

Araújo, N.P.D.S., de Matos, N.A., Oliveira, M., de Souza, A.B.F., Castro, T.D.F., Machado-Júnior, P.A., … & Bezerra, F.S. (2022). Quercetin improves pulmonary function and prevents emphysema caused by exposure to cigarette smoke in male mice. *Antioxidants*, *11*(2), 181.

Bano, A., Ahmad, M., Hadda, T.B., Saboor, A., et al. (2014). Quantitative ethnomedicinal study of plants used in the skardu valley at high altitude of Karakoram-Himalayan range, Pakistan. *Journal of Ethnobiology and Ethnomedicine*, *10*(1), 1–18.

Bibi, S., Sultana, J., Sultana, H., & Malik, R.N. (2014). Ethnobotanical uses of medicinal plants in the highlands of Soan Valley, Salt Range, Pakistan. *Journal of Ethnopharmacology*, *155*(1), 352–361.

Bibi, T., Ahmad, M., Tareen, R.B., Tareen, N.M., Jabeen, R., Rehman, S.U., … & Yaseen, G. (2014). Ethnobotany of medicinal plants in district Mastung of Balochistan province-Pakistan. *Journal of Ethnopharmacology*, *157*, 79–89.

Darbandi, A., Asadi, A., Ghanavati, R., Afifirad, R., Emamie, A.D., & Talebi, M. (2021). The effect of probiotics on respiratory tract infection with special emphasis on COVID-19: Systemic review 2010–20. *International Journal of Infectious Diseases*, *105*, 91–104.

Dua, K., Nammi, S., Chang, D., Chellappan, D.K., Gupta, G., & Collet, T. (Eds.). (2021). *Medicinal Plants for Lung Diseases: A Pharmacological and Immunological Perspective*. Springer.

Global Initiative for Chronic Obstructive Lung Disease. (2010). Global Strategy for the Diagnosis, Management, and Prevention of Chronic Obstructive Pulmonary Disease. Available from: http://www.goldcopd.org/guidelinesresources

Hussain, K., Shahazad, A., & Zia-ul-Hussnain, S. (2008). An ethnobotanical survey of important wild medicinal plants of Hattar district Haripur, Pakistan. *Ethnobotanical Leaflets*, *2008*(1), 5.

Ibrar, M., Hussain, F., & Sultan, A. (2007). Ethnobotanical studies on plant resources of Ranyal hills, District Shangla, Pakistan. *Pakistan Journal of Botany*, *39*(2), 329.

Infusino, F., Marazzato, M., Mancone, M., & Fedele, F. (2020). Diet supplementation, probiotics, and nutraceuticals in SARS-CoV-2 infection: A scoping review. *Nutrients*, *12*(6), 1718.

Ishtiaq, M., Mahmood, A., & Maqbool, M. (2015). Indigenous knowledge of medicinal plants from Sudhanoti district (AJK), Pakistan. *Journal of Ethnopharmacology*, *168*, 201–207.

Jabeen, A., Khan, M.A., Ahmad, M., Zafar, M., & Ahmad, F. (2009). Indigenous uses of economically important flora of Margallah Hills National Park, Islamabad, Pakistan. *African Journal of Biotechnology* *8*(5), 763–784.

Jain, V., Vashisht, R., Yilmaz, G., et al. (2023). Pneumonia Pathology. [Updated 2022 Aug 1]. In: StatPearls [Internet]. Treasure Island (FL): StatPearls Publishing; 2023 Jan. Available https://www.ncbi.nlm.nih.gov/books/NBK526116/

Kasper, D., Fauci, A., Hauser, S., Longo, D., et al. (2015). *Harrison's Principles of Internal Medicine*. McGraw-Hill 19 (1,2).

Kawai, M., Hirano, T., Higa, S., et al. (2007). Flavonoids and related compounds as anti-allergic substances. *Allergology International*, *56*(2), 113–123.

Khan, I., & Razzaq Islam, M. (2007). Ethnobotanical studies of some medicinal and aromatic plants at higher altitudes of Pakistan. *American-Eurasian Journal of Agricultural & Environmental Sciences*, *2*, 470–473.

Kumar, S., & Pandey, A.K. (2013). Chemistry and biological activities of flavonoids: an overview. *The Scientific World Journal*, *2013*, 16. http://dx.doi.org/10.1155/2013/162750

MacNee, W. (2006). Pathology, pathogenesis, and pathophysiology. *BMJ*, *332*(7551), 1202–1204.

Mercader-Barcelo, J., Truyols-Vives, J., Rio, C., Lopez-Safont, N., Sala-Llinas, E., & Chaplin, A. (2020). Insights into the role of bioactive food ingredients and the microbiome in idiopathic pulmonary fibrosis. *International Journal of Molecular Sciences*, *21*(17), 6051.

Murad, W., Azizullah, A., Adnan, M., Tariq, A., Khan, K.U., Waheed, S., & Ahmad, A. (2013). Ethnobotanical assessment of plant resources of Banda Daud Shah, district Karak, Pakistan. *Journal of Ethnobiology and Ethnomedicine*, *9*, 1–10.

Nelson, S., Mason, C.M., Kolls, J., & Summer, W.R. (1995). Pathophysiology of pneumonia. *Clinics in Chest Medicine*, *16*(1), 1–12.

Ni, L., Li, Z., Ren, H., Kong, L., Chen, X., Xiong, M., … & Li, J. (2022). Berberine inhibits non-small cell lung cancer cell growth through repressing DNA repair and replication rather than through apoptosis. *Clinical and Experimental Pharmacology and Physiology*, *49*(1), 134–144.

Potter, J., & Higginson, I.J. (2004). Pain experienced by lung cancer patients: a review of prevalence, causes and pathophysiology. *Lung Cancer*, *43*(3), 247–257.

Qureshi, R., Waheed, A., Arshad, M., & Umbreen, T. (2009). Medico-ethnobotanical inventory of tehsil Chakwal, Pakistan. *Pakistan Journal of Botany*, *41*(2), 529–538.

Rivers, M.C., & Mark, J. (2017). Tamarindus indica. IUCN Red List of Threatened Species. 2017: e.T62020997A62020999.

Saikia, D., & Deka, S.C. (2011). Cereals: from staple food to nutraceuticals. *International Food Research Journal*, *18*(1), 21–30.

Shaheen, H., Qureshi, R., Akram, A., & Gulfraz, M. (2014). Inventory of medicinal flora from Thal desert, Punjab, Pakistan. *African Journal of Traditional Complementary and Alternative Medicines*, *11*(3), 282–290.

Sinyor, B., & Concepcion Perez, L. (2023). Pathophysiology of Asthma. [Updated 2022 May 8]. In: StatPearls [Internet]. Treasure Island (FL): StatPearls Publishing; 2023 Jan. Available https://www.ncbi.nlm.nih.gov/books/NBK551579/

Soriano, J.B., Kendrick, P.J., Paulson, K.R., Gupta, V., Abrams, E.M., Adedoyin, R.A., … & Moradi, M. (2020). Prevalence and attributable health burden of chronic respiratory diseases, 1990–2017: a systematic analysis for the Global Burden of Disease Study 2017. *The Lancet Respiratory Medicine*, *8*(6), 585–596.

Subbarao, P., Mandhane, P.J., & Sears, M.R. (2009). Asthma: epidemiology, etiology and risk factors. *CMAJ*, *181*(9), E181–E190.

Taur, D.J., & Patil, R.Y. (2011). Some medicinal plants with antiasthmatic potential: a current status. *Asian Pacific Journal of Tropical Biomedicine*, *1*(5), 413–418.

Ullah, S., Khan, M.R., Shah, N.A., Shah, S.A., et al. (2014). Ethnomedicinal plant use value in the Lakki Marwat District of Pakistan. *Journal of Ethnopharmacology*, *158*, 412–422.

Upaganlawar, A., & Ghule, B. (2009). Pharmacological activities of Boswellia serrata Roxb. -mini review. *Ethnobotanical Leaflets*, *13*, 766–774.

Venkatesan, N., Punithavathi, D., & Babu, M. (2007). Protection from acute and chronic lung diseases by curcumin. *The Molecular Targets and Therapeutic Uses of Curcumin in Health and Disease*, 379–405.

Vestbo, J., Hurd, S.S., Agustí, A.G., Jones, P.W., Vogelmeier, C., Anzueto, R., … & Rodriguez-Roisin, R. (2013). Global strategy for the diagnosis, management, and prevention of chronic obstructive pulmonary disease: GOLD executive summary. *American Journal of Respiratory and Critical Care Medicine*, *187*(4), 347–365.

Xu, L., Song, Q., Ouyang, Z., Zheng, M., Zhang, X., & Zhang, C. (2021). Efficacy of silymarin in treatment of COPD via P47phox signaling pathway. *Food Science and Technology*, *42*. https://doi.org/10.1590/fst.52821

Yusuf, A.A., Lawal, B., Abubakar, A.N., Berinyuy, E.B., et al. (2018). In-vitro antioxidants, antimicrobial and toxicological evaluation of Nigerian Zingiber officinale. *Clinical Phytoscience*, *4*(1), 1–8.

9 Nutraceuticals

Fine Tuning of Food and Nutrition for Cancer Treatment and Prevention

Yamini Tiwari, Parul Johri, and Mala Trivedi

9.1 INTRODUCTION

The last two decades have seen a rise in the importance of a healthy diet as a basic need due to the rapid transformation of modern lifestyles and the lack of time for physical care, exercise, and desk occupations. As people have become more health-concerned, the factors that matter most when making food decisions have shifted. The public's focus on going above and beyond RDAs in terms of food to lower their risk of chronic diseases is growing. Today, many people struggle with obesity, diabetes, high blood pressure, stress, allergies, cardiovascular disease, and cancer. The new health and wellness paradigm encourages people to eat healthily in order to live longer. Individuals strive for a healthier body and a more youthful appearance in order to improve their quality of life. Natural healing elements can improve a wide range of health conditions, including those related to women's health, skin, eyes, cardiovascular health, joint health, mental health, bone health, sleep quality, cancer prevention, weight management, and athletic performance. The way of nature teaches us to look at health from a more holistic angle. Customers are more concerned about their health, so companies must provide scientific evidence to back up their health claims about new bioactive chemicals and cutting-edge methods of administration. With improved medical and pharmacological advancements and longer life expectancies, we can now see further into the future. Nutritional, organoleptic, and protective roles can all be played by the foods we eat. The pharmaceutical industry has made extensive use of bioactive dietary components (pills, capsules, solutions, gels, liquors, powders, granules, etc.). The term "nutraceuticals" is used to describe the goods that have been shown to have positive effects on human health. They help the body physiologically, protect against chronic diseases, boost health, and slow down the ageing process. A great amount of work has gone into this review to introduce novel ideas concerning nutraceuticals. And to acquire a new perspective on bioactive substances, we learn how to classify them. The law and emerging

DOI: 10.1201/9781003392934-9

technologies inform our analysis. Here we introduce some of the most well-known bioactive chemicals now in use as nutraceuticals and disease-modifying drugs (Shahgholian 2022).

The promotion of general health and wellness, the management of symptoms, and the prevention of malignant processes are all possible using nutraceuticals, which are regarded as non-specific biological therapies.

9.1.1 Definition of Nutraceutical

The word "nutraceutical" is a portmanteau of "nutrient," meaning a healthy food additive, and "pharmaceutical," meaning pharmaceutical medicine. In 1989, an American entrepreneur and current head of the Foundation for Innovation in Medicine Stephen DeFelice came up with the term.

Hippocrates, the father of medicine, was a Greek physician, and he is credited with coining the phrase "let food be your medicine," which is central to the theory underpinning nutraceuticals. One of the most pressing questions is their effect on human nutrition. This has far-reaching consequences for consumers, healthcare professionals, regulators, food producers, and distributors (Figure 9.1).

A nutraceutical is a food or dietary component with medicinal or health benefits for the body, such as promoting health or reducing the risk of disease. The discovery and production of nutraceuticals have mushroomed into a multibillion-dollar industry as a result of the widespread belief that they offer a safer, more all-natural route to therapeutic efficacy (Rana et al. 2016).

Types of Nutraceuticals: More and more individuals are paying close attention to what goes into their bodies as the findings of modern science emphasise the value of maintaining a healthy, well-rounded diet. Since obesity has become a global problem, proper nutrition is more important than ever. Unfortunately, most conventional therapies for disorders related to poor nutrition, such as medications, merely mask the symptoms rather than addressing the underlying cause.

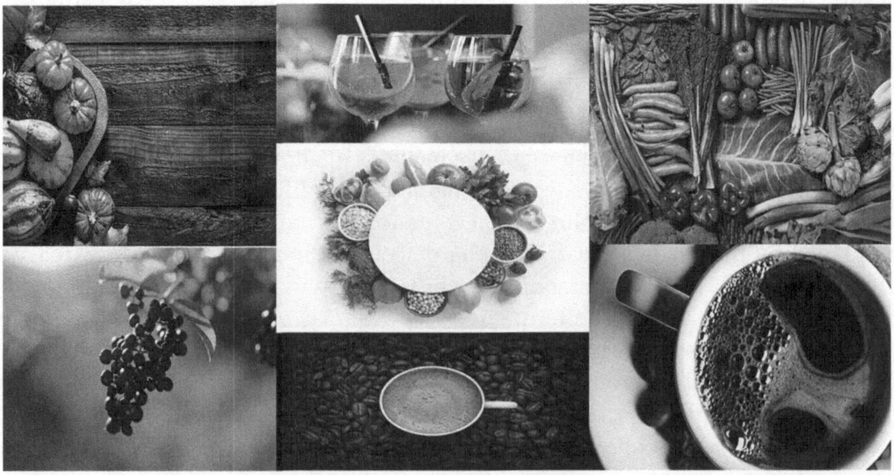

FIGURE 9.1 Food items part of daily life and important source of nutraceuticals.

Nutraceuticals are a class of dietary supplements that operate on the principle that food and medicine are interchangeable. Due to its natural makeup and foundational principles in healthy eating, nutraceuticals have become a popular choice for those looking to improve their nutritional status.

Nutritional supplements that also have medicinal effects are called nutraceuticals. Nutraceuticals come in many forms, from prebiotic and probiotic dietary fibre to vitamins with antioxidant properties. Nutraceuticals include everything from complex polyunsaturated fatty acids and polyphenols to simple kitchen cupboard staples like spices, making them one of the most inclusive umbrella words for nutritional therapy.

If you're unfamiliar with nutraceuticals and want to find an alternate way to improve your diet, you should do some reading and compile a list of goods that will work for you.

9.1.2 Role of Nutraceuticals

Nutraceuticals have a straightforward objective, they aim to treat and prevent serious diseases. Probiotics, for instance, are dietary supplements used to reduce the risk of dangerous gastrointestinal conditions like yeast infections that can develop when bacteria are abundant in the gut.

In addition, probiotics promote healthy bacteria, which assists digestion and nutrition absorption and helps keep you energised and alert. Certain nutraceutical goods, like polyphenols, have components with antioxidant capabilities that can shield your tissues and joints from inflammation, keeping you robust and mobile no matter what you're doing.

Certain other goods, like dietary fibre, are helpful in regulating cholesterol and blood pressure. As you can see, these are only a few of the many advantages of using nutraceuticals.

9.2 NUTRACEUTICALS IN CANCER PREVENTION

Nutraceuticals, often known as "functional foods," are food additives, extracts, or derivatives that have health benefits beyond what they provide nutritionally (Santini et al. 2017) Dietary supplements are a source of nutrients (carbohydrates, proteins, lipids) and non-nutrients (fillers, binders, etc). (e.g., prebiotics, probiotics, phytochemicals, enzymatic regulators) (Bergamin et al. 2019). Recent years have seen many scientific studies demonstrating that food is a very potent means at our disposal for protecting the body and maintaining a state of well-being. In fact, nutrition has both sound and adverse effects on the development of degenerative, autoimmune, and neoplastic disorders. The interaction between nutrients and organisms may determine a person's lifetime health or sickness.

One-third of cancer deaths may be averted via better nutrition and other lifestyle choices (Kerschbaum and Nussler 2019).

Although encouraging in vitro findings with multiple cell types, no mechanistic preclinical studies have been conducted. have been done up to this point. Because of a paucity of preclinical data, the first large-scale clinical studies of phytochemicals conducted in the 1990s were unsuccessful.

Herbal remedies have been used to combat cancer for centuries. The alkaloids of the Vinca species (vincristine and vinblastine) and the Pacific yew *Taxus brevifolia* are only a couple examples of the many plants used in the development of chemotherapy medications used to treat cancer (Taxol).

A wide variety of approaches were utilised by ancient societies all throughout the world to diagnose and treat illness, as well as to promote and sustain long and healthy lives. Plant extracts are one type of this methodology. When the same or comparable plants are utilised by other cultures to treat the same symptoms or ailments, it's good evidence that they're helpful as medicines. Many plant extracts are utilised in the treatment and prevention of cancer, which despite modern advancements remains a global health problem. Cancer patients who undergo nutritional modification may benefit from this approach to care (Weisburger 1999). Foods intermediate in high-quality protein, fibre, and fat (particularly lipids of the omega-3 fatty acid series) have been shown to affect cancer patients while having a low-carbohydrate profile positively (Tuomisto et al. 2004). Nutraceuticals can improve quality of life by lowering the risk of cancer cachexia and decreasing the toxicity of chemotherapy and radiation therapy (Grimble 2003).

Phytochemicals have been found to affect multiple cell levels in various ways. Most of them have come to be recognised as a diverse antioxidant source that can modulate redox-mediated transcription factor signalling. In addition, they influence the endocrine system, the immune system, and inflammatory enzymes directly. Some have been found to have an immediate impact on the DNA cleavage and repair procedure.

Research conducted in vitro suggests that phytochemicals may aid tumorigenic effects of carcinogens by inhibiting mutagenic activity and reducing cell proliferation (Surh 2003). The term "chemoprevention" refers to the employment of chemicals, either natural or manufactured, to interrupt, slow down, or stop the carcinogenic process. Most early-stage solid tumours are found as intraepithelial neoplasia or carcinoma in situ, which are equivalent to the promoting and progressing stages, respectively. Agents that inhibit "promotion" or "progression" could thus be of considerable clinical interest. Bioactive chemicals in the diet may have a significant effect on gene expression regulation even at modest doses. Further studies on the impact of nutraceuticals on gene expression will hopefully shed light on the mechanisms by which diseases including obesity, diabetes, atherosclerosis, hypertension, and cancer might be prevented through dietary changes.

Phytochemicals were also shown to prevent lipid peroxidation and to regulate the body's natural inflammatory and defence mechanisms (Issa et al. 2006). Plant extracts, because of their anti-cancer activities and low toxicity, are a promising new tool in the war against the disease.

Yet, in order to apply the right chemical to a suitable clinical circumstance, it is necessary to study each compound's mechanism of action and its effectiveness in a particular form of cancer. The study of plant biochemistry, genetics, and human nutrition is known as "nutritional genomics" (Della Penna 1999).

There have been a few studies on the effect of some nutraceuticals on activity, and these have led the way for much more in-depth research into these compounds, employing a wide range of animal models for various hereditary diseases (Orzechowski et al. 2002). Food supplements as an adjunctive therapy to improve cancer patients' quality of life are an area of urgent research and development. Nutraceuticals and functional foods play an important role in slowing the spread of cancer (Ogilvie 1998).

Cachexia, which can be described as severe abnormalities in glucose, protein, and lipid metabolism, is actually present in some cancer patients and is associated with a poor quality of life, a diminished response to therapy, and a shortened lifespan. Cancer patients may benefit from nutritional modification to correct these metabolic changes. To reduce the side effects of cancer treatments like chemotherapy and radiation, nutritional therapy can be an effective weapon (McCullough and Giovannucci 2004). In addition, nutraceuticals can considerably improve NK cell function and TNF levels in patients with advanced cancer.

9.3 MAIN PHYTOCHEMICALS STUDIED FOR CANCER CARE

Chemical structures, botanical origin, biological properties, biosynthesis, etc., are all criteria that can be used to categorise dietary phytochemicals (Table 9.1).

9.3.1 Polyphenols

Plants produce polyphenols, secondary metabolites with hydroxyl groups connected to benzene rings. The average human diet contains around 8,000 distinct polyphenols (found primarily in wine, tea, coffee, cocoa, vegetables, and grains) (Lecour and Lamont 2011). They can be separated into many categories according to the number of phenol rings and the structure that connects these rings. Here, the most significant groupings are the phenolic acids, flavonoids, stilbenes, and curcuminoids due to their ability to prevent the onset of carcinogenic processes and slow the development of cancer.

9.3.2 Epigallocatechin-3-Gallate

The primary catechin in green tea is known as EGCG (epigallocatechin-3-gallate) (Camellia sinensis). Drinking green tea regularly has been linked to several health advantages, and it is widely acknowledged as the most potent cancer-preventative beverage in Asia.

EGCG's anticancer activities have been confirmed across several cancer cell lines, including those of rarer cancers such as anaplastic thyroid carcinoma (De Amicis et al. 2013) and malignant mesothelioma (Ranzato et al. 2012).

For a more nuanced understanding of EGCG's anticancer effects, clinical trials should be carefully planned.

Low bioavailability and conversion to inactive methylated metabolites are problems for clinical applications of green tea. The polyphenols in green tea are biotransformed differently in humans than in rats and mice, which may account for the species-based

TABLE 9.1
List of Important Phytochemicals Carrying Nutraceutical Properties

S. No.	Phytochemicals	Source	Chemical properties	Medicinal properties
1	Curcumin	*Curcuma longa*	Curcumin-I Curcumin-II Curcumin-III	Antioxidant, anti-inflammatory, and anticancer properties (Reuter et al. 2011)
2	Resveratrol	Grapes (*Vitis vinifera* L.), Blueberries (*Vaccinium corymbosum* L.), Raspberries (*Rubus idaeus* L.), Mulberries (*Morus alba* Hort. ex Loudon L.), and peanuts (*Arachis hypogaea* L.). *Polygonum cuspidatum*	*Cis*-Stilbenoid Trans-Stilbenoid	Antioxidant, anti-inflammatory, and anticancer properties (Singh et al. 2013)
3	Astaxanthin	Synthesised in appropriate quantities by microalgae—Haematococcus lacustris (Gir.-Chantr.) Rostaf., Chromochloris zofingiensis (Donz) Fucikova and L. A. Lewis, Chlorococcum sp., and Phaffia rhodozyma, Salmon	xanthophyll carotenoid	Antioxidant, anti-inflammatory, and anticancer properties Higuera-Ciapara et al. 2006)
4	Sulforaphane, indole-3-carbinol	Broccoli (*Brassica oleracea* var. italica Plenck), Cabbage (*Brassica oleracea* var. capitata L.), Brussels sprouts (*Brassica oleracea* var. gemmifera Zenker), Cauliflower (*Brassica oleracea* var. botrytis L.), Kale (*Brassica oleracea* var. viridis DC. L.)	Glucosinolates	Antioxidant, anti-inflammatory, and anticancer properties (Connolly et al. 2021)
5	Quercetin	Apples (*Malus domestica* (Suckow) Borkh.), Grapes (*Vitis vinifera* L.), Olives (*Olea europaea* Hoffmanns. and Link L.), Oranges (*Citrus sinensis* (L.) Osbeck), and Raspberries (*Rubus idaeus* L.)—vegetables—tomatoes (*Solanum lycopersicum* L.), onions (*Allium cepa* L.), broccoli (*Brassica oleracea* var. italica Plenck), and capers (*Capparis spinosa* L.)—drinks (tea and red wine), and herbal extracts	flavonoid belonging to the flavonols group	Antioxidant, anti-inflammatory, and anticancer properties (Zhang et al. 2012)

6	Epigallocatechin-3-gallate (EGCG)-	Green tea (*Camellia sinensis* L.). Carob (*Ceratonia siliqua* L.) flour, Apples (*Malus domestica* (Suckow) Borkh.), blackberries (*Rubus plicatus* L. Weihe and Nees), raspberries (*Rubus idaeus* L.), pistachios (*Pistacia vera* L.), prunes (*Prunus domestica* L.), peaches (Prunus persica (L.) Batsch), and avocados (*Persea americana* Mill.).	Catechin	Antioxidant, anti-inflammatory, and anticancer properties (Ranzato et al., 2012)
7	Lycopene	Tomatoes (*Solanum lycopersicum* L.), Apricots (*Prunus armeniaca* S. X. Sun L.), Guava (*Psidium guajava* L.), Papaya (*Carica papaya* L.), watermelon (*Citrullus lanatus* subsp. vulgaris (Schrad.) Fursa), and pink grapefruit (Citrus × paradisi Macfad.).	Carotenoid	Antioxidant, anti-inflammatory, and anticancer properties (Muller et al. 2016)

variation in their anti-cancer effects (Clifford et al. 2013). Also, while planning studies on the efficacy of green tea, it is essential to account for genetic polymorphisms in genes involved in the biotransformation of EGCG, such as catechol-O-methyltransferase (COMT) (Moyers and Kumar 2004). In contrast, EGCG's multiple antitumor effects imply that it may be helpful in cancer prevention and therapy, either alone or in conjunction with other anticancer medicines or phytochemicals.

9.3.3 Resveratrol

In terms of cancer, resveratrol is the most significant stilbene. As a phytoalexin, it has a natural ability to inhibit cell proliferation (plant antibiotic). Anti-cancer, anti-carcinogenesis, and anti-inflammatory actions are just a few of the many bioactivities attributed to it (Singh et al. 2013). Uncertainty surrounds the molecular processes by which resveratrol might induce these effects; however, activation of sirtuin proteins appears to be central. The potential of resveratrol as a cancer-preventative and -curing agent is receiving a lot of attention (Ranzato et al. 2014). Repeated daily dosages of resveratrol have been found to be safe and well-tolerated, and the drug's plasma pharmacokinetics in humans are now fairly well-established (Gescher et al. 2013).

In contrast, resveratrol has been demonstrated in pharmacokinetics studies to have a low bioavailability (only 1%) due to significant glucuronidation and sulfation as well as processing by gut bacterial enzymes (Scott et al. 2012).

9.3.4 The Antioxidant Quercetin

Quercetin, an example of a flavonoid, is a chemical found in plants and consumed by humans at doses between 16 and 25 milligrammes per day (Hertog et al. 1993).

Researchers believe quercetin's actions are linked to the triggering of cell death through a variety of pathways. Studies of quercetin's anticancer effects in living organisms have shown that it can prevent induced carcinogenesis, particularly in the colon, and that it can also reduce the growth, invasion, and metastasis of melanoma (Zhang et al. 2012). The fundamental issue with quercetin, as with resveratrol, is its limited bioavailability (Dajas 2012).

9.4 NUTRIENTS AND MINERALS IN THE TREATMENT OF CANCER

Several studies point to the potential importance of vitamins A, C, and E and trace minerals like selenium in cancer prevention. There is some evidence that micro-nutrient supplements used as adjuvants in cancer patients can improve their prognosis (Misotti and Gnagnarella 2013). Ascorbate, or vitamin C, is not only a vital component of a healthy diet but also a popular over-the-counter and alternative medicine treatment for a wide range of illnesses (Levine et al. 1999). Cell cycle arrest, activation of the apoptotic factors, and inhibition of iron uptake have all been implicated in the studies of ascorbate toxicity that have focused on its mechanism. Because of its position as an electron donor in redox processes, ascorbate is often thought to play a significant part in the mechanism of ascorbate toxicity in tumour cells (Ranzato et al. 2011). Ascorbate's true potential is being investigated in other in vitro and in vivo investigations, which also involve mixing it with chemotherapy medicines (Martinotti et al. 2011).

9.5 THE WAY FORWARD

Natural environments may provide practical active principles for combating cancer cells. The biological effects of phytochemicals on human cells are diverse and exciting. The rising popularity of using phytochemicals in cancer treatment has spurred the development of many phytochemical-containing nutraceuticals. Now, the goal must be to create nutritional supplements to help specific populations avoid or postpone the beginning of diseases related to poor eating. Insight into the molecular mechanisms by which these factors influence human health will make this a reality.

REFERENCES

Bergamin, A., Mantzioris, E., Cross, G., Deo, P., Garg, S., & Hill, A.M. (2019). Nutraceuticals: Reviewing their role in chronic disease prevention and management. *Pharmaceutical Medicine*, *33*(4), 291–309. 10.1007/S40290-019-00289-W

Clifford, M.N., van der Hooft, J.J., & Crozier, A. (2013). Human studies on the absorption, distribution, metabolism, and excretion of tea polyphenols. *Am J Clin Nutr*, *98*, 1619S–1630S. 10.3945/ajcn.113.058958

Connolly, E.L., Sim, M., Travica, N., Marx, W., Beasy, G., Lynch, G.S., Bondonno, C.P., Lewis, J.R., Hodgson, J.M., & Blekkenhorst, L.C. (2021). Glucosinolates from cruciferous vegetables and their potential role in chronic disease: Investigating the preclinical and clinical evidence. *Front. Pharmacol*, *12*, 2964.

Dajas, F. (2012). Life or death: Neuroprotective and anticancer effects of quercetin. *Ethnopharmacol*, *143*, 383–396. 10.1016/j.jep.2012.07.005

De Amicis, F., Perri, A., Vizza, D., Russo, A., Panno, M.L., Bonofiglio, D., … Ando, S. (2013). Epigallocatechin gallate inhibits growth and epithelial-to-mesenchymal transition in human thyroid carcinoma cell lines. *J Cell Physiol*, *228*, 2054–2062. 10.1002/jcp.24372

Della Penna, D. (1999). Nutritional genomics: Manipulating plant micronutrients to improve human health. *Science*, *285*, 375–379. 10.1126/science.285.5426.375

Gescher, A., Steward, W.P., & Brown, K. (2013). Resveratrol in the management of human cancer: How strong is the clinical evidence? *Ann N Y Acad Sci*, *1290*, 12–20. 10.1111/nyas.12205

Grimble, R.F. (2003). Nutritional therapy for cancer cachexia. *Gut*, *52*, 1391–1392. 10.1136/gut.52.10.1391

Hertog, M.G., Feskens, E.J., Hollman, P.C., Katan, M.B., & Kromhout, D. (1993). Dietary antioxidant flavonoids and risk of coronary heart disease: The Zutphen Elderly Study. *Lancet*, *342*, 1007–1011. 10.1016/0140-6736(93)92876-U

Higuera-Ciapara, I., Félix-Valenzuela, L., & Goycoolea, F.M. (2006). Astaxanthin: A review of its chemistry and applications. *Crit. Rev. Food Sci. Nutr*, *46*, 185–196.

Issa, A.Y., Volate, S.R., & Wargovich, M.J. (2006). The role of phytochemicals in inhibition of cancer and inflammation: New directions and perspectives. *J Food Compos Anal*, *19*, 405–419. 10.1016/j.jfca.2006.02.009

Kerschbaum, E., & Nüssler, V. (2019). Cancer prevention with nutrition and lifestyle. *Visc Med.* Aug, *35*(4), 204–209. doi: 10.1159/000501776. Epub 2019 Jul 23. PMID: 31602380; PMCID: PMC6738231.

Lecour, S., & Lamont, K.T. (2011). Natural polyphenols and cardioprotection. *Mini Rev Med Chem*, *11*, 1191–1199. 10.2174/138955711804586766

Levine, M., Rumsey, S.C., Daruwala, R., Park, J.B., & Wang, Y. (1999). Criteria and recommendations for vitamin C intake. *JAMA*, *281*, 1415–1423. 10.1001/jama.281.15.1415

Martinotti, S., Ranzato, E., & Burlando, B. (2011). In vitro screening of synergistic ascorbate-drug combinations for the treatment of malignant mesothelioma. *Toxicol In Vitro*, *25*, 1568–1574. 10.1016/j.tiv.2011.05.023

McCullough, M.L., & Giovannucci, E.L. (2004). Diet and cancer prevention. *Oncogene*, *23*, 6349–6364. 10.1038/sj.onc.1207716

Misotti, A.M., & Gnagnarella, P. (2013). Vitamin supplement consumption and breast cancer risk: A review. *Ecancermedicalscience*, *7*, 365.

Moyers, S.B., & Kumar, N.B. (2004). Green tea polyphenols and cancer chemoprevention: Multiple mechanisms and endpoints for phase II trials. *Nutr Rev*, *62*, 204–211. 10.1111/j.1753-4887.2004.tb00041.x

Müller, L., Caris-Veyrat, C., Lowe, G., & Böhm, V. (2016). Lycopene and its antioxidant role in the prevention of cardiovascular diseases - A critical review. *Crit. Rev. Food Sci. Nutr*, *56*, 1868–1879.

Ogilvie, G.K. (1998). Interventional nutrition for the cancer patient. *Clin Tech Small Anim Pract*, *13*, 224–231. 10.1016/S1096-2867(98)80007-8

Orzechowski, A., Ostaszewski, P., Jank, M., & Berwid, S.J. (2002). Bioactive substances of plant origin in food - impact on genomics. *Reprod Nutr Dev*, *42*, 461–477. 10.1051/rnd:2002037

Ranzato, E., Biffo, S., & Burlando, B. (2011). Selective ascorbate toxicity in malignant mesothelioma: A redox Trojan mechanism. *Am J Respir Cell Mol Biol*, *44*, 108–117. 10.1165/rcmb.2009-0340OC

Ranzato, E., Martinotti, S., Magnelli, V., Murer, B., Biffo, S., Mutti, L., & Burlando, B. (2012). Epigallocatechin-3-gallate induces mesothelioma cell death via H2O2-dependent T-type Ca2+ channel opening. *J Cell Mol Med*, *16*, 2667–2678. 10.1111/j.1582-4934.2012.01584.x

Rana, J.C., Singh, M., Chauhan, R.S., Chahota, R.K., Sharma, T.R., Yadav, R., & Archak, S. (2016). Genetic resources of buckwheat in India. *Molecular Breeding and Nutritional Aspects of Buckwheat*, 109–129. 10.1016/B978-0-12-803692-1.00009-2

Ranzato, E., Martinotti, S., Calabrese, C.M., & Calabrese, G. (2014). Role of nutraceuticals in cancer therapy. *Journal of Food Research*, *3*(4), 18. 10.5539/JFR.V3N4P18

Reuter, S., Gupta, S.C., Park, B., Goel, A., & Aggarwal, B.B. (2011). Epigenetic changes induced by curcumin and other natural compounds. *Genes Nutr*, *6*, 93.

Santini, A., Tenore, G.C., & Novellino, E. (2017). Nutraceuticals: A paradigm of proactive medicine. *European Journal of Pharmaceutical Sciences: Official Journal of the European Federation for Pharmaceutical Sciences*, *96*, 53–61. 10.1016/J.EJPS.2016.09.003

Shahgholian, N. (2022). Introduction to nutraceuticals and natural products. *Handbook of Nutraceuticals and Natural Products*, 1–14. 10.1002/9781119746843.CH1

Scott, E., Steward, W.P., Gescher, A.J., & Brown, K. (2012). Resveratrol in human cancer chemoprevention - choosing the 'right' dose. *Mol Nutr Food Res*, *56*, 7–13. 10.1002/mnfr.201100400

Singh, C.K., George, J., & Ahmad, N. (2013). Resveratrol-based combinatorial strategies for cancer management. *Ann N Y Acad Sci*, *1290*, 113–121. 10.1111/nyas.12160

Surh, Y.J. (2003). Cancer chemoprevention with dietary phytochemicals. *Nat Rev Cancer*, *3*, 768–780. 10.1038/nrc1189

Tuomisto, J.T., Tuomisto, J., Tainio, M., Niittynen, M., Verkasalo, P., Vartiainen, T., … Pekkanen, J. (2004). Risk-benefit analysis of eating farmed salmon. *Science*, *305*, 476–477.

Weisburger, J.H. (1999). Antimutagens, anticarcinogens, and effective worldwide cancer prevention. *J Environ Pathol Toxicol Oncol*, *18*, 85–93.
Zhang, X., Chen, L.X., Ouyang, L., Cheng, Y., & Liu, B. (2012). Plant natural compounds: Targeting pathways of autophagy as anti-cancer therapeutic agents. *Cell Prolif*, *45*, 466–476. 10.1111/j.1365-2184.2012.00833.x

10 Nutraceuticals Explored

Safety, Toxicity, and Contaminant Concerns

Mustansir Bhori, Ameyota De, Shreya Das, Vaishnavi Kesarkar, Aayushi Kadam, and Kanchanlata Tungare

10.1 INTRODUCTION TO NUTRACEUTICALS

Nutraceutical is a combination of "nutrition" and "pharmaceutical," the term applies to products produced from isolated plant products: nutrients in processed foods such as cereals, soups, and beverages (Kalra 2003). Dietary supplements, regulated as pharmaceuticals, and medicinal food ingredients, are defined as the substances that provide either a physiological benefit or protection against chronic disease (Nasri et al. 2014).

Specifically, the supplements consist of whole food sources classified into subgroups which are probiotics, prebiotics, polyunsaturated fatty acids, antioxidant vitamins, polyphenols, spices, and fibre. They even include both digestible and indigestible carbohydrates that are native to plants. There are also functional fibres that are separated from natural sources and added to processed products. Total fibre is the sum of diet and function supplements used for improving health, slowing aging, and preventing chronic disease, extending life expectancy, and supporting body structure and function (Zhao 2007). Nutrient supplements, unlike pharmaceuticals, are substances that are usually not patented, although both pharmaceutical and nutraceutical compounds can be used to prevent and treat disease (Chauhan et al. 2013). They have products that carry or contain one or more nutritional ingredients, such as by increasing the daily intake of ingredients, and their combinations of the ingredients, used for health purposes other than nutrition (Nasri et al. 2014).

Nowadays, nutraceuticals are growing with exponential nutritional, safety, and therapeutic benefits, and the nutraceuticals global market grew to US$250 billion in 2018 and it is still growing (Hardy 2000). Diabetes (Baradaran et al. 2013), Atherosclerosis (Madihi et al. 2013; Setorki et al. 2013), Cardiovascular disease (CVD) (Khosravi-Boroujeni et al. 2012), Cancer (Shirzad et al. 2013) and Neurological diseases (Akhlaghi et al. 2011) are some disorders that include

 DOI: 10.1201/9781003392934-10

extensive treatments. These states are accompanied by many changes, including changes in the redox state, they have antioxidant activity capable of combating this situation (Parsaei et al. 2013; Baradaran et al. 2014) and are particularly useful in diabetes (Mirhoseini et al. 2013), infectious diseases (Bahmani et al. 2013), kidney disease (Rafieian-Kopaie 2013), and gastrointestinal disease (Kiani et al. 2013).

Nutritional supplements would have a safer profile with better bioavailability if supported by clinical evidence. Nutraceuticals encompass probiotics, prebiotics, and medical-purpose foods, while food supplements include minerals, vitamins, proteins, and herbal items. Some spices and herbs in food may lower disease risks and enhance quality of life (Helal et al. 2019). Nutraceuticals offer potential benefits in preventing and treating complex disorders but require strict regulation to prevent misuse and side effects (Puri et al. 2022). Researchers aim to enhance the efficacy and bioavailability of drug-based nutraceuticals, with safety assessments similar to pharmaceuticals, involving in-vivo, ex-vivo, and in-vitro evaluations of tissue, physiological, and cellular effects.

Non-invasive optical imaging technology, including three-dimensional fluorescent tomographic imaging, has advanced significantly, enabling the identification and localisation of deep tissues and quantitative fluorescence measurements within the body. Fluorescence imaging (FLI) allows real-time assessment of tissue biology with targeted probes and nonradioactive contrast agents, offering safety, multiplexing capabilities, and quick acquisition times (Bu et al. 2014). Limitations include the use of limited infusion data and small fields of view, but recent optical imaging systems offer deep tissue tomographic capabilities for studying various diseases (Hussain et al. 2022).

Zebrafish (*Danio rerio*) are favoured for evaluating health effects, ecotoxicology, and DNA damage compared to traditional mammals due to their similarities in physiology, development, and genetics. Their advantages include small size, transparent embryos, short reproductive cycles, and external embryo development. Zebrafish are used to assess the safety and toxicity of nutraceuticals (Chahardehi et al. 2020). These studies explore caffeine's impact on development, quercetin's therapeutic potential, resveratrol's anti-inflammatory effects, and spirulina as a dietary source for zebrafish, offering valuable insights into various health-related aspects.

10.2 APPLICATIONS

Nutraceuticals are used in most therapeutic areas, including anti-arthritis, colds and coughs, sleep disorders, digestion, and the prevention of certain types of cancer, osteoporosis, blood pressure, cholesterol control, pain relievers, depression, and diabetes (Das et al. 2012). A healthy diet is important for good health. So, dietary supplements and functional foods offer opportunities to reduce healthcare costs and help to improve human health (Cencic and Chingwaru 2010). There has been a lot of work in the production of nutraceuticals and functional foods. Recent advances in dietary supplements and functional foods for health benefits are being applied to disease prevention applications (Boggia et al. 2020). Nutraceuticals have played an important role in combating such diseases to provide health benefits to people (Nasri et al. 2014) they are used as dietary supplements to assist nutritional, immunological, and physiological functions in the prevention or treatment of disorders, such as gastrointestinal (GI) disorder (Shahidi 2012). There is a wide variety of herbal products, including natural products synthesised by various Indian or other industries around the globe, and more people are enjoying their health benefits (Ekor 2014). Prebiotics and probiotics (which help develop a healthy micro-environment in humans to treat chronic diseases), lycopene (which has powerful antioxidant properties), and plant sterols (which lower blood cholesterol levels and can be used to lower blood pressure) have been discussed for their health benefits.

10.3 TOXICITY

Pharmacokinetic/toxicokinetic research expertise appears to be crucial for determining the safety and toxicity of nutraceuticals. Due to their accessibility, affordability, tolerance, and high margin of safety, the usage of nutraceuticals in both humans and animals has grown in popularity by the turn of the 21st century. Although some nutraceuticals are risk-free, some may be poisonous. Due to a dearth of toxicological and pharmacological research, many nutraceuticals lack toxicity/safety evidence. Certain nutraceuticals may become unsafe due to contamination by poisonous plants, metals, mycotoxins, pesticides, fertilisers, illegal medicines, etc. In order to assess the safety, and toxicity of the usage of therapeutic medications and nutraceuticals, interaction studies are crucial.

10.3.1 Toxicity Studies – *In-vitro and In-vivo*

10.3.1.1 Adverse Reaction Prediction – Statistical Analysis

Online access to the Connectivity Map (CMap) database is available at http://www.broadinstitute.org/cmap/. CMap is essentially a collection of transcriptome data from 6,100 human cell cultures that were exposed to 1,309 different bioactive compounds together with vehicle controls. A small set of gene probes with the highest fold change (for example, the 250 most up- and down-regulated gene probes) may be used as "signatures" for certain medications. For instance, the Gene Set Enrichment Analysis methodology can be used to examine various signatures and compare the genomic expression of two drugs (Lamb et al. 2006). The majority of a drug's effects are controlled by the linked genes, and a drug's signature can reveal both its pharmacological and toxicological characteristics. The majority of a drug's effects are controlled by the linked genes, and a drug's signature can reveal both its pharmacological and toxicological characteristics. Recent studies have demonstrated that drugs with comparable side effects frequently have similar CMap expression profiles (the raw data) (Wang et al. 2013). They used the drug-specific genomic expression profile as a guilt-by-association predictor of negative effects to develop a "risk score" model. The risk score (RS) of the test drug will be determined using the average similarity score across all reference medications. If N (N>0) reference medications (designated as R1, R2, R3, … , RN) are known to have certain hazardous effects, then the RS for the test drug D will be calculated as follows.

$$RS_D = S_1 + S_2 + S_3 \ldots + S_N N$$

The expression "similarity" between the test drug and the reference drug is represented by Si (1 I N). If a supplement or medication displays a high RS in comparison to other CMAP chemicals, then the possible risk may need to be taken into consideration. For example, for renal injury and folic acid RS discovery according to genomic expression signatures, the systematic assessment of the safety of nutraceuticals may be made easier by utilising effective computational approaches in conjunction with drug-induced changes in gene expression (Stallons et al. 2014).

10.3.1.2 Evaluation of the Toxicity of Nutraceuticals Using Gene Expression Profiling

A number of genomics applications, such as transcriptome sequencing, whole-genome sequencing, and chromatin immunoprecipitation sequencing (ChIP-seq) (RNA-seq), have been made possible by the development of next-generation sequencing (NGS) technology (Chi 2008). The accuracy, repeatability, and informational content of RNA-seq have recently undergone a thorough review by the FDA-led Sequencing Quality Control (SEQC) project. The identification of specific gene expression patterns induced by a chemical or dietary supplement could shed light on the toxicologically harmful mechanisms of action. Over the past ten years, we have carried out numerous toxicogenomic studies to evaluate a range of herbal dietary supplements. Examples of ways to evaluate the toxicity and safety of dietary supplements using gene expression profiling According to reports, kava consumption can harm the liver (Campo et al. 2002; Clough et al. 2003; Humberston et al. 2003) Patients who consume kava may experience acute liver failure and perhaps pass away. Hepatic necrosis and cholestatic hepatitis have both been seen clinically. According to reports, kava products can cause acute liver failure in humans. As a result, regulatory bodies in several countries have taken action, warning consumers and even banning kava products from the market. For instance, CYP1A1 is involved in metabolising the reactive metabolites that are responsible for the carcinogenicity of the polycyclic aromatic hydrocarbon (PAH) class of compounds (Whitlock 1999). Reactive metabolites of PAHs can produce more when CYP1A1 activity is increased. As a result, any substance that stimulates CYP1A1 activity may also increase the toxicity of PAHs, raising safety issues. In the livers of rats given kava extract, a considerable elevation of CYP1A1 gene expression was discovered using microarray analysis (Guo et al. 2007). To further this work, the active kavalactones involved in CYP1A1 induction as well as the molecular and biochemical mechanisms by which kava extract induces CYP1A1 were investigated in cultured cells (Li et al. 2011).

10.3.1.3 Zebrafish Model for Toxicity Testing of Nutraceutical

Comparative evolutionary analysis of the human and fish genomes has revealed reveals that the neurological, cardiovascular, and digestive systems share a lot of the same structure and physiology (Han et al. 2018). According to Mizgirev et al. (2010), the zebrafish *(Danio rerio)* is a viable model for testing drugs that may be used to treat human illnesses. The complete zebrafish genome has been sequenced (Pham et al. 2016). They are a quick model for investigating genetic and spontaneous alterations. Zebrafish embryos are a useful model for drug testing and assessing the teratogenic effects of exposure to hazardous substances (Bailey et al. 2013) since they can swiftly absorb small molecules as well. Zebrafish larvae and embryos make excellent models for determining how harmful compounds are, especially when they're present in small amounts. Existing studies have screened the toxicity of Nutraceuticals using the zebrafish model. According to Lee et al., zebrafish were made to exhibit seizure-like behaviour after being exposed to ginkgo toxin for two hours. Their findings showed that an in vivo model of epileptic seizures caused by ginkgo toxin could be used in future studies. It has been proposed that the naturally occurring neurotoxic ginkgo toxin found in ginkgo Biloba inhibits the synthesis of the neurotransmitter gamma-aminobutyric acid (GABA). In adult zebrafish, Bernardi et al. (2013) investigated the neurotoxic effects of neem. Following exposure to 20 or 40 L/L of neem extract, they used a passive avoidance test to gauge general activity,anxiety-like effects, learning, and memory. Neem extract made zebrafish less active overall and exhibited anxiety-like behaviour. Zebrafish learning and memory, however, were unaffected.

10.3.1.4 *Caenorhabditis Elegans*: A Model Organism for Assessing the Toxicity of Dietary Supplements

A tiny, translucent, free-living nematode called *Caenorhabditis elegans* inhabits dirt. Particularly in investigations addressing the potential biological activity of natural compounds, the organism has drawn interest for its usage as an alternative in vivo model. *Eleutherococcus* and *Rhodiola* have been shown to boost stress tolerance in a variety of model species (previous research has evaluated the toxicity of nutraceuticals utilising the *C. elegans* model (Wiegant et al. 2009). Despite being poisonous to *C. elegans* at greater levels, many ethnobotanical substances seem to be protective at lower concentrations. The Asiatic plant Daphne genkwa, also known by its dried flower bud as gen Kwa flos (GF), is utilised in traditional Chinese medicine (TCM). Studies of this plant's effects on C. elegans have also been done. The outcomes in this model organism have not been as encouraging as those of other nutraceuticals. In general, the worms' mortality was not increased by exposure to different GF concentrations. However, it was discovered that the highest investigated concentration (0.24 g/mL) reduced lifespan, while lower amounts had little impact on this endpoint either negatively or positively. There was a significant decrease in body length, as well as deformation of the vulva (Qiao et al. 2014).

10.3.2 Nutraceuticals and Their Toxic Effects

10.3.2.1 Aloe Vera

The "plant of immortality," commonly known as aloe vera, is grown all over the world. This stemless plant contains more than 200 compounds, including amino acids, vitamins, minerals, lignin, and phytosterols in its whole leaf extract (WLE: gel and latex) (Gupta and Malhotra 2012). Although oral administration of aloe vera may result in gastrointestinal pain and diarrhoea and impair medicine absorption, aloe vera is not known to have any serious adverse effects. According to the IARC,2006, ingesting non-decolorised liquid aloe vera causes cancer in animals and may do the same to humans. After two years of oral administration of Aloe vera WLE in drinking water, evidence of carcinogenic activity was shown in F344/N rats. Numerous anthraquinones have been reported to be mutagenic in the majority of In-vitro and In-vivo test systems, and they are mainly focused on studies on the genotoxicity of aloe latex.

10.3.2.2 Bitter Melon

In the 14th century, the bitter melon plant (*Momordica charantia*), which is native to India, was brought to China. It is currently utilised on a global scale as both a food and a treatment. Bitter melon is used as a natural diabetes treatment because it can lower blood sugar levels by improving the liver's ability to utilise glucose and reducing its ability to produce it (Joseph and Jini 2013). The side effects are Diarrhoea, abdominal pain, headaches, fever, hypoglycemia, atrial fibrillation of the heart, urine incontinence, and chest pain are some of the adverse effects of bitter melon. It is not advised for pregnant women to consume bitter melon. Since it can lead to miscarriage, bleeding, contractions, and menstrual stimulation Additionally, due to the presence of vicine in the seed, those who lack the gene for glucose-6-phosphate dehydrogenase should refrain from consuming bitter melon products.

10.3.2.3 Green Coffee/Bean

Green coffee beans from the Coffea canephora and Coffea arabica species are mature or immature coffee beans that haven't been roasted (GCB). Caffeine is the most important component of the coffee bean, even though it contains more than 1,000 other phytochemicals from a nutraceutical perspective. Although caffeine is a functional food and has GRAS certification from the US FDA, its risk assessment seems difficult. Caffeine concentrations that are toxic are far higher than those needed to inhibit adenosine receptors. Caffeine concentrations must be 20 times greater to prevent cyclic nucleotide breakdown by PDE inhibition, 40 times higher to block GABA, and 100 times higher to mobilise intracellular calcium depots (Fredholm et al. 1999). Clinical indications of intoxication, such as anxiety, restlessness, and tachycardia, are linked to blood caffeine levels above 30 g/mL. The symptoms of acute and chronic caffeine intoxication that follow high dosages (300–800 mg/person/day) are referred to as caffeinism. These symptoms include restlessness, agitation, anxiety, and irritability. They also include muscular tremors, hyperventilation, arrhythmia, tachycardia, and hypertension, followed by hypotension, diuresis, gastrointestinal problems, renal failure, and respiratory failure. An excessive intake of caffeine can result in rhabdomyolysis, hypokalaemia, hyponatremia, decreased iron and zinc absorption, hyponatremia, and, ultimately, cardiac collapse (Campana et al. 2014).

10.3.2.4 Goldenseal

The perennial herb known as goldenseal (*Hydrastis canadensis*), sometimes known as orangeroot or yellow puccoon, is indigenous to Canada and the eastern United States. Isoquinoline alkaloids, including hydrastine, berberine, canadine, canalidine, and many others, are present in the plant. Both internally and externally, goldenseal is used to treat mouth, skin, and for the treatment of urinary and gastrointestinal illnesses as well as ocular infections. Only a few possible adverse effects include mouth ulcers, gastrointestinal distress (constipation or diarrhoea), nausea, vomiting, nervousness, CNS depression, tachycardia, and seizures. High doses may result in mortality, paralysis, and respiratory issues. Long-term use can result in hallucinations, delirium, and vitamin B deficiency. Goldenseal toxicity appears to be caused by berberine and hydrastine (Gurley et al. 2005).

10.3.2.5 Pennyroyal

People have used fresh and dried pennyroyal (*Mentha pulegium*) for ages despite the fact that the oil is exceedingly toxic. 85% of the ketone pulegone is found in pennyroyal oil. The oil has long been employed in traditional medicine as an inducer of menstruation and as an abortifacient. The uterus's irritation and subsequent contractions are assumed to be the cause of the oil's abortive impact. In two cases of pennyroyal oil use for abortion, Sullivan et al. 1979 detected shock, disseminated intravascular coagulation, and significant hepatic dysfunction. deaths and necrosis Pulegone and menthofuran were found to cause hepatotoxicity and mortality in patient serum, according to Anderson et al. 1996. Hepatotoxicity, gastrointestinal distress and bleeding, haematuria, vaginal haemorrhage, renal failure, and coma are all recognised side effects of the oil.

10.3.3 Toxic Contamination in Nutraceuticals

10.3.3.1 Pyrrolizidine Alkaloids

Pyrolizidine alkaloids (PAs) are the most harmful toxins that may be discovered in a variety of plant species, such as Crotalaria, Senecio, Heliotropium, Symphytum, Cynoglossum, Amsinckia, and Echitum (Preliasco et at. 2017). There are more than 150 PAs that are now recognised, and some of them often contaminate foods and herbal nutraceuticals. The fundamental structures of senecionine and heliotrope can be used to illustrate the PAs, which have the pyrrolizidine nucleus. Although their potency varies as a result of their bioactivation in the liver to hazardous metabolites known as pyrroles, the toxic effects of PAs are comparatively comparable (Panter et al. 2012). These pyrroles are strong DNA cross-linkers and alkylating agents that interact with cellular proteins to cause cellular malfunction, aberrant mitosis, and tissue necrosis. Hepatotoxicity in both people and animals is one of the harmful health effects that many PAs can have (Winship 1991; Fu et al. 2017). Numerous PAs may possibly be cytotoxic and carcinogenic in the future. The chronic carcinogenicity of certain PAs is currently the basis for the risk evaluation of these alkaloids. Application to rats using the total of the detected PAs as a dose metric.

10.3.3.2 Heavy Metals

Although nutritional supplements are generally thought to be harmless, they may become dangerous if they become contaminated with specific metals. In actuality, heavy metal contamination in conventional drugs contains a lot of evidence (Meena et al. 2010). Due to their toxicity and cumulative nature, heavy metal concentrations may conceivably reach levels that have detrimental effects on both human and animal health. Cadmium (Cd), mercury (Hg), lead (Pb), and arsenic (As) are non-essential hazardous metals of particular concern because of their toxicity even in small amounts (Gil et al. 2016). Renal cancers, impaired cognitive growth, elevated blood pressure, and cardiovascular damage have all been linked to lead exposure. Traditional and folk treatments were discovered to contain dangerous levels of Pb in a recent retrospective-observational study, causing symptoms such as abdominal pain, constipation, hypertension, anaemia, neurological problems, and kidney damage. The reproductive and developmental system, bones, kidneys, lungs, and cadmium may become toxic. Arsenic can have harmful effects on the nervous, haematological, gastrointestinal, cardiovascular, and cutaneous systems. Cd and As both cause cancer. Hg intoxication can have toxic consequences on the neurological, renal, cardiovascular, reproductive, and immunological systems (Bridges and Zalpus 2017).

10.3.3.3 Pesticides

Pesticides must be used when growing food and medicinal plants on a large scale. Pesticide residues have frequently been found in crude herbal material after analysis (Ahmed et al. 2001; Wong et al. 2007). Herbicides and insecticides are the two types of pesticides that are most commonly used, and naturally, insecticides are far more hazardous than any other kind of pesticide. There are many different kinds of insecticides, including carbamates (aldicarb, bendiocarb, carbaryl, carbofuran, methomyl, etc., organophosphates (chlorpyrifos, diazinon, malathion, methyl parathion, etc., and other substances. Overexposure to pesticide residue can cause a number of harmful health impacts, from short-term problems like skin rashes and asthma attacks to long-term problems including cancer, neurological, reproductive, and developmental illnesses. It is anticipated that compared to other types of insecticides, the residue of organochlorines will last longer in dietary supplements and components. Organophosphates and carbamates have higher harmful effects after acute exposure, while organochlorines have more toxic effects after chronic exposure(Sarkhail et al. 2012; Tong et al. 2017).

10.3.3.4 Mycotoxins

Plants and dietary supplements may be contaminated by mycotoxins, secondary compounds that fungi create. When transferring raw plant materials and during plant growth, mycotoxins might develop. A substance, as well as during supplement storage. Aflatoxin A, citrinin, and other mycotoxins are frequently detected in nutraceuticals and food additives. When Raman et al. (Raman et al. 2004) examined a variety of botanical supplements, they discovered mould in many of the samples. Penicillium, Aspergillus, and Fusarium were the most often isolated moulds found in therapeutic plants (Abou-Arab et al. 1999). Due to increased humidity inside the pack and improper preservation techniques, packed samples of herbal plants are more likely to have mould than unpacked samples. Aflatoxin B1 contamination was found in various spices, aromatic herbs, and therapeutic plants from Italy. Aspergillus flavus is the principal producer of aflatoxin B1, and its harmful effects include hepatotoxicity, hepatocarcinogencity, and immunosuppressive, mutagenic, teratogenic, and effects (Prado et al. 2012). It is interesting that a nutraceutical can include numerous mycotoxins, and from a regulatory standpoint, an additive or synergistic interaction should be taken into account.

10.4 CONCLUSION

Nutraceuticals are compounds with physiological advantages or those that offer defence against chronic diseases. They can be used to boost wellbeing, slow down ageing, stop chronic diseases from occurring, lengthen life expectancy, or support the body's structure or functions. Due to their potential for having nutritional, safe, and therapeutic impacts, nutraceuticals have recently attracted a lot of attention. These supplements have demonstrated promising outcomes for a variety of problems, according to recent investigations. Nutraceuticals are being consumed more and more frequently on a global scale, which is attributed to their stated efficacy and safety. Recently, attention has been drawn to the use of cutting-edge nanosized drug delivery systems as a platform for nutraceutical composition. This is driven by the encouraging findings about the nutraceuticals tested's bioavailability, safety, targeting, and stability. This led to the adoption of a variety of drug delivery technologies, including nanoparticles, liposomes, dendrimers, phytosomes, nanoemulsions, and others.

A rigorous review of the literature on the advantages and safety of nutraceuticals is required in light of the regulatory frameworks that now govern them and the growing public interest in this market. Future research must pinpoint potential and limitations in the therapeutic capabilities of nutraceuticals, as well as important target markets, and suggest strategies for enhancing health using these products. Epidemiological and observational studies can provide information on how effectively these medications work and create a secure profile for future clinical evaluations. In this view, comparing the efficacy of two or more nutraceutical formulations can be accomplished through the use of meta-analysis of the accessible clinical trials and/or pilot research. When taken as a whole, these studies can serve as the basis for solid guidelines and clinical recommendations for marketing nutraceuticals.

REFERENCES

Abou-Arab, A.A.K., Soliman Kawther, M., El Tantawy, M.E., Ismail Badeaa, R., & Naguib Khayria, N. (1999). Quantity estimation of some contaminants in commonly used medicinal plants in the Egyptian market. *Food Chemistry*, *67* (4), 357–363.

Ahmed, M.T., Loutfy, N., & Yousef, Y. (2001). Contamination of medicinal herbs with organophosphorus insecticides. *Bulletin of Environmental Contamination and Toxicology*, *66* (4), 421–426.

Akhlaghi, M., Shabanian, G., Rafieian-Kopaei, M., Parvin, N., Saadat, M., & Akhlaghi, M. (2011). Citrus aurantium blossom and preoperative anxiety. *Revista Brasileira de Anestesiologia 2011*, *61*(6), 702–712.

Anderson, I.B., Mullen, W.H., Meeker, J.E., Khojasteh-Bakht, S.C., Oishi, S., Nelson, S.D., & Blanc, P.D. (1996). Pennyroyal toxicity: Measurement of toxic metabolite levels in two cases and review of the literature. *Annals of Internal Medicine*, *124*(8), 726–734.

Bahmani, M., Vakili-Saatloo, N., Maghsoudi, R., Momtaz, H., Saki, K., Kazemi-Ghoshchi, B., et al. (2013). A comparative study on the effect of ethanol extract of wild Scrophularia deserti and streptomycin on Brucellla melitensis. *Journal of HerbMed Pharmacol.Pharmacology 2013*, *2*, 17–20.

Bailey, J., Oliveri, A., & Levin, E.D. (2013). Zebrafish model systems for developmental neurobehavioral toxicology. Zebrafish model systems for developmental neurobehavioral toxicology. *Birth Defects Research. Part C, Embryo Today: Reviews: Reviews*, *99*(1), 14–23.

Baradaran, A., Madihi, Y., Merrikhi, A., Rafieian-Kopaei, M., & Nasri, H. (2013). Serum lipoprotein (a) in diabetic patients with various renal function not yet on dialysis. *PakPakistan JJournal of MedMedical Sci.Sciences 2013*, *29*(1(Suppl))(SupplSuppl.), 354–357.

Baradaran, A., Nasri, H., Nematbakhsh, M., & Rafieian-Kopaei, M. (2014). Antioxidant activity and preventive effect of aqueous leaf extract of Aloe Vera on gentamicin-induced nephrotoxicity in male Wistar rats. *Clinical Terapeutica 2014*, *165*(1), 7–11.

Bernardi, M.M., Dias, S.G., & Barbosa, V.E. (2013). Neurotoxicity of neem commercial formulation (azadirachta indica A. juss) in adult zebrafish (Danio Rerio). *Environmental Toxicology and Pharmacology*, *36*(3), 1276–1282.

Boggia, R., Zunin, P., & Turrini, F. (2020). Functional foods and food supplements. *Applied Sciences*, *10*(23), 8538. MDPI AG.

Bridges, C.C., & Zalups, R.K. (2017). The Aging kidney and the nephrotoxic effects of Mercury. *Journal of Toxicology and Environmental Health. Part B, Critical Reviews*, *20*(2), 55–80.

Bu, L., Shen, B., & Cheng, Z. (2014). Fluorescent imaging of cancerous tissues for targeted surgery. *Advanced drug delivery reviews*, *76*, 21–38.

Campana, C., Griffin, P.L., & Simon, E.L. (2014). Caffeine overdose resulting in severe rhabdomyolysis and acute renal failure. *The American Journal of Emergency Medicine*, 32(1), 111.e3–111.e4.

Campo, J.V., McNabb, J., Perel, J.M., Mazariegos, G.V., Hasegawa, S.L., & Reyes, J. (2002). Kava-induced fulminant hepatic failure. *Journal of the American Academy of Child and Adolescent Psychiatry*, *41*(6), 631–632.

Cencic, A., & Chingwaru, W. (2010). The role of functional foods, nutraceuticals, and food supplements in intestinal health. *Nutrients*, *2*(6), 611–625.

Chahardehi, A.M., Arsad, H., & Lim, V. (2020). Zebrafish as a successful animal model for screening toxicity of medicinal plants. *Plants (Basel, Switzerland)*, *9*(10), 1345.

Chauhan, B., Kumar, G., Kalam, N., & Ansari, S.H. (2013). Current concepts and prospects of herbal nutraceutical: A review. *Journal of Advanced Pharmaceutical Technology and Research*, *4*(1), 4–8.

Chi, K.R. (2008). The year of sequencing. *Nature Methods*, *5*(1), 11–14.

Clough, A.R., Bailie, R.S., & Currie, B. (2003). Liver function test abnormalities in users of aqueous kava extracts. *Journal of Toxicology. Clinical Toxicology*, *41*(6), 821–829.

Das, L., Bhaumik, E., Raychaudhuri, U., & Chakraborty, R. (2012). Role of nutraceuticals in human health. *Journal of Food Science and Technology*, *49*(2), 173–183.

Ekor M. (2014). The growing use of herbal medicines: Issues relating to adverse reactions and challenges in monitoring safety. *Frontiers in pharmacology*, *4*, 177.

Fredholm, B.B., Bättig, K., Holmén, J., Nehlig, A., & Zvartau, E.E. (1999). Actions of caffeine in the brain with special reference to factors that contribute to its widespread use. *Pharmacological Reviews*, *51*(1), 83–133.

Fu, P.P., Xia, Q., He, X., Barel, S., Edery, N., Beland, F.A., & Shimshoni, J.A. (2017). Detection of pyrrolizidine alkaloid DNA adducts in livers of cattle poisoned with heliotropium europaeum. *Chemical Research in Toxicology*, *30*(3), 851–858.

Gil, F., Hernández, A.F., & Martín-Domingo, M.C. (2016). Chapter 58 - Toxic contamination of nutraceuticals and food ingredients. In R.C. Gupta (Ed.) *Nutraceuticals* (pp. 825–837). Boston: Academic Press.

Guo, L., Mei, N., Dial, S., Fuscoe, J., & Chen, T. (2007). Comparison of Gene expression profiles altered by comfrey and Riddelliine in Rat Liver. *BMC Bioinformatics*, *8*(7): S22(Suppl. 7), S22.

Gupta, V.K., & Malhotra, S. (2012). Pharmacological Attribute of Aloe Vera: Revalidation through Experimental and Clinical Studies. *Ayu*, *33*(2), 193–196.

Gurley, B.J., Gardner, S.F., Hubbard, M.A., Williams, D.K., Gentry, W.B., Khan, I.A., & Shah, A. (2005). In vivo effects of goldenseal, kavakava, black cohosh, and valerian on human cytochrome P450, 1A2, 2D6, 2E1, and 3A4/5 phenotypes. *Clinical Pharmacology and Therapeutics*, *77*(5), 415–426.

Han, H. S., Hyung-SeopJang, Gun Hyuk G. H. JangJ., Indong Jun, Indong, Hyunseon Seo, Hyunseon, Jimin Park, J., Sion Glyn-Jones, S., Hyun-Kwang Seok, et al., … Edwards, J. R. (2018).

Hardy, G. (2000). Nutraceuticals and functional foods: Introduction and meaning. *Nutrition*. 2000.

Helal, N.A., Eassa, H.A., Amer, A.M., Eltokhy, M.A., Edafiogho, I., & Nounou, M.I. (2019). Nutraceuticals' novel formulations: The good, the bad, the unknown and patents involved. *Recent Patents on Drug Delivery and Formulation*, *13*(2), 105–156.

Humberston, C.L., Akhtar, J., & Krenzelok, E.P. (2003). Acute hepatitis induced by kava kava. *Journal of Toxicology. Clinical Toxicology*, *41*(2), 109–113.

Hussain, S., Mubeen, I., Ullah, N., Shah, S.S.U.D., Khan, B.A., Zahoor, M., Ullah, R., Khan, F.A., & Sultan, M.A. (2022). Modern diagnostic imaging technique applications and risk factors in the medical field: A review. *BioMed Research International*, *2022*, 5164970.

Joseph, B., & Jini, D. (2013). Antidiabetic effects of Momordica charantia (bitter melon) and its medicinal potency. *Asian Pacific Journal of Tropical Disease*, *3*(2), 93–102.

Kalra, E.K. (2003). Nutraceutical – Definition and introduction. *AAPS PharmSci*, *5*(3), E25.

Khosravi-Boroujeni, H., Mohammadifard, N., Sarrafzadegan, N., Sajjadi, F., Maghroun, M., Khosravi, A., … Azadbakht, L. (2012). Potato consumption and cardiovascular disease risk factors among Iranian population. *International Journal of Food Sciences and Nutrition*, *63*(8), 913–920.

Kiani, M.A., Khodadad, A., Mohammadi, S., Ghayour Mobarhan, M., Saeidi, M., Jafari, S.A. et al. (2013). Effect of peppermint on pediatrics' pain under endoscopic examination of the large bowel. *Journal of HerbMed Pharmacology*, *2*, 41–44.

Lamb, J., Crawford, E.D., Peck, D., Modell, J.W., Blat, I.C., Wrobel, M.J., … Golub, T.R. (2006). The connectivity map: Using gene-expression signatures to connect small molecules, genes, and disease. *Science*, *313*(5795), 1929–1935.

Li, Y., Mei, H., Wu, Q., Zhang, S., Fang, J.L., Shi, L., & Guo, L. (2011). Methysticin and 7,8-dihydromethysticin are two major kavalactones in kava extract to induce CYP1A1. *Toxicological Sciences*, *124*(2), 388–399.

Madihi, Y., Merrikhi, A., Baradaran, A., Rafieian-Kopaei, M., Shahinfard, N., Ansari, R. et al. (2013). Impact of sumac on postprandial high-fat oxidative stress. *Pakistan Journal of Medical Sciences*, *29*, 340–345.

Meena, A.K., Bansal, P., Kumar, S., Rao, M.M., & Garg, V.K. (2010). Estimation of heavy metals in commonly used medicinal plants: A market basket survey. *Environmental Monitoring and Assessment*, *170*(1–4), 657–660.

Mizgirev, I.V., & Revskoy, S. (2010). A new zebrafish model for experimental leukemia therapy. *Cancer Biology and Therapy*, *9*(11), 895–902.

Mirhoseini, M., Baradaran, A., & Rafieian-Kopaei, M. (2013). Medicinal plants, diabetes mellitus and urgent needs. *Journal of HerbMed Pharmacology*, *2*, 53–54.

Nasri, H., Baradaran, A., Shirzad, H., & Rafieian-Kopaei, M. (2014). New concepts in nutraceuticals as alternative for pharmaceuticals. *International Journal of Preventive Medicine*, *5*(12), 1487–1499.

Panter, K.E., Welch, K.D., Gardner, D.R., Lee, S.T., Green, B., Pfister, J., … Stegelmeier, B. (2012). Poisonous plants of the United States. In *Veterinary toxicology* (pp. 1031–1079).

Parsaei, P., Karimi, M., Asadi, S.Y., & Rafieian-Kopaei, M. (2013). Bioactive components and preventive effect of green tea (Camellia sinensis) extract on post-laparotomy intra-abdominal adhesion in rats. *International Journal of Surgery*, *11*(9), 811–815.

Pham, D.-H., De Roo, B., Nguyen, X.-B., & Mattias V., Kecskés, A., Annelii Ny, Copmans, D. et al.(2016). Use of zebrafish larvae as a multi-endpoint platform to characterize the toxicity profile of silica nanoparticles. *Scientific Reports*, *6*(November), 37145.

Prado, G., Altoé, A.F., Gomes, T.C.B., Leal, A.S., Morais, V.A.D., Oliveira, M.S., … Cruz Madeira, J.E. (2012). Occurrence of aflatoxin b1 in natural products. *Brazilian Journal of Microbiology. Publication of the Brazilian Society for Microbiology*, *43*(4), 1428–1436.

Preliasco, M., Gardner, D., Moraes, J., González, A.C., Uriarte, G., & Rivero, R. (2017). Senecio grisebachii baker: Pyrrolizidine alkaloids and experimental poisoning in calves. *Toxicon: Official Journal of the International Society on Toxinology*, *133*(July), 68–73.

Puri, V., Nagpal, M., Singh, I., Singh, M., Dhingra, G.A., Huanbutta, K., … Sangnim, T. (2022). A comprehensive review on nutraceuticals: Therapy support and formulation challenges. *Nutrients*, *14*(21).

Qiao, Y., Zhao, Y., Wu, Q., Sun, L., Ruan, Q., Chen, Y., …Wang, D. (2014). Full toxicity assessment of Genkwa Flos and the underlying mechanism in nematode *Caenorhabditis elegans*. *PLOS ONE*, *9*(3), e91825.

Rafieian-Kopaei, M., Baradaran, A., Merrikhi, A., Nematbakhsh, M., Madihi, Y., & Nasri, H. (2013). Efficacy of co-administration of garlic extract and metformin for prevention of gentamicin-renal toxicity in Wistar rats: A Biochemical Study. *International Journal of Preventive Medicine*, *4*(3), 258–264.

Raman, P., Patino, L.C., & Nair, M.G. (2004). Evaluation of metal and microbial contamination in botanical supplements. *Journal of Agricultural and Food Chemistry*, *52*(26), 7822–7827.

Sarkhail, P., Yunesian, M., Ahmadkhaniha, R., Sarkheil, P., & Rastkari, N. (2012). Levels of organophosphorus pesticides in medicinal plants commonly consumed in Iran. *Daru*, *20*(1), 9.

Setorki, M., Rafieian-Kopaei, M., Merikhi, A., Heidarian, E., Shahinfard, N., Ansari, R., … Baradaran, A. (2013). Suppressive impact of Anethum graveolens consumption on biochemical risk factors of atherosclerosis in hypercholesterolemic rabbits. *International Journal of Preventive Medicine*, *4*(8), 889–895.

Shahidi, F. (2012) Nutraceuticals, functional foods and dietary supplements in health and disease. *Journal of Food and Drug Analysis*, 20(1), Article 78.

Shirzad, H., Kiani, M., & Shirzad, M. (2013). Impacts of tomato extract on the mice fibrosarcoma cells. *Journal of HerbMed Pharmacology*, *2*, 13–16.

Stallons, L.J., Whitaker, R.M., & Schnellmann, R.G. (2014). Suppressed mitochondrial biogenesis in folic acid-induced acute kidney injury and early fibrosis. *Toxicology Letters*, *224*(3), 326–332.

Sullivan, J.B. Jr., Rumack, B.H., Thomas Jr. H., Jr. Peterson, R.G., & Bryson, P. (1979). Pennyroyal oil poisoning and hepatotoxicity. *JAMA*, *242*(26), 2873–2874.

Tong, M., Gao, W., Jiao, W., Zhou, J., Li, Y., He, L., & Hou, R. (2017). Uptake, translocation, metabolism, and distribution of glyphosate in nontarget tea plant (Camellia sinensis L.). *Journal of Agricultural and Food Chemistry*, *65*(35), 7638–7646.

"Toxicology and Carcinogenesis Studies of Ginkgo Biloba Extract (CAS No. 90045-36-6) in F344/N Rats and B6C3F1/N Mice (Gavage Studies)." 2013. United States.

"Toxicology and Carcinogenesis Studies of Goldenseal Root Powder (Hydrastis Canadensis) in F344/N Rats and B6C3F1 Mice (Feed Studies)." 2010. United States.

Wang, K., Sun, J., Zhou, S., Wan, C., Qin, S., Li, C., ...Yang, L. (2013). Prediction of drug-target interactions for drug repositioning only based on genomic expression similarity. *PLOS Computational Biology*, *9*(11), e1003315.

Wiegant, F.A.C., Surinova, S., Ytsma, E., Langelaar-Makkinje, M., Wikman, G., & Post, J.A. (2009). Plant adaptogens increase lifespan and stress resistance in *C. elegans*. *Biogerontology*, *10*(1), 27–42.

Winship, K.A. (1991). Toxicity of comfrey. *Adverse Drug Reactions and Toxicological Reviews*, *10*(1), 47–59.

Whitlock, J.P. (1999). Induction of cytochrome P4501A1. *Annual Review of Pharmacology and Toxicology*, *39*(1), 103–125.

Wong, T.C., Lee, F. S.-C., Hu, G.L., Chang, L., Wang, X., & Fu, P.P. (2007). A survey of heavy metal and organochlorine pesticide contaminations in commercial Lingzhi products. *Journal of Food and Drug Analysis*, 15(4).

Zhao, J. (2007). Bentham Science Publisher.

11 State of the Art on Polyphenols as Nutraceuticals

Focus on Cancer Preventive and Immuno-Fortifying Properties

Parul Johri, Rajesh K. Tiwari, and Mala Trivedi

11.1 INTRODUCTION

Polyphenols are a group of compounds found naturally in plants that contain multiple phenol groups, or molecules with a hydroxyl group (-OH) attached to an aromatic ring. They are known for their antioxidant and anti-inflammatory properties, and are believed to play a role in preventing chronic diseases, such as cancer and cardiovascular disease. Polyphenols are of particular interest due to their ability to scavenge free radicals and modulate inflammatory processes. They have been shown to reduce the risk of cardiovascular disease, cancer, and diabetes, as well as improve cognitive function (Pandey and Rizvi 2009). Polyphenols are a group of compounds found in plants that are characterised by their phenolic structures. These compounds are classified into two major groups, flavonoids and non-flavonoids. Flavonoids are the most abundant polyphenols and are found in a wide variety of fruits, vegetables, and other plant foods. They are divided into six subclasses: flavonols, flavones, isoflavones, flavanones, anthocyanins, and proanthocyanidins. Non-flavonoids are less common and include phenolic acids, lignans, stilbenes, and tannins.

11.2 POLYPHENOLS AS A FORTIFYING AGENT

Polyphenols are a group of plant-derived compounds that have been identified as having beneficial health effects. They are found in a variety of fruits, vegetables, and beverages, including tea, wine, and cocoa. Polyphenols are known for their antioxidant activity, which helps in protecting cells from damage caused by free

DOI: 10.1201/9781003392934-11

radicals. They also have anti-inflammatory and anti-carcinogenic properties. In recent years, polyphenols have been studied for their potential use as nutraceuticals. Nutraceuticals are dietary supplements designed to provide health benefits beyond basic nutrition (Scarano et al. 2020). They are divided into two major classes: flavonoids and non-flavonoids. Flavonoids are the most abundant type of polyphenols example-catechins, anthocyanins, and flavonols found in fruits, vegetables, tea, and wine (Manach et al. 2004). Non-flavonoids are less abundant and include phenolic acids, stilbenes, lignans, and tannins.

Polyphenols are naturally occurring compounds found in a variety of natural products we consume as our routine diet (Manach et al. 2004). Polyphenols have been shown to reduce inflammation, which can have a positive effect on overall health. Additionally, they are believed to have anti-oncogenic properties, as they have been shown to inhibit the growth of cancerous cells in laboratory studies (Rothwell et al. 2017). Polyphenols have been used for centuries in traditional medicine to treat a variety of ailments. However, in recent years, they have been studied more extensively and have been found to have several potential benefits. For example, polyphenols are believed to help reduce cholesterol levels, as well as improve blood sugar control, reduce the risk of heart disease, and reduce the risk of certain types of cancer (Asensi et al. 2011). Additionally, polyphenols may improve cognitive function and help to protect against age-related cognitive decline. Besides beneficial effects, they also have some hazards, too, for example, polyphenols may cause gastrointestinal upset, or even allergic reactions in some individuals, as they form some toxic complexes with chemical compounds taken as medicines, therefore, it is always advisable to take them as supplements with the advice of physician only (Han et al. 2007).

11.3 ROLE OF POLYPHENOLS IN CANCER PREVENTION

Polyphenols are compounds packed with potent antioxidant and anti-inflammatory qualities. Recent research has suggested that polyphenols may play a role in the prevention and treatment of cancer. Cancer is a complex disease that is caused by a variety of factors, including genetics, lifestyle, and environmental factors. Cancer cells are characterised by uncontrolled growth and the ability to spread throughout the body. The goal of cancer treatment is to stop the growth and spread of cancer cells. Polyphenols have been studied for their potential anti-cancer properties. Abotaleb et al. 2020 in their studies have found that polyphenols have the ability to inhibit the growth of cancer cells, as well as induce apoptosis (cell death). They can also modulate the activity of certain proteins that are involved in cell growth and the spread of cancer. They can also reduce inflammation, which has been linked to an increased risk of cancer. In addition to their potential anti-cancer properties, polyphenols may also help to reduce the side effects of cancer treatments. Studies have found that polyphenols can reduce the side effects of chemotherapy, such as nausea, vomiting, and hair loss. In conclusion, polyphenols are compounds found in plants that are packed with potent antioxidant and anti-inflammatory qualities. They may play a role in the prevention and treatment of cancer by inhibiting the growth of cancer cells and modulating the activity of certain proteins involved in the spread of cancer (Abbas et al. 2017; Spatafora and Tringali 2012).

11.4 ROLE OF POLYPHENOLS IN LIVER CANCER

Davinelli et al. 2020 in their recently concluded studies suggested that polyphenols play an important role in preventing and treating liver cancer.

Liver cancer is the fifth most common type of cancer and the third leading cause of cancer death worldwide. The liver is an important organ in the body and performs a variety of essential functions, including the breakdown of toxins and other harmful substances. When the liver is damaged or impaired, toxic levels of certain substances can accumulate and lead to the formation of tumours. Polyphenols are believed to protect the liver from damage caused by toxins and other carcinogens. Polyphenol-rich diets were found to reduce the risk of liver cancer by up to 40%. They reduce oxidative damage to the liver, which can lead to the formation of cancer cells. Additionally, polyphenols have been shown to inhibit the growth of cancer cells and reduce the risk of metastasis.

Polyphenols may also help to reduce inflammation, which is a major risk factor for liver cancer. Chronic inflammation can damage the liver and lead to the formation of tumours. Polyphenols are believed to reduce inflammation by modulating the activity of certain genes involved in the inflammatory process. They treat liver cancer by reducing the blood supply to tumours, thus slowing their growth. It is important to note that polyphenols are not a substitute for medical treatment and should not be used in place of conventional therapies. They are believed to reduce oxidative damage to the liver and inhibit the growth of cancer cells. Additionally, these compounds may reduce inflammation and have anti-angiogenic properties.

11.5 POLYPHENOL IN ORAL CANCER PREVENTION

Studies have found that polyphenols may reduce the risk of oral cancer by directly attacking cancer cells, reducing the activity of carcinogens, and influencing the expression of genes related to cancer. One of the ways that polyphenols may reduce the risk of oral cancer is by directly attacking cancer cells (Ding et al. 2013).

Fukai et al. 2000 reported that polyphenols have properties of inducing cell cycle arrest, inducing apoptosis (programmed cell death), and inhibiting angiogenesis (the formation of new blood vessels). By attacking cancer cells, polyphenols may be able to stop the growth and spread of cancer. Polyphenols have been found to induce the expression of tumour suppressor genes, which can inhibit the growth of cancer cells. Polyphenols are also used as adjuncts to conventional cancer treatments, such as chemotherapy and radiation therapy. In addition, polyphenols have been found to induce apoptosis (programmed cell death), which can further reduce the size of tumours and make them more susceptible to treatment (Fukai et al. 2000). They also reduce side effects of cancer therapy such as fatigue, nausea, and hair loss. Polyphenols are known to have various anti-cancer properties, which may reduce the risk of developing cancer and enhance the effectiveness of cancer treatments. (Fukai et al. 2000).

TABLE 11.1
Types of Polyphenols and their Source and Cancer Targets

S. No.	Polyphenols	Fruit / Plant Source	Cancer Type
1	Resveratrol	Blueberries, berries, red grapes	Prostrate, Breast, colon
2	Curcumin	Turmeric	Breast
3	Licopen	Strawberries, cherries, tomatoes, papaya, watermelon	Prostrate, Breast,
4	Epigallocatenin	Hazelnuts, peaches, blackberries, tea, apple, etc.	Prostrate, Breast, colon
5	Oleuropein	Olives, olive oil	Breast

11.6 POLYPHENOL IN BREAST CANCER

Breast cancer is the most commonly diagnosed cancer among women worldwide. While it is not yet clear what causes breast cancer, lifestyle factors such as diet and physical activity are known to play a role in the risk of developing the disease (Abdal et al. 2016). Many studies have suggested that a diet rich in polyphenols may reduce the risk of breast cancer. One way in which polyphenols may reduce the risk of breast cancer is by inhibiting the growth and spread of cancer cells. Polyphenols have been shown to inhibit the activity of certain enzymes, such as aromatase, which are involved in the production of oestrogen. Oestrogen is a hormone that can stimulate the growth of certain types of breast cancer cells. By inhibiting the activity of aromatase, polyphenols may reduce the risk of breast cancer (Zabaleta et al. 2020). Several studies have suggested that a diet rich in polyphenols may reduce the risk of breast cancer by modulating the immune system. Polyphenols may also reduce the risk of breast cancer by eliminating free radicals. Free radicals are unstable molecules that can damage cells and DNA and are believed to play a role in the development of certain cancers. These chemicals have a strong antioxidant activity, which may help to eliminate free radicals and reduce the risk of cancer (Alsamri et al. 2019). Polyphenols also reduce the risk of metastasis, which is the spread of cancer to other parts of the body. In conclusion, polyphenols may play a role in the prevention and treatment of breast cancer. They may inhibit the growth and spread of cancer cells, modulate the immune system, eliminate free radicals, and reduce the side effects of chemotherapy (Zan et al. 2019). For these reasons, a diet rich in polyphenols may reduce the risk of developing breast cancer and may also improve the chances of successful treatment. (Table 11.1)

11.7 POLYPHENOLS IN LUNG CANCER TREATMENT

Lung cancer is one of the leading causes of death worldwide, it is rated as the second largest killer disease in both the sex. Recent research has highlighted the potential role of polyphenols in the treatment of lung cancer, a leading cause of cancer death worldwide (Zhou et al. 2019). The antioxidant properties of polyphenols may be beneficial in treating lung cancer. These compounds are able to scavenge free radicals, which are reactive molecules that can cause damage to DNA, proteins, and lipids. Some polyphenols have been found to inhibit the growth of cancer cells in laboratory studies. For example, resveratrol, a polyphenol found in red wine, has been shown to inhibit the growth of breast and colon cancer cells, as well as lung cancer cells (Horgan et al. 2019). The anti-inflammatory properties of polyphenols may also be beneficial in lung cancer treatment. Chronic inflammation is linked to an increased risk of cancer, and polyphenols may be able to reduce this risk by reducing inflammation (Amararathna et al. 2020). Studies have shown that polyphenols can reduce inflammation by inhibiting the production of pro-inflammatory molecules, such as cytokines and chemokines. Another important property of polyphenols is anti-angiogenic properties, where they inhibit the formation of new blood vessels that can supply tumours with oxygen and nutrients. Wan et. al. 2019 in their studies have shown that polyphenols can reduce the risk of developing lung cancer by altering gene expression and reducing the activity of certain molecules involved in cancer development. Additionally, polyphenols may reduce the risk of lung cancer by reducing inflammation and oxidative stress. Zan et al. 2019 reported anti-inflammatory, anti-angiogenic properties, as well as their ability to modulate the activity of certain genes involved in cancer development.

11.8 POLYPHENOLS AS THERAPEUTIC AGENTS IN CERVICAL CANCER

Cervical cancer is one of the leading causes of death among women worldwide. It is responsible for over 250,000 deaths annually. Treatment options for cervical cancer include surgery, chemotherapy, and radiation therapy, but these treatments have significant side effects. Therefore, there is an urgent need for alternative treatments that are effective and have fewer side effects. One such promising therapy is the use of polyphenols as therapeutic agents for cervical cancer. Polyphenols have antioxidant, anti-inflammatory, and anti-carcinogenic properties, making them attractive candidates for treating cervical cancer (Moga et al. 2016).

Several studies have shown that polyphenols can reduce the risk of cervical cancer. For example, a study conducted by He et al. 2012 found that regular consumption of polyphenol-rich foods reduced the risk of cervical cancer by 33%. Other studies have shown that polyphenols can inhibit the growth and spread of cervical cancer cells. Polyphenols can be used alone or in combination with other therapies to treat cervical cancer. They can be administered orally, intravenously, or topically. Several studies have demonstrated the efficacy of polyphenols in combination with chemotherapy or radiation therapy. For example, a study conducted in China found that a combination of polyphenols and chemotherapy increased the response rate of cervical cancer cells to chemotherapy by 30%. Polyphenols have also been shown to reduce the side effects of chemotherapy and radiation therapy. Singh et al. 2013 found that polyphenols reduced the risk of gastrointestinal side effects by 50%. They also reduced the risk of leukopenia and thrombocytopenia, two common side effects of chemotherapy. In addition to their use as therapeutic agents, polyphenols can also be used to prevent cervical cancer. Several studies have demonstrated that polyphenols can reduce the risk of developing cervical cancer. For example, a study conducted in China found that polyphenol-rich foods reduced the risk of cervical cancer by 50% (He et al. 2012). Polyphenols have the potential to be an effective and safe therapy for cervical cancer. They have been shown to reduce the risk of developing cervical cancer and increase the response rate of cervical cancer cells to chemotherapy and radiation therapy.

11.9 POLYPHENOLS AS THERAPEUTIC AGENTS IN HEAD AND NECK CARCINOMA

They also have anti-inflammatory properties, which can reduce inflammation associated with cancer and help reduce tumour growth (Kim et al. 2010). Polyphenols can modulate the activity of enzymes and proteins involved in the growth and development of cancer cells. Recent research has shown that polyphenols may be beneficial in the treatment of head and neck carcinoma. Studies have demonstrated that polyphenols can inhibit the growth of head and neck carcinoma cells in vitro. Polyphenols can reduce the expression of certain proteins involved in the growth and proliferation of head and neck carcinoma cells. In addition to their potential therapeutic effects, polyphenols may also be beneficial in the prevention of head and neck carcinoma (Nimbalkar 2020). Studies have suggested that polyphenols can reduce the risk of head and neck carcinoma by decreasing the production of reactive oxygen species and preventing the damage to DNA that is associated with carcinogenesis.

11.10 IMMUNO-FORTIFYING PROPERTIES OF POLYPHENOLS

Immuno-fortifying properties, also known as immunomodulatory properties, are the ability of certain substances to enhance the body's natural immune system. They can also be found in certain pharmaceutical products. Immuno-fortifying properties can help protect the body from a variety of illnesses and diseases, including cancer, heart disease, and other chronic illnesses. Immuno-fortifying properties are different from traditional treatments for illnesses and diseases (Shakoor 2021). Instead of treating the disease, immuno-fortifying properties help to strengthen the body's natural defenses against disease. This can be a more effective approach, as it can help prevent the onset of a more serious illness or disease. The most common form of immuno-fortifying properties are antioxidants. Free radicals are molecules that can damage the body's cells, leading to disease and aging. Polyphenols are plant-based compounds that can help protect the body against oxidative stress. Oxidative stress is caused by an imbalance in the body's antioxidant system. Polyphenols can help balance the body's antioxidant system, thus helping to protect the body against oxidative stress. Probiotics are live bacteria that can help strengthen the body's natural defenses against disease. They can help improve digestion and absorption of nutrients, as well as boost the body's immune system. Probiotics can also help protect the body from infections and other illnesses. Finally, certain vitamins and minerals can also help to strengthen the body's natural defenses against disease. Vitamins A, C, and E, for example, are essential for a healthy immune system. Minerals such as zinc and selenium can also help to boost the body's immune system. Immuno-fortifying properties can be beneficial for those looking to boost their immune system.

Introduction Polyphenols are a group of compounds found in plants that are known to possess a variety of biological activities, including antioxidant, anti-inflammatory, and immunomodulatory properties (Cassidy et al. 2011; Chiva-Blanch et al. 2013; Hanhineva et al. 2010). These compounds have been studied extensively in recent years and are believed to have the potential to play an important role in the prevention and treatment of a number of diseases, including cancer, cardiovascular disease, and inflammatory and autoimmune diseases (Hooper et al. 2012; Ahtesh et al. 2020). Polyphenols are believed to possess the potential to modulate the activity of the immune system, which could be beneficial in the prevention and treatment of a number of immune-mediated diseases. The most studied immuno-fortifying property of polyphenols is their ability to modulate the activity of T and B cells (Medzhitov and Janeway 2000). In particular, polyphenols have been found to enhance the proliferation and differentiation of T cells, as well as to increase their production of cytokines, such as interleukin This could potentially lead to an improved response to infection and/or vaccination. In addition, polyphenols have been found to increase the production of antibodies and modulate the activity of B cells, which could potentially lead to a better response to pathogens and allergens (Wong et al. 2011). Polyphenols have also been found to modulate the activity of macrophages and natural killer cells. Macrophages are important immune cells that play a key role in the recognition and destruction of pathogens. Polyphenols have been found to enhance the production of pro-inflammatory cytokines by macrophages, which could potentially lead to an improved response to infection. They are also responsible for enhancing the activity of natural killer cells, which are important for the destruction of tumour cells. Their anti-inflammatory properties, help in reducing the risk of inflammatory and autoimmune diseases. Polyphenols have been found to inhibit the production of pro-inflammatory cytokines, such as tumour necrosis factor-alpha and interleukin 1beta. The immuno-fortifying properties of polyphenols make them promising candidates for therapeutic interventions in various immune-mediated diseases. In particular, polyphenols could potentially be used to enhance the efficacy of vaccines and to improve the response to infection. In addition, polyphenols could potentially be used to reduce the risk of inflammatory and autoimmune diseases, as well as to reduce the risk of tumour formation. Finally, polyphenols could potentially be used to improve the efficacy of treatments for cancer, cardiovascular disease, and other chronic diseases.

REFERENCES

Abbas, M., Saeed, F., Anjum, F.M., et al. (2017). Natural polyphenols: An overview. *Int J Food Prop*, 20, 1689–1699.

Abdal Dayem, A., Choi, H.Y., Yang, G.M., Kim, K., Saha, S.K., & Cho, S.G. (2016 Sep 21). The anti-cancer effect of polyphenols against breast cancer and cancer stem cells: Molecular mechanisms. *Nutrients*, 8(9), 581. doi: 10.3390/nu8090581. PMID: 27657126; PMCID: PMC5037565.

Abotaleb, M., Liskova, A., Kubatka, P., & Büsselberg, D. (2020). Therapeutic potential of plant phenolic acids in the treatment of cancer. *Biomolecules*, 10(2), 221.

Ahtesh, F.B., Stojanovska, L., Feehan, J., de Courten, M.P., Flavel, M., Kitchen, B., & Apostolopoulos, V. (2020). Polyphenol rich sugar cane extract inhibits bacterial growth. *Prilozi.*, 41, 49–57.

Alsamri, H., El Hasasna, H., Al Dhaheri, Y., Eid, A.H., Attoub, S., & Iratni, R. (2019). Carnosol, a natural polyphenol, inhibits migration, metastasis, and tumor growth of breast cancer via a ROS-dependent proteasome degradation of STAT3. *Front Oncol.*, 9(743).

Amararathna, M., Hoskin, D.W., & Rupasinghe, H.P.V. (2020). Anthocyanin-rich haskap (*Lonicera Caerulea* L.) berry extracts reduce nitrosamine-induced DNA damage in human normal lung epithelial cells in vitro. *Food Chem Toxicol.*, 141(111404).

Asensi, M., Ortega, A., Mena, S., et al. (2011). Natural polyphenols in cancer therapy. *Crit Rev Clin Lab Sci*, 48, 197–216.

Cassidy, A., O'Reilly, É.J., Kay, C., Sampson, L., Franz, M., Forman, J.P., Curhan, G., & Rimm, E.B. (2011). Habitual intake of flavonoid subclasses and incident hypertension in adults. *Am. J. Clin. Nutr.*, 93, 338–347.

Chiva-Blanch, G., Urpi-Sarda, M., Ros, E., Valderas-Martinez, P., Casas, R., Arranz, S., Guillén, M., Lamuela-Raventós, R.M., Llorach, R., & Andres-Lacueva, C. (2013). Effects of red wine polyphenols and alcohol on glucose metabolism and the lipid profile: A randomized clinical trial. *Clin. Nutr.*, 32, 200–206.

Davinelli, S., De Stefani, D., De Vivo, I., & Scapagnini, G. (2020). Polyphenols as caloric restriction Mimetics regulating mitochondrial biogenesis and mitophagy. *Trends Endocrinol Metab.*, 31(7), 536–550.

Ding, Y., Yao, H., Yao, Y., Fai, L.Y., & Zhang, Z.(2013 Jun 14). Protection of dietary polyphenols against oral cancer. *Nutrients.*, 5(6), 2173–2191. doi: 10.3390/nu5062173. PMID: 23771133; PMCID: PMC3725499.

Fukai, T., Sakagami, H., Toguchi, M., Takayama, F., Iwakura, I., Atsumi, T., Ueha, T., Nakashima, H., Nomura, T. (2000). Cytotoxic activity of low molecular weight polyphenols against human oral tumor cell lines. *Anticancer Res.*, 20, 2525–2536.

Han, X., Shen, T., & Lou, H. (2007). Dietary polyphenols and their biological significance. *Int. J. Mol. Sci.*, 8, 950–988. doi: 10.3390/i8090950.

Hanhineva, K., Törrönen, R., Bondia-Pons, I., Pekkinen, J., Kolehmainen, M., Mykkänen, H., & Poutanen, K. (2010) Impact of dietary polyphenols on carbohydrate metabolism. *Int. J. Mol. Sci.*, 11, 1365–1402.

He, F., Wang, Q., Zheng, X.L., Yan, J.Q., Yang, L., Sun, H., Hu, N., Lin, Y., & Wang X. (2012). Wogonin potentiates cisplatin-induced cancer cell apoptosis through accumulation of intracellular reactive oxygen species. *Oncol. Rep.*, 28, 601–605.

Hooper, L., Kay, C., Abdelhamid, A., Kroon, P.A., Cohn, J.S., Rimm, E.B., & Cassidy, A. (2012). Effects of chocolate, cocoa, and flavan-3-ols on cardiovascular health: A systematic review and meta-analysis of randomized trials. *Am. J. Clin. Nutr.*, 95, 740–751.

Horgan, X.J., Tatum, H., Brannan, E., Paull, D.H., & Rhodes, L.V. (2019). Resveratrol analogues surprisingly: Effective against triple-negative breast cancer, independent of ERα. *Oncol Rep.*, 41, 3517–3526.

Kim, J.W., Amin, A.R., & Shin, D.M. (2010 Aug). Chemoprevention of head and neck cancer with green tea polyphenols. *Cancer Prev Res (Phila).*, 3(8), 900–909. doi: 10.1158/1940-6207.CAPR-09-0131. Epub 2010 Jul 27. PMID: 20663981; PMCID: PMC2917478.

Manach, C., Scalbert, A., Morand, C., Rémésy, C., & Jiménez, L. (2004). Polyphenols: Food sources and bioavailability. *Am. J. Clin. Nutr.*, 79, 727–747. doi: 10.1093/ajcn/79.5.727.

Medzhitov, R., & Janeway, C. (2000). Innate immunity. *N. Engl. J. Med.*, 343, 338–344.

Moga, M.A., Dimienescu, O.G., Arvatescu, C.A., Mironescu, A., Dracea, L., & Ples, L. (2016 Aug 17). The role of natural polyphenols in the prevention and treatment of cervical cancer - An overview. *Molecules.*, 21(8), 1055. doi: 10.3390/molecules21081055. PMID: 27548122; PMCID: PMC6274328.

Nimbalkar, V.K., Manna, S., Maru, G.B., & Mahimkar, M.B. (2020). Head and neck cancer prevention by phytochemicals: Current status and challenges. *Curr. Pharmacol. Rep.*, 6, 85–102. 10.1007/s40495-020-00213-w

Pandey, K.B., & Rizvi, S.I. (2009). Plant polyphenols as dietary antioxidants in human health and disease. *Oxid. Med. Cell Longev.*, 2, 270–278. doi: 10.4161/oxim.2.5.9498

Rothwell, J.A., Knaze, V., & Zamora-Ros, R. (2017). Polyphenols: dietary assessment and role in the prevention of cancers. *Curr Opin Clin Nutr Metab Care*, 20, 512–521.

Scarano, A., Chieppa, M., & Santino, A. (2020 Dec 3). Plant polyphenols-biofortified foods as a novel tool for the prevention of human gut diseases. *Antioxidants (Basel).*, 9(12), 1225. doi: 10.3390/antiox9121225. PMID: 33287404; PMCID: PMC7761854.

Shakoor, H., Feehan, J., Apostolopoulos, V., Platat, C., Al Dhaheri, A.S., Ali, H.I., Ismail, L.C., Bosevski, M., & Stojanovska, L. (2021 Feb 25). Immunomodulatory effects of dietary polyphenols. *Nutrients.*, 13(3), 728. doi: 10.3390/nu13030728. PMID: 33668814; PMCID: PMC7996139.

Singh, M., Bhui, K., Singh, R., & Shukla, Y. (2013). Tea polyphenols enhance cisplatin chemosensitivity in cervical cancer cells via induction of apoptosis. *Life Sci.*, 93, 7–16. doi: 10.1016/j.lfs.2013.02.001

Spatafora, C., & Tringali, C. (2012). Natural-derived polyphenols as potential anticancer agents. *Anticancer Agents Med Chem*, 12, 902–918.

Wan Mohd Tajuddin, W.N.B., Lajis, N.H., Abas, F., Othman, I., & Naidu, R. (2019). Mechanistic understanding of curcumin's therapeutic effects in lung cancer. *Nutrients.*, 11(2989).

Wong, C.P., Nguyen, L.P., Noh, S.K., Bray, T.M., Bruno, R.S., & Ho, E. (2011). Induction of regulatory T cells by green tea polyphenol EGCG. *Immunol. Lett.*, 139, 7–13.

Zabaleta, M.E., Forbes-Hernández, T.Y., Simal-Gandara, J., Quiles, J.L., Cianciosi, D., Bullon, B., Giampieri, F., & Battino, M. (2020). Effect of polyphenols on HER2-positive breast cancer and related miRNAs: Epigenomic regulation. *Food Research International*, 137, 109623, ISSN 0963-9969, 10.1016/j.foodres.2020.109623.

Zan, L., Chen, Q., Zhang, L., & Li, X. (2019). Epigallocatechin gallate (EGCG) suppresses growth and tumorigenicity in breast cancer cells by down regulation of miR-25. *Bioengineered.*, 10, 374–382.

Zhou, Q., Pan, H., & Li, J. (2019). Molecular insights into potential contributions of natural polyphenols to lung cancer treatment. *Cancers (Basel).*, 11(1565).

12 Nanotechnology and Its Role in Nutraceuticals Towards Human Health

S. Lakshmana Prabu, A. Umamaheswari, S. Barath Raj, and M. Dhivya Sree

12.1 INTRODUCTION

Nutraceuticals are functional food supplements made with the goal of enhancing human health, well-being, and performance. The term "nutraceuticals" refers to a wide range of natural substances, such as polyunsaturated fatty acids, herbal products, prebiotics, probiotics, antioxidants, and prebiotics, which are considered to achieve the therapeutic objectives from nature (Das et al. 2012). Recent lifestyle changes among human beings increased the prevalence of various diseases like obesity, type-2 diabetes, cardiovascular diseases, etc. They simultaneously grow more health and nutrition-conscious as customers. Also, they are better equipped to choose foods from a variety of sources that either naturally include functional components that promote health or have food supplements added through fortification. As a result, there is a growing demand for a balanced diet and nutraceuticals formulated to deliver health benefits. These factors stimulated researchers to research the possible health benefits of nutraceuticals and their mechanisms of action; lately, they have been encouraged to generate novel products that would catch the attention of customers (Daliu et al. 2019).

Researchers working on dietary supplement delivery systems for nutraceuticals frequently encounter problems with inadequate water solubility and bioavailability. Poor bioavailability, or the portion of the dose that is ultimately not available at the site of action (in this case, the amount that can enter the bloodstream), is caused by functional ingredients' poor dissolution in water, which is the primary route for their administration, transport, and reaching their target sites.

Nanotechnology is an interdisciplinary area where more research is focused in the biomedical field with a highly ordered particle of nano-size and shape. Products made by this nanotechnology can be utilised to improve the absorption, bioavailability, and regulated release of nutrients and health supplements to get new therapeutic agents in treating different diseases. Nanoscience is expanding its scope and impact in various fields, including biology, food, nutrition, dietetics, and nutraceuticals. Nanotechnology can transform the nutraceutical sector by enabling the manipulation and self-assembly of materials with unique properties

 DOI: 10.1201/9781003392934-12

on nanoscales. This technology has the potential to revolutionise scientific, technological, and economic advancements, affecting macroscale aspects of food, such as texture, taste, processability, and shelf-life stability (Chen et al. 2006; Sanguansri and Augustin 2006).

12.2 NANOTECHNOLOGY IN FOOD INDUSTRY

Food that has been grown, created, processed, or packed using nanotechnology tools or processes is referred to as "nanofood." Nanofoods are distinguished from regular food when nanoparticles or nanotechnology techniques and tools are utilised during the cultivation, production, processing, or packaging of the product. Neither of these ambitious options appears viable in the foreseeable future, so we are not referring to food atomically altered or created by nanomachines. Due to its broad definition, this is a field of nanoscience and has been extensively studied for applications in fields such as agriculture, food processing, food packaging, and nutraceutical manufacturing. Scientists have found that using nanoscale structures in food can change its colour, odour, nutritional function, and other properties. The development of these products promises increased efficiency, enhanced flavour, customizability, and many other benefits. As a result of the fact that many food structures are naturally found at the nanoscale, nanofood has really been a part of food preparation for ages. The role of Nanomaterials in nutraceuticals is shown in Figure 12.1.

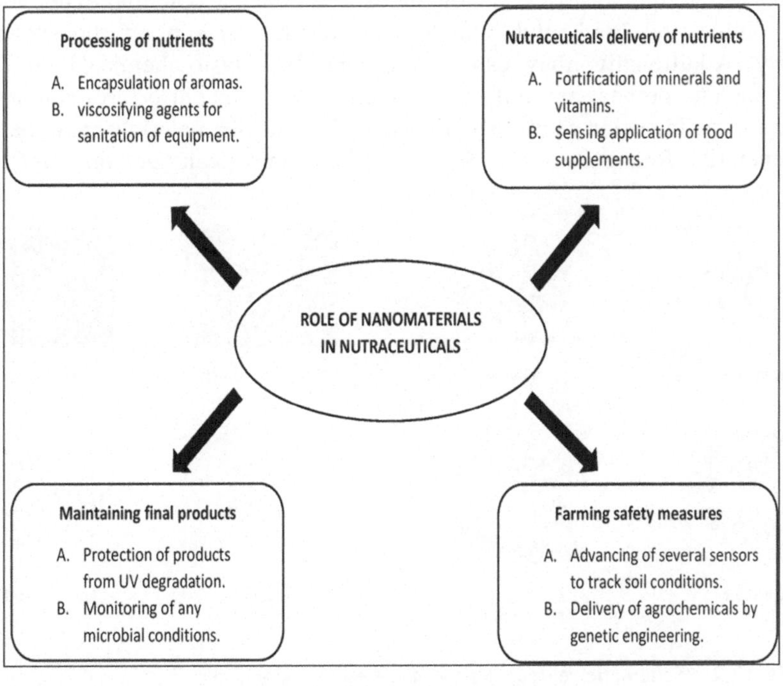

FIGURE 12.1 The role of nanomaterials in nutraceutical products.

12.3 NANOENCAPSULATION TECHNIQUES

Numerous attempts have been made to use nanotechnology for the encapsulation of functional food supplements as a result of the growing body of experimental evidence supporting the effectiveness of nutraceuticals in preventing and/or treating a variety of pathological diseases. Encapsulation technology is a highly promising strategy in the delivery of nutritional supplements due to several advantages.

The ability to protect the chemical composition of nutraceuticals from environmental factors like pH, light, temperature, radicals, or oxygen is made possible by the nanoencapsulation technique. It also increases the bioavailability of the products, enables targeted delivery to specific locations, and permits a controlled release of the encapsulated substance (Assadpour and Mahdi Jafari 2019). The ability of nanosystems to control the release of delivered drugs, consisting of specific concentration/time release profiles at the desired site of action, is a major challenge in nutraceutical encapsulation. Therefore, an ideal delivery system should be able to release its contents at different biological environments as well as specific stimuli such as pH, enzymes, and temperature while protecting the nutraceutical from the same stimuli. Various nanocarriers used are depicted in Figure 12.2.

Furthermore, encapsulation of nutraceutical compounds leads to improve its solubility, as the properties depend on the physicochemical properties of the vesicles rather than the encapsulated compounds when the nutraceutical compound is loaded into a carrier. Nanosystems also offer the potential to deliver both water-soluble and lipid-soluble molecules together to support the synergistic property. Additionally, they can also ensure the physio-chemical stability of food items and prevent any unfavourable changes in flavour or aroma that could arise from the inclusion of nutraceuticals. As long as the materials have the status of Generally Recognised as Safe (GRAS), they can be of any nature

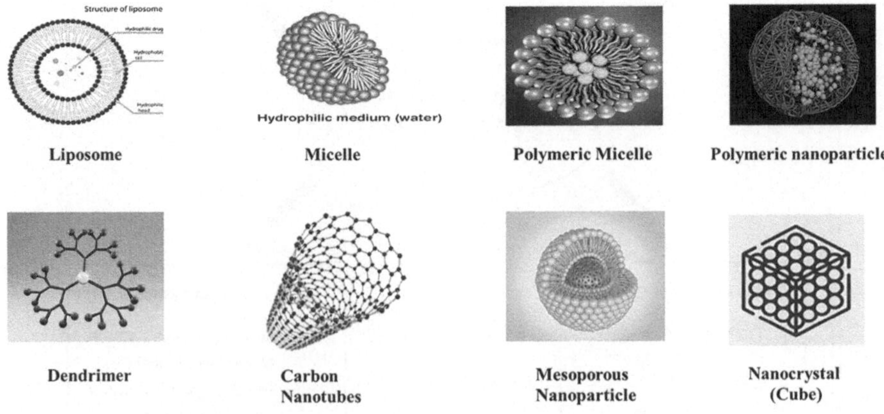

FIGURE 12.2 Schematic representation of different nanocarriers.

(lipid, polymeric, or protein) and be employed to create drug delivery systems. Finally, the type of drug delivery system to be developed and its chemical and physical properties are decided upon in accordance with the chemical-physical characteristics of the substance to be encapsulated, the target to be attained, and the type of ultimate application. Thus, nanoencapsulation of nutraceuticals may increase their beneficial benefits on human health while minimising their negative consequences (Grumezescu and Oprea 2017). Table 12.1 illustrates how nanotechnology is used in several nutraceuticals.

TABLE 12.1
Application of Nanotechnology in Nutraceuticals

S.No.	Nutraceuticals	Delivery System	Applications
1.	Curcumin	Organogel based nanoemulsion	The dissolution of nanoemulsions is very fast and complete. Enhanced oral bioavailability of curcumin. Can be used in functional food, dietary supplement, and pharmaceutical industries
2.	β-carotene, folic acid, curcumin and ergocalciferol	Protein-polysaccharide soluble nanocomplex	To increase the antioxidant activity
3.	Omega-3-fatty acids and oil-soluble vitamins	Biopolymeric nanogels	It encapsulates and protects bioactive substances. Made exclusively from food-grade raw materials, this system improves the quality of the food and beverages
4.	Hydrophobins (Hyd)-Vitamin D3	Nanoencapsulation	Promising hydrophobic nutraceutical nano vehicles for food and beverage enhancement. Vitamin D3 provides excellent protection against deterioration
5.	Folic acid with whey protein and commercial-resistant starch	Nanoencapsulation	Higher encapsulation efficiency. Improved folic acid stability. Increases stabilisation of biological activity
6.	α-tocopherol	Supercritical assisted nanosuspension	Increases the dissolution rate. Boosts bioavailability. Increases the stability.
7.	Carotenoids	Lipid nanocarriers	Great potential for clinical applications. A new delivery system for lipophilic plant extracts.
8.	Folic acid and calcium	Dual nutraceutical nanomaterial	To provide a high content of essential nutrients for human health.

12.4 NANOPARTICLES

Biopolymer nanoparticles consist of a matrix of biopolymers that can be attached to solid particles by intermolecular attractive forces or covalent chemical bonds. Nanoparticles consist of a single biopolymer or have a core-shell structure. The versatility of encapsulated compounds and to an extent these particles can be manipulated to tune their surface properties to make them the most promising delivery systems in the pharmaceutical and cosmetic industries.

To encapsulate and distribute substances, a wide range of natural and synthetic polymers have been utilised. Synthetic polymers such as D, L-polylactic acid (PLA), polyglycolic acid (PGA), polylactic-co-glycolic acid (PLGA), and polycaprolactic acid (PCL), as well as the naturally occurring polymer chitosan derived from the shells of crustaceans which has antibacterial as well as antioxidant properties. Additionally, copolymers made from combinations of the monomers lactide, galactide, and caprolactone are being employed more frequently (Shahidi and Abuzaytoun 2005).

Soy proteins have caught the interest of researchers to be employed in the creation of nanocarriers for the delivery of bioactives, including nutraceuticals, because of their biodegradability, bioavailability, and potential to encapsulate hydrophobic chemicals. A storage globulin from soy called β-conglycinin was used to create nanoparticles that contained hydrophobic curcumin, a polyphenol with anti-inflammatory and antioxidant properties. The vicilin storage protein of soybeans, β-conglycinin, was disassembled and then reassembled using urea as the solvent, and the resulting nanoparticles are more natural-looking and have higher encapsulation efficiency (by about 80%) than those produced in earlier studies. Curcumin's bioaccessibility was discovered to be 40% or so (as opposed to 20% or so for free curcumin). A promising biocompatible delivery strategy for hydrophobic chemicals is represented by β-conglycinin nanostructures (Liu et al. 2019).

Sanna and her colleagues used the nanoprecipitation method to create white tea extract-loaded polymeric nanoparticles using a mixture of poly(ε-caprolactone) and alginate. The acquired results demonstrate how this polymeric structure enables the preservation of polyphenolic extract, its regulated release in the gastrointestinal tract, and the conservation of antioxidant properties.

Jain et al., developed a nanosystem to research its potential application in breast cancer. It consists of zein nanoparticles that have been loaded with beta-carotene. The resulting system showed higher anticancer activity with respect to free beta-carotene both in vitro (MCF-7 cells) and in vivo (rat-induced breast cancer). This may be due to increased cellular uptake of zein nanoparticles. It is also worth noting that the association of beta-carotene-loaded nanoparticles with free methotrexate, the most widely used anticancer drug, showed dual beneficial effects. A synergistic effect has been observed through *in vitro* anticancer activity against MCF-7 cells (breast cancer cell line) and also reduced side effects of methotrexate on the liver and kidneys.

12.5 SOLID LIPID NANOPARTICLES AND NANOSTRUCTURED LIPID CARRIERS

One of the most effective lipid-based nanocarriers for the delivery of pharmaceuticals and nutraceuticals is solid lipid nanoparticles (SLNs) which have a structure comparable to that of an oil-in-water nanoemulsion. The "double face" of the SLNs refers to many benefits, including the ability to control drug release, medium stability, good biodegradability, biocompatibility, and high loading capacity for lipophilic drugs. On the other hand, when poorly soluble drugs are in the melted lipids, the SLNs' have low loading capacity and the potential for core expulsion during phase transition. This confirms that SLN components should be selected based on the chemical-physical properties of the dietary supplement to be encapsulated (Shin et al. 2015).

Nanostructured lipid carriers (NLCs) were fabricated to address the instability problem of SLNs due to lipid crystallisation and subsequent ejection of the encapsulated drug. NLCs consist of a mixture of solid and liquid lipids. They are characterised by a matrix and have higher stability and elasticity when compared to SLN (Gordillo-Galeano and Mora-Huertas 2018).

Mehrad et al., have shown that the contents of SLNs have a significant impact on both their applicability and effectiveness in the delivery of β-carotene as a nutraceutical component. The authors of this study examined how the lipid makeup of SLNs affected their capacity to stabilise the physicochemical properties of β-carotene. Whey protein isolate was used as a stabilising factor together with palmitic acid and corn oil to create the SLNs. The combination of palmitic acid and corn oil reduced the likelihood that the encapsulated nutraceutical would be expelled from the solid matrix, and whey protein isolate improved the oxidative stability of the carotene. Palmitic acid also allowed the formation of a solid shell on the lipid droplets and protected the encapsulated nutraceutical.

SLNs and NLCs have been shown to be suitable carriers for oral administration of resveratrol. The experimental study performed by Neves and his team, that these two lipid nanocarriers have encapsulation efficiency of about 80%, protected the resveratrol. In addition, in vitro studies on Caco-2 cells showed that SLN has impaired absorption whereas NLCs have significantly increased intestinal permeability of resveratrol, and the developed formulations were well tolerated in the intestinal mucosa. The outcome of the study demonstrated that NLC is a convenient carrier for oral administration of resveratrol; further, it can be used in the purpose of a supplement as well as a nutraceutical (Neves et al. 2016).

12.6 LIPOSOMES

Liposomes or lipid vesicles are formed from naturally abundant polar lipids, mainly phospholipids derived from soybeans and eggs. They can be used to encapsulate both water-soluble and fat-soluble compounds.

Liposomes are spherical multimolecular assemblies with a bilayer shell structure. Depending on the manufacturing process, lipid vesicles can be unilamellar or multilamellar and contain one or more bilayer envelopes. The size of the liposomes typically varies from 20 nm to hundreds of microns. Their core is aqueous in nature and its chemical composition corresponds to the aqueous solution in which the vesicles are produced. Polar lipids are used to prepare the liposomes, which have an electrical charge; hence, water-soluble ionic species can be trapped within the liposomes. Thus, the pH and ionic strength of the liposome core can differ from that of the continuous phase in which the liposomes are subsequently dispersed (Nsairat et al. 2022).

Lee and Tsai developed a liposomal topical formulation using soybean phosphatidylcholine and α-tocopherol as lipid components to encapsulate Coenzyme Q10 (CoQ_{10}), an endogenous cellular antioxidant and the study results demonstrated that the liposomal CoQ10 can be used as a topical application of CoQ_{10} (Lee and Tsai 2010). Amri et al. reviewed the administration of resveratrol in different formulations and they highlighted that incorporating the resveratrol into the liposomal carrier systems can improve its stability, bioavailability, and provide significant anti-tumour activity.

Despite being viewed as waste, pomace a phenolic compound from red grape has very good antioxidant properties. Manconi and team developed liposomes to protect the pomace from the gastric environment by incorporating the grape extract into the liposomal vesicular system which was stabilised by two natural polysaccharides (Arabic gum or sodium alginate). The developed liposomes have good stability and also protected pomace in the gastric environment and showed better antioxidant properties in Caco-2 cells against oxidative stress. They have concluded that, in the near future, polymer-associated liposome formulations can be used in the nutraceutical field (Manconi et al. 2016).

12.7 NANO EMULSIONS

Nanoemulsions are very fine oil-in-water (O/W) emulsions with average droplet diameters between 50 and 200 nm. An emulsion is described as a mixture of two liquids that are totally or partially incompatible with one another, such as oil and water, with the droplets of one liquid spread throughout the other.

In contrast to these well-known O/W emulsions, nanoemulsions are sufficiently small that they do not scatter light in the visible range of the spectrum. Therefore, it appears transparent rather than optically opaque. Creaming is the process by which oil droplets migrate to the top of the emulsion to form a concentrated layer of oil droplets. This is often followed by a complete breakdown of the emulsion, leaving a clearly visible layer of oil on top of the emulsion.

Achieving bioavailability of bioactive food compounds on oral dosage forms is crucial, influenced by factors like the food matrix effect, molecular structure, bioacessibility, transporters, and enzymes. Nanotechnology offers potential methods for potent, better bioavailability, enhancing solubilisation and absorption in the gastrointestinal tract. Nanoemulsion (NE) and macroemulsions can similarly be prepared using high-pressure homogenisers or membrane and microfluidic channels. Note that the appropriate selection of surfactants and/or polymers and their quantity play a significant role in the preparation of nanoemulsions.

Oil-in-water and water-in-oil nanoemulsions are used for encapsulation and protection of active ingredients and are suitable for encapsulation of nutraceuticals to improve the efficacy of hydrophobic and hydrophilic active ingredients and food ingredients. Applications of nanoemulsion in nutraceuticals are shown in Table 12.2.

TABLE 12.2
Applications of Nanoemulsion in Nutraceuticals

Nutraceutical Compund	Emulsification Method	Objective	Outcome
Vitamin E	Phase Inversion	The emulsified phase inversion (EPI) technique is used to create the food-grade nanoemulsion that is abundant in vitamin E acetate.	The EPI approach, in comparison to the high-energy method, may create smaller droplets at greater surfactant levels to encapsulate oil-soluble vitamins in food, beverages, cosmetics, and pharmaceutical items.
Fish oil	High-speed homogenisation/ ultrasonication	Oil-in-water nanoemulsions (NE) and conventional emulsions (CE) were created using fish fat oil containing EPA and DHA as raw ingredients, and their absorption in the small intestine of rats was studied.	The rat small intestine's emulsion system greatly increases lipid absorption when exposed to NE.
Capsaicin (CAP)	Self-assembly method	A food-grade nanoemulsion was created to improve the bioavailability and solubility of CAP and lessen its irritability.	Organogel CAP nanoemulsion had increased biological accessibility and dissolution rate. The inflammation of the gastric mucosa was better relieved by it.
Ginger essential oil (GEO)	Ultrasonication	A nano emulsion-based edible coating containing ginger essential oil was studied for its antimicrobial and antioxidant effectiveness.	The durability of chicken breast was increased by GEO nano emulsion more so than by traditional emulsion.
Demethyltangeretin (5DT)	High-pressure homogenisation	Emulsion-based delivery strategy to increase the bioavailability of 5DT and its absorption in intestinal cancer cells	A higher rate of cell absorption and a lower percentage of cancer cell survival can result from 5DT wrapped in nanoemulsion.

12.8 NANOCRYSTALS

A surfactant, or polymeric stabiliser, surrounds a crystallised medication or bioactive that makes up a nanocrystal (NC). This NC can increase the bioavailability of medications or bioactives that are difficult to dissolve in water. In NC the bioactive itself can act as the solid matrix of the nanoparticles, in contrast to lipid and polymeric nanoparticles where a bioactive is encapsulated. Therefore, a nanocrystal's main benefit is that it has a 100% bioactive loading. However, this kind of nanoencapsulation functions very well for the bioactives that have high melting points or the ability to crystallise at room temperature, such as bioactives from the carotenoid family. Because they are often created in a liquid dispersion media where they are suspended in the liquid (nanocrystals are also known as nanosuspension). Because of their straightforward structure and composition, NCs have drawn a lot of attention from the pharmaceutical industry. Bioactive NCs have not been the subject of as much research as medication NCs, nevertheless. The food industry can greatly benefit from NCs, which also increase formulation performance by increasing the saturation solubility and rate of dissolution of bioactive particles. Additionally, because of their large loading capacities, bioactives can be transported to/into cells with a high degree of efficiency, enabling them to have a high enough therapeutic concentration to produce the required pharmacological effects (Junghanns and Müller 2008).

12.9 CONCLUSION

With recent increased public awareness about their health and nutritional issues, there is a growing desire for specialty foods that may offer some additional health benefits beyond those of basic nutrition. Various pathologies, including inflammation, cancer, and cardiovascular disorders, can be prevented, or treated with the use of nutraceuticals.

Nanotechnology is a recent scientific and technological innovation in the 21st century that has been considered a promising one in the delivery of nutraceuticals, improved bioavailability in terms of the preservation and stability of nutrients, the improvement of solubility and dissolution rate, the improvement of intestinal permeability, the targeting of intracellular and subcellular organelles, and prolonged circulation time. To avoid undesirable effects like transporting or depositing active ingredients or excipients in cells or tissues where they are not intended to be, or increasing the absorption of substances that are not intended to transport, the nanocarriers for nutraceuticals (nanoparticles, nanoemulsions, nanoliposomes, etc.) should be fabricated with food-grade ingredients. The precise mechanism of action by which some nanocarriers can increase the effects of nutraceuticals is one area that is still not completely understood. To maximise the potential of these natural substances in preventing and/or curing diseases, it is vital to step up scientific studies focused on elucidating the precise mechanism of action of nutraceutical-loaded nanocarriers. Future investment in nutraceutical research will be crucial to make their industrial application more and more realistic given how harmful diseases like obesity, cancer, diabetes, and other cardiovascular diseases have increased due to changes in lifestyle.

REFERENCES

Assadpour, E., & Mahdi Jafari, S. (2019). A systematic review on nanoencapsulation of food bioactive ingredients and nutraceuticals by various nanocarriers. *Critical Reviews in Food Science and Nutrition*, 59(19), 3129–3151.

Chen, H., Weiss, J., & Shahidi, F. (2006). Nanotechnology in nutraceuticals and functional foods. *Food Technology*.

Daliu, P., Santini, A., & Novellino, E. (2019). From pharmaceuticals to nutraceuticals: Bridging disease prevention and management. *Expert Review of Clinical Pharmacology*, 12(1), 1–7.

Das, L., Bhaumik, E., Raychaudhuri, U., & Chakraborty, R. (2012). Role of nutraceuticals in human health. *Journal of Food Science and Technology*, 49, 173–183.

Gordillo-Galeano A., & Mora-Huertas, C.E. (2018). Solid lipid nanoparticles and nanostructured lipid carriers: A review emphasizing on particle structure and drug release. *European Journal of Pharmaceutics and Biopharmaceutics*, 133, 285–308.

Grumezescu, A.M., & Oprea, A.E. (Eds.). (2017). *Nanotechnology Applications in Food: Flavor, Stability, Nutrition and Safety*. Academic Press.

Junghanns, J.U.A.H., & Müller, R.H. (2008). Nanocrystal technology, drug delivery and clinical applications. *International Journal of Nanomedicine*, 3(3), 295.

Lee, W., & Tsai, T. (2010). Preparation and characterization of liposomal coenzyme Q10 for in vivo topical application. *International Journal of Pharmaceutics*, 395, 78–83.

Liu, L., Liu, P., Li, X., Zhang, N., & Tang, C. (2019). Novel soy β-conglycinin core-shell nanoparticles as outstanding ecofriendly nanocarriers for curcumin. *Journal of Agricultural and Food Chemistry* 67, 6292–6301.

Manconi, M., Marongiu, F., Castangia, I., Manca, M.L., Caddeo, C., Tuberoso, C.I.G., et al. (2016). Polymer-associated liposomes for the oral delivery of grape pomace extract. *Colloids and Surfaces B: Biointerfaces*, 146, 910–917.

Neves, A.R., Martins, S., Segundo, M.A., & Reis, S. (2016). Nanoscale delivery of resveratrol towards enhancement of supplements and nutraceuticals. *Nutrients*, 8, 131.

Nsairat, H., Khater, D., Sayed, U., Odeh, F., Al Bawab, A., & Alshaer, W. (2022). Liposomes: Structure, composition, types, and clinical applications. *Heliyon*, 8(5), e09394.

Sanguansri, P., & Augustin, M.A. (2006). Nanoscale materials development - A food industry perspective. *Trends in Food Science and Technology*, 17(10), 547–556.

Shahidi, F., & Abuzaytoun, R. (2005). Chitin, chitosan, and co-products: Chemistry, production, applications, and health effects. *Advances in Food and Nutrition Research*, 49, 93–135.

Shin, G.H., Kim, J.T., & Park, H.J. (2015). Recent developments in nanoformulations of lipophilic functional foods. *Trends in Food Science and Technology*, 46, 114–157.

13 Computational Strategies for the Discovery of Nutraceuticals against Lifestyle Diseases

A. Umamaheswari, N. Tamilselvan, S. Sowntharya, Trudi Collet, and A. Puratchikody

13.1 INTRODUCTION

The manifestation of nutraceuticals is growing tremendously in this modern era owing to their immense nutritional benefits and is considered as a holistic approach to attain complete physical and mental well-being in accordance with the conventional medicinal systems. According to Hippocrates philosophy, food is considered as medicine, with a well-known quote "Let food be the medicine and medicine be the food" (Helal et al. 2019). Hence, it can be overwhelmed by the use of computational approaches which are proficient with the integration of advanced analytical tools and techniques to facilitate the discovery of novel bioactive constituents from the large libraries of nutritional supplements (Murugan et al. 2022).

Computational strategies are considered as an innovative technology intended for the high-throughput bioactive compounds screening and to speed up the designing novel nutraceuticals economically with very less side effects. In the field of discovery of nutraceuticals against lifestyle diseases, *in silico* approaches are still in their initial stages, offering an exceptional prospect for further extensive study and examination (Kumar et al. 2019).

13.2 NUTRACEUTICALS

Ever since the introduction of the term nutraceuticals, food supplements are substances used to compensate the micro and macro nutritional deficits, while on the other hand "nutraceuticals" are specifically designed preparations which aids in the treatment of widespread pathological ailments with robust technical evidence (Santini and Novellino 2018).

 DOI: 10.1201/9781003392934-13

Nutraceutical compounds are found in various forms like food supplements, dietary supplements and isolated compounds. Hence, every nutraceutical supplements are not dietary supplements and also not all the dietary supplements are nutraceuticals.

13.3 ROLE OF NUTRACEUTICALS IN LIFESTYLE DISEASES

Nutraceuticals aids in enhancing the health and wellbeing of human beings by modulating the immunity, therefore preventing and treating numerous diseases. Role of nutraceuticals in the disease prevention and well-being are indicated in Figure 13.1 and various diseases which can be treated by means of several nutraceuticals are:

13.3.1 Alzheimer's Disease (AD)

Dementia is a syndrome is considered as a major influencing factor in causing specific brain disease known as Alzheimer's disease. Oxidative stress plays a leading role in this neurodegenerative disease. Phosphatidylserine is a very stimulating nutraceutical complex, a vital phospholipid in CNS making up the elementary arrangement of the plasma membrane. It plays a major role in cell-to-cell transduction and transport of biochemicals between other cells (Lokhande 2018).

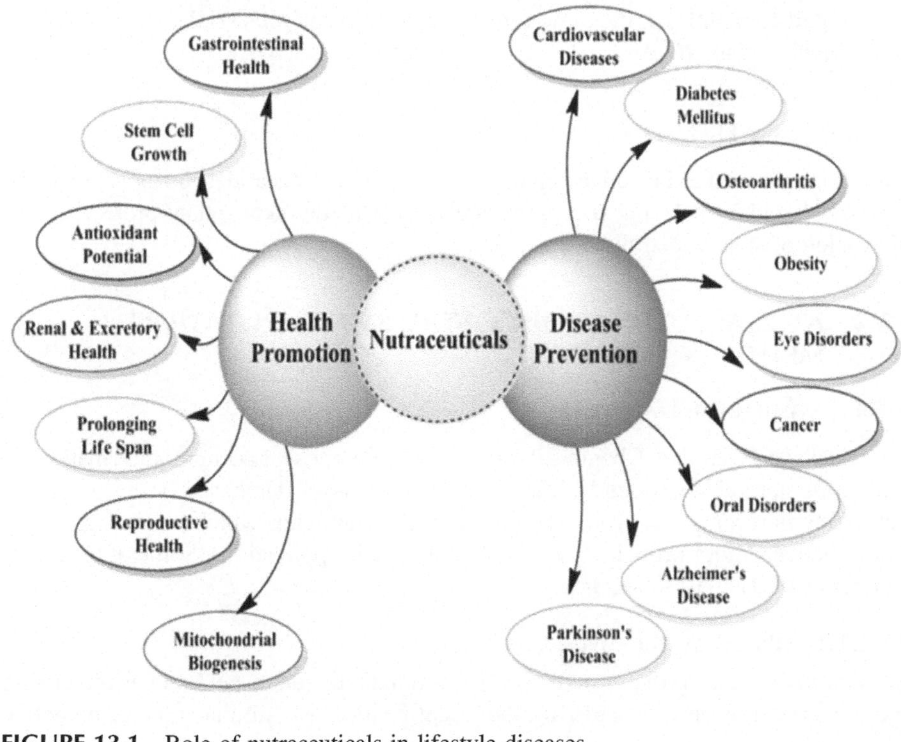

FIGURE 13.1 Role of nutraceuticals in lifestyle diseases.

13.3.2 Cardiovascular Diseases (CVD)

Damage of blood vessels and impairment in the functioning of the heart are acquiescent to nutraceutical interference.

- Ischaemic heart diseases and Atherosclerosis – Allicin and Allin from *Allium sativum* possess antihyperlipidemic activity (Chakraborty and Roy 2021).
- Cardiac arrhythmias – Omega-3 fatty acids from marine sources aid in the prevention of Cardiac arrhythmias (Manson et al. 2019).
- Hypertension – Casein and whey protein derivatives of milk are potential ACE inhibitors (antihypertensive effects) (Liao et al. 2021).

13.3.3 Cancer

Uncontrolled proliferation of cells with various complications is treated by conventional Radio and Chemotherapies, but they can cause serious side effects (Saldanha and Tollefsbol 2012).

- Pancreatic, Colorectal, Prostate, Gastric, and Hepatic cancers – Curcumin (Diferuloyl-Methane) from Turmeric (*Curcuma Longa*) inhibits carcinogenesis and it is more effective when combined with the radio and chemotherapies (Yoshida et al. 2018).
- Ginger, Genistein, and Silibinin from Silybummarianum seeds possess significant anti-carcinogenic effects against cancer cells (Hsiao et al. 2019; Mahira et al. 2019).

13.3.4 Skin Diseases

Nutraceuticals such as bioactive peptides, bioactive polysaccharides, botanical extracts, carotenoids aid in delaying the premature ageing of the skin, photo-protection and alleviation of skin-related disorders.

13.4 NUTRACEUTICALS DISCOVERY BY COMPUTATIONAL METHODS

13.4.1 Chemical Databases

Chemical databases are Chemo-Libraries which comprise structural information of numerous natural compounds. The evolution of these databases is continuously advancing in recent years from simple chemical compounds which play a significant role in both chemoinformatic as well as bioinformatic applications. Some of the major categories of databases used are:

13.4.1.1 Based on the Structure

Structurally similar or the same functional group compounds can be identified using these chemo-libraries. It aids in the identification of similar potent bioactive compounds with higher binding profiles and is highly beneficial in ligand-based modelling.

13.4.1.2 Based on the Target

Precise chemical molecules can be identified based on the information regarding the desired target site.

13.4.1.3 Based on the Properties

An enormous dataset of molecules can also be identified based on the desired physicochemical properties which are highly beneficial in the post modelling studies (Ojeda-Montes et al. 2019).

A list of major chemical databases widely for the computational applications in nutraceutical research are depicted in Table 13.1.

Moreover, these chemical databases are classified into two major modules based on the nature of chemical compounds.

TABLE 13.1
Chemical Databases for Nutraceuticals Research

S.No	Database Name	No. of Compounds	Website	Reference
1.	PubChem	>100 million – small and large molecules	https://pubchem.ncbi.nlm.nih.gov	Kim et al. (2019)
2.	ChEMBL	>2 million compounds with bioactivity	https://www.ebi.ac.uk/chembl/	Mendez et al. (2019)
3.	NCI	275.000 – small molecules for cancer/AIDS	https://cactus.nci.nih.gov/ncidb2.2/	NCI
4.	ChemDB	5 million datasets – small molecules (physicochemical properties)	http://cdb.ics.uci.edu	Chen et al. (2007)
5.	ChemSpider	>67 million datasets of free chemical structures	http://www.chemspider.com	Chem Spider
6.	BindingDB	1 million binding data – >6000 protein targets for 400.000 small molecules	https://www.bindingdb.org/bind/index.jsp	Gilson et al. (2016)
7.	PDB-Bind	21.000 datasets – protein–ligand complexes	http://www.pdbbind.org.cn	Su et al. (2018)
8.	PDBeChem	30.000 entries – small molecules, ligands and monomers	https://www.ebi.ac.uk/pdbe-srv/pdbechem/	Dimitropoulos et al. (2006)
9.	SMPDB	50.000 datasets – Small Molecule Pathway Database	https://smpdb.ca	Frolkis et al. (2010)
10.	DrugBank	>13.000 entries – nutraceutical molecules	https://www.drugbank.ca	Xing et al. (2012)

a. ***Virtual Natural product Libraries*** – Chemical datasets are extensively available in the retrievable format suitable for several *in silico* applications.
b. ***Physical Natural product Libraries*** – These Chemo-libraries aid in providing the suitable format of chemical compounds for various *in silico* applications which are also readily purchasable constituents (Chen et al. 2017).

Some of the most significant physical and virtual chemo-Databases available with open access are represented in Table 13.2.

13.4.2 Virtual Screening (VS) Techniques

Generally, identification of bioactive compounds via laborious process is very expensive and time-consuming. To overwhelm the traditional method of discovery of nutraceuticals, innovative approaches are developed which aims to optimise the research methodology. Amongst them, virtual screening is one of the major techniques used for the determination of potent bioactive molecules to incorporate in nutraceuticals. This methodology aids in increasing the effectiveness of the discovery process and rationalising the discovered compounds (da Silva Rocha et al. 2019).

TABLE 13.2
List of Some Leading Virtual and Physical Databases

S.No	Name of the Databases	Available No. of Compounds	Format	Web-Link	Reference
			Virtual Natural compounds databases		
1.	COCONUT	406,747	.SMILES and.SDF	https://coconut.naturalproducts.net/	Sorokina et al. (2021)
2.	CMNPD	Greater than 31,000	.SDF	https://www.cmnpd.org/	Lyu et al. (2021)
3.	NPAtlas	24,594	.SMILES and.SDF	https://www.npatlas.org/	Van Santen et al. (2019)
4.	FooDB	23,883	.MOL,.SDF,.PDB, and.SMILES	https://foodb.ca/	Chen et al. (2007)
5.	TCM database@Taiwan	>20,000	.MOL2	http://tcm.cmu.edu.tw/	Chen (2011)
			Physical Natural compounds databases		
6.	ZINC 15	>80,000	.MOL2.SDF.SMILES	https://zinc15.docking.org/	Sterling and Irwin (2015)
7.	MolPort	>10,000	.SDF.SMILES	https://www.molport.com/	Chen et al. (2007)

The most prevalently used common methods for the identification and discovery of potent nutraceutical substances are,

- Quantitative Structure-Activity Relationship (QSAR)
- Molecular and Pharmacophore Modelling
- Molecular Docking

These methodologies are very useful in reducing the number of experimental trials, an expensive laboratory process for the selection of nutraceuticals (Lin et al. 2020). Predominantly in the field of nutraceuticals, these approaches are utilised to unravel the bioactive food constituents with health-enhancing, disease-preventing, and treatment aspects (Carpio et al. 2021). Some of the widely used molecular descriptor calculation and molecular docking freely available software are listed in Table 13.3.

13.4.3 Quantitative Structure-Activity Relationship (QSAR)

QSAR study is a ligand-based *in silico* approach which aids in the correlation of structural properties of various chemical compounds and their bioactivity

TABLE 13.3
List of Some Freely Available Software with Commercial Use

S.No	Name	Availability	Link	Reference
			Molecular descriptor calculations	
1.	Open Babel	Free	http://openbabel.org	Cherkasov et al. (2014)
2.	RDKit	Free	http://www.rdkit.org/	Cherkasov et al. (2014)
			Molecular Docking Softwares	
1.	AutoDock	Free	http://autodock.scripps.edu/	Morris et al. (2009)
2.	AutoDock Vina	Free	https://vina.scripps.edu/	Trott and Olson (2010)
3.	PyRx	Free	https://pyrx.sourceforge.io/downloads	Dallakyan and Olson, (2015)
4.	Dock	Free	http://dock.compbio.ucsf.edu/	Allen et al. (2015)
5.	Haddock	Free	https://wenmr.science.uu.nl/	Dominguez et al. (2003)
6.	SwissDock	Free	http://www.swissdock.ch/	Grosdidier et al. (2011)
7.	PyDock	Free	https://life.bsc.es/pid/pydock	Jiménez-García et al. (2013)
8.	DockingServer	Free	https://www.dockingserver.com/web	Bikadi and Hazai, (2009)
			Pharmacophore modelling	
1.	Pharmer	Free for academic use	http://pharmer.sourceforge.net	Koes and Camacho (2011)
2.	Pharmmaker	Free	http://prody.csb.pitt.edu/pharmmaker/	Lee et al. (2020)
3.	PharmaGist	Free	https://bioinfo3d.cs.tau.ac.il/PharmaGist/php.php	Schneidman-Duhovny et al. (2008)

(Neves et al. 2018). Generally, QSAR models are created by linking equations which relates a number of dependent variables with a numeral of calculated descriptors, together with the physicochemical and topological properties (Rybińska-Fryca et al. 2020). The generation and building of the model dataset, validation process are carried out for the stability and accuracy of analysis. Then, the produced model aids as a prediction and identification tool to arrange and select the compounds which possess potent biological activity and decreases the number of components for further processing to invitro and in vivo investigation (Cherkasov et al. 2014).

13.4.4 Molecular and Pharmacophore Modelling

The molecular modelling (MM) technique encompasses both theoretical as well as computational approaches to model and mimics the behaviour of naturally available molecules. The MM methods are used to elucidate the various chemical and biological response mechanisms and their interaction approaches linking the molecular structures, to predict the physicochemical, and biological properties. These methods are very much beneficial in the field of nutraceuticals, cosmeceuticals, and functional food constituents research (Tao et al. 2020).

Furthermore, pharmacophore modelling is a three-dimensional arrangement of chemical topographies, which are vital for the molecular recognition of a small molecule against a specific target protein. It affords a higher binding affinity towards various structurally varied ligand molecules to a specific target. Pharmacophore modelling can be done in two different ways as given below:

Structure-based – Prediction of possible interactions between the target protein receptor and the varied active ligand molecules.

Ligand-based – Overlapping a cluster of active ligand molecules and generating a new compound with specific chemical topographies which aids in enhancing the bioactivity against the receptor protein macromolecule (Yang 2010).

Presently, there are numerous 3D pharmacophore modelling generators available for both commercial as well as academic purposes (Schaller et al. 2020). After the generation of a pharmacophore model, they are retrieved for further screening process is generally referred to as Pharmacophore-based Virtual Screening (Grabowski et al. 2020).

A homology model of tyrosinase receptor protein carried out via Swiss model web server was visualised using Chimera and represented in Figure 13.2. It is considered as a major target protein in treating various skin ailments like melasma, ephelis, and patches, owing to their crucial role in modulating the synthesis of melanin pigment which prevents the skin from ultraviolet damage.

13.4.5 Molecular Docking

It is the most frequently used *in silico* technique, which aids in the prediction of small molecule (ligand) interaction with protein (receptor) at the nuclear level. This method allows for classification of small molecules based on the nature of binding

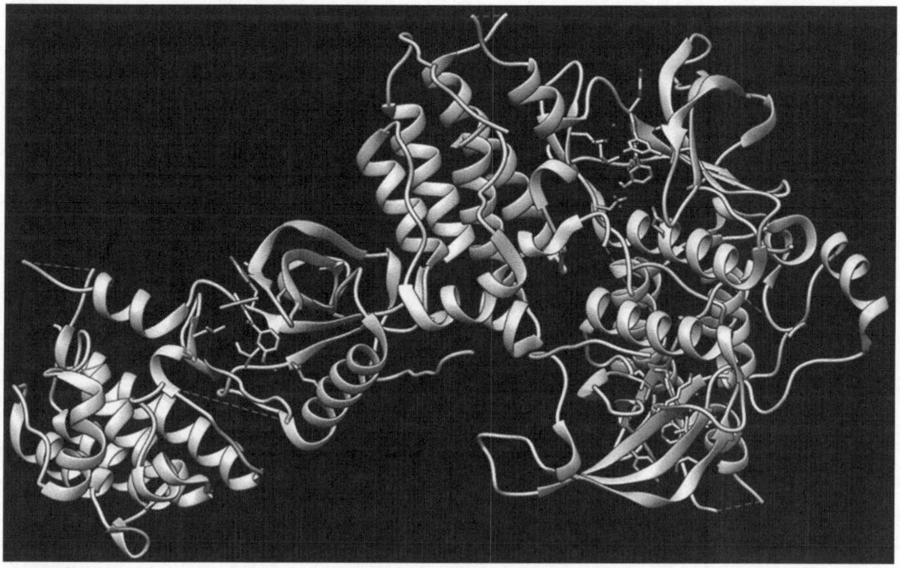

FIGURE 13.2 Example of a homology modelled tyrosine protein (PDB ID: 3GQL).

energy to the target proteins. Furthermore, it aids in the illumination of vital biological processes behind this interaction. It is known as the structure-based method that requires a 3D design with very high resolution of the scrutinised target resulting from

1. X-ray crystallography
2. Nuclear Magnetic Resonance Spectroscopy and
3. Cryo-Electron Microscopy

There is a steep increase in the usage of these techniques in the field of nutrition and dietary sciences (Tao et al. 2020).

For instance, to examine the possible interaction between the Tyrosinase receptor protein and nutraceutical ligand compound ginsenoside Re from ginseng plant roots is analysed and visualised using the Chimera software. According to the docking study, the ginsenoside Re effectively inhibits the Tyrosinase protein, and further in vitro studies prove the ligand as a potential compound against various skin ailments (Briganti and Picardo 2003). An example of a docking pose of the natural compound is visualised via Chimera visualisation software which is shown in Figure 13.3.

13.5 CURRENT TRENDS AND FUTURE PROSPECTS OF NUTRACEUTICALS

In this modern era, the development of computational strategies aids in overcoming the challenges associated with the discovery, nutraceutical development, and even in clinical trials for the evaluation of safety, efficacy, and toxicity. Subsequently, the

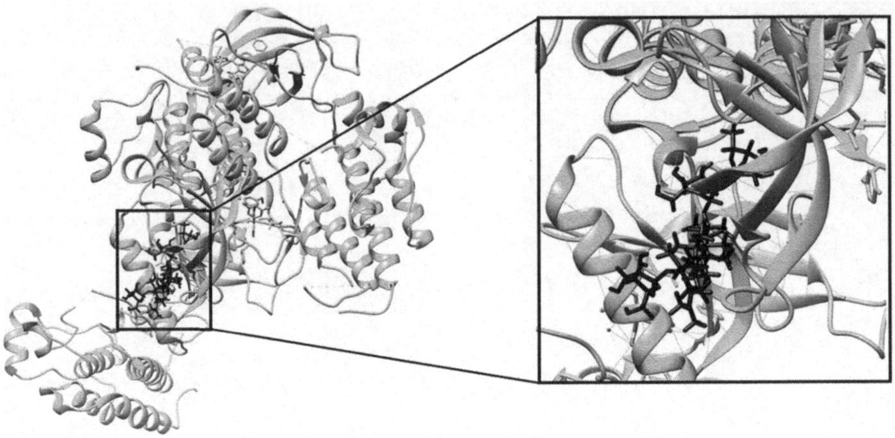

FIGURE 13.3 Binding poses of ginsenoside Re (Ligand) with tyrosine protein.

progress in these approaches is 'Nutrigenetics' and 'Nutrigenomics' which aids in scrutinising the nutrition and their gene expressions by signifying the dietary supplements in relation with the human genomic arrangements, modification in the gene expression and gene transcripts (Pandita et al. 2022).

13.6 CONCLUSION

Nutraceuticals exhibited potential health benefits against various lifestyle disease pathologies with improved therapeutic efficiency than the traditional formulations. Owing to the increase in the requisite of nutraceutical compounds databases for the natural compound and chemoinformatic applications aids in facilitating the design and development of new nutraceuticals with improved bioactivity profiles with the help of various *in silico* screening approaches. Moreover, the mechanism of actions of bioactive molecules is also studied easily by means of computational techniques. There is a boundless prospect for the advancement of novel strategies and methods that might improve the possibility of identification as well as optimisation of novel nutraceutical compounds via docking. At present, with abundant intelligent approaches existing in the literature, researchers are facing complications in selecting the best method that could be functional for a specific dataset. Computational strategies can pave the way for new and interesting avenues of research in nutraceuticals and denote a significant challenge for researchers in developing novel nutraceutical compounds with less toxicity. Nowadays, computational methods aid in the approval process of novel nutraceuticals by consolidation of the existing data on their mechanism of action, which assists in evaluating the effectiveness and safety of the launched foodstuffs in the market. Also, several associated limitations of computational approaches when applied to food supplements are future challenges to be unravelled and prospects to advance the utility of computational strategies in a broader milieu.

REFERENCES

Allen, W.J., Balius, T.E., Mukherjee, S., Brozell, S.R., Moustakas, D.T., Lang, P.T., & Rizzo, R.C. (2015). DOCK 6: Impact of new features and current docking performance. *Journal of Computational Chemistry*, 36(15), 1132–1156.

Briganti, S.C., & Picardo, M. (2003). Chemical and instrumental approaches to treat hyperpigmentation. *Pigment Cell Research*, 16(2), 101–110.

Bikadi, Z., & Hazai, E. (2009). Application of the PM6 semi-empirical method to modeling proteins enhances docking accuracy of AutoDock. *Journal of Cheminformatics*, 1, 15.s

Carpio, L.E., Sanz, Y., Gozalbes, R., & Barigye, S.J. (2021). Computational strategies for the discovery of biological functions of health foods, nutraceuticals and cosmeceuticals: A review. *Molecular Diversity*, 25, 1425–1438.

Chakraborty, R., & Roy, S. (2021). Angiotensin-converting enzyme inhibitors from plants: a review of their diversity, modes of action, prospects, and concerns in the management of diabetes-centric complications. *Journal of Integrative Medicine*, 19(6), 478–492.

Chen, C.Y.C. (2011). TCM Database@ Taiwan: The world's largest traditional Chinese medicine database for drug screening in silico. *PloS One*, 6(1), e15939.

Chen, G., Huang, K., Miao, M., Feng, B., & Campanella, O.H. (2019). Molecular dynamics simulation for mechanism elucidation of food processing and safety: State of the art. *Comprehensive Reviews in Food Science and Food Safety*, 18(1), 243–263.

Chen, J.H., Linstead, E., Swamidass, S.J., Wang, D., & Baldi, P. (2007). ChemDB update—full-text search and virtual chemical space. *Bioinformatics*, 23(17), 2348–2351.

Chen, Y., de Bruyn Kops, C., & Kirchmair, J. (2017). Data resources for the computer-guided discovery of bioactive natural products. *Journal of Chemical Information and Modeling*, 57(9), 2099–2111.

Cherkasov, A., Muratov, E.N., Fourches, D., Varnek, A., Baskin, I.I., Cronin, M., & Tropsha, A. (2014). QSAR modeling: where have you been? Where are you going to. *Journal of Medicinal Chemistry*, 57(12), 4977–5010.

da Silva Rocha, S.F., Olanda, C.G., Fokoue, H.H., & Sant′Anna, C.M. (2019). Virtual screening techniques in drug discovery: Review and recent applications. *Current Topics in Medicinal Chemistry*, 19(19), 1751–1767.

Dallakyan, S., & Olson, A.J. (2015). Small-molecule library screening by docking with PyRx. *Chemical Biology: Methods and Protocols*, 243–250.

Dimitropoulos, D., Ionides, J., & Henrick, K. (2006). Using MSD chem to search the PDB ligand dictionary. *Current Protocols in Bioinformatics*, 15(1), 14-3.

Dominguez, C., Boelens, R., & Bonvin, A.M. (2003). HADDOCK: a protein–protein docking approach based on biochemical or biophysical information. *Journal of the American Chemical Society*, 125(7), 1731–1737.

Frolkis, A., Knox, C., Lim, E., Jewison, T., Law, V., Hau, D.D., & Wishart, D.S. (2010). SMPDB: The small molecule pathway database. *Nucleic Acids Research*, 38(1), D480–D487.

Gilson, M.K., Liu, T., Baitaluk, M., Nicola, G., Hwang, L., & Chong, J. (2016). BindingDB in 2015: A public database for medicinal chemistry, computational chemistry and systems pharmacology. *Nucleic Acids Research*, 44(D1), D1045–D1053.

Grabowski, M., Murgueitio, M.S., Bermudez, M., Wolber, G., & Weindl, G. (2020). The novel small-molecule antagonist MMG-11 preferentially inhibits TLR2/1 signaling. *Biochemical Pharmacology*, 171, 113687.

Grosdidier, A., Zoete, V., & Michielin, O. (2011). SwissDock, a protein-small molecule docking web service based on EADock DSS. *Nucleic Acids Research*, 39(2), W270–W277.

Helal, N.A., Eassa, H.A., Amer, A.M., Eltokhy, M.A., Edafiogho, I., & Nounou, M.I. (2019). Nutraceuticals' novel formulations: The good, the bad, the unknown and patents involved. *Recent Patents on Drug Delivery & Formulation*, 13(2), 105–156.

Hsiao, Y.C., Peng, S.F., Lai, K.C., Liao, C.L., Huang, Y.P., Lin, C.C., & Chung, J.G. (2019). Genistein induces apoptosis in vitro and has antitumor activity against human leukemia HL-60 cancer cell xenograft growth in vivo. *Environmental Toxicology*, 34(4), 443–456.

Jiménez-García, B., Pons, C., & Fernández-Recio, J. (2013). pyDockWEB: A web server for rigid-body protein–protein docking using electrostatics and desolvation scoring. *Bioinformatics*, 29(13), 1698–1699.

Kim, S., Chen, J., Cheng, T., Gindulyte, A., He, J., He, S., & Bolton, E.E. (2019). PubChem 2019 update: Improved access to chemical data. *Nucleic Acids Research*, 47(D1), D1102–D1109.

Koes, D.R., & Camacho, C.J. (2011). Pharmer: efficient and exact pharmacophore search. *Journal of Chemical Information and Modeling*, 51(6), 1307–1314.

Kumar, R., Singh, A.K., Gupta, A., & Pandey, A.K. (2019). In-silico approaches to study therapeutic efficacy of nutraceuticals. *Phytochemistry: An In-silico and In-vitro Update: Advances in Phytochemical Research*, 479–490.

Lee, J.Y., Krieger, J.M., Li, H., & Bahar, I. (2020). Pharmmaker: Pharmacophore modeling and hit identification based on drug ability simulations. *Protein Science*, 29(1), 76–86.

Liao, W., Sun, G., Xu, D., Wang, Y., Lu, Y., Sun, J., & Wang, S. (2021). The blood-pressure-lowering effect of food-protein-derived peptides: A meta-analysis of recent clinical trials. *Foods*, 10(10), 2316.

Lin, X., Li, X., & Lin, X. (2020). A review on applications of computational methods in drug screening and design. *Molecules*, 25(6), 1375.

Lokhande, S.S. (2018). Role of nutraceuticals in various diseases: A comprehensive review. *Asian Journal of Pharmaceutical Research*, 8(4), 236–240.

Lyu, C., Chen, T., Qiang, B., Liu, N., Wang, H., Zhang, L., & Liu, Z. (2021). CMNPD: A comprehensive marine natural products database towards facilitating drug discovery from the ocean. *Nucleic Acids Research*, 49(D1), D509–D515.

Mahira, S., Kommineni, N., Husain, G.M., & Khan, W. (2019). Cabazitaxel and silibinin co-encapsulated cationic liposomes for CD44 targeted delivery: A new insight into nanomedicine based combinational chemotherapy for prostate cancer. *Biomedicine & Pharmacotherapy*, 110, 803–817.

Manson, J.E., Cook, N.R., Lee, I.M., Christen, W., Bassuk, S.S., Mora, S., & Buring, J.E. (2019). Marine n–3 fatty acids and prevention of cardiovascular disease and cancer. *New England Journal of Medicine*, 380(1), 23–32.

Mendez, D., Gaulon, A., Bento, A.P., Chambers, J., DeVeij, M., Félix, E., Magariños, M.P., Mosquera, J.F., Mutowo, P., Nowotka, M., Gordillo-Marañón, M., HunterF, F., *et al.* (2019). ChEMBL: Towards direct deposition of bioassay data. *Nucleic acids research*, 47(D1), D930–D940.

Morris, G.M., Huey, R., Lindstrom, W., Sanner, M.F., Belew, R.K., Goodsell, D.S., & Olson, A.J. (2009). AutoDock4 and AutoDockTools4: Automated docking with selective receptor flexibility. *Journal of Computational Chemistry*, 30(16), 2785–2791.

Murugan, N.A., Podobas, A., Gadioli, D., Vitali, E., Palermo, G., & Markidis, S. (2022). A review on parallel virtual screening softwares for high-performance computers. *Pharmaceuticals*, 15(1), 63.

Neves, B.J., Braga, R.C., Melo-Filho, C.C., Moreira-Filho, J.T., Muratov, E.N., & Andrade, C.H. (2018). QSAR-based virtual screening: Advances and applications in drug discovery. *Frontiers in Pharmacology*, 9, 1275.

Ojeda-Montes, M.J., Casanova-Martí, A., Gimeno, A., Tomás-Hernández, S., Cereto-Massagué, A., Wolber, G., & Garcia-Vallvé, S. (2019). Mining large databases to find new leads with low similarity to known actives: Application to find new DPP-IV inhibitors. *Future Medicinal Chemistry*, 11(12), 1387–1401.

Pandita, D., & Pandita, A. (2022). Omics Technology for the Promotion of Nutraceuticals and Functional Foods. *Frontiers in Physiology*, 680.

Rybińska-Fryca, A., Sosnowska, A., & Puzyn, T. (2020). Representation of the structure—A key point of building QSAR/QSPR models for ionic liquids. *Materials*, 13(11), 2500.

Saldanha, S.N., & Tollefsbol, T.O. (2012). The role of nutraceuticals in chemoprevention and chemotherapy and their clinical outcomes. *Journal of Oncology*, 2012, 192464.

Santini, A., & Novellino, E. (2018). Nutraceuticals-shedding light on the grey area between pharmaceuticals and food. *Expert Review of Clinical Pharmacology*, 11(6), 545–547.

Schaller, D., Šribar, D., Noonan, T., Deng, L., Nguyen, T.N., Pach, S., & Wolber, G. (2020). Next generation 3D pharmacophore modeling. *Wiley Interdisciplinary Reviews: Computational Molecular Science*, 10(4), e1468.

Schneidman-Duhovny, D., Dror, O., Inbar, Y., Nussinov, R., & Wolfson, H.J. (2008). PharmaGist: A webserver for ligand-based pharmacophore detection. *Nucleic Acids Research*, 36(2), W223–W228.

Sorokina, M., Merseburger, P., Rajan, K., Yirik, M.A., & Steinbeck, C. (2021). COCONUT online: Collection of open natural products database. *Journal of Cheminformatics*, 13(1), 1–13.

Sterling, T., & Irwin, J.J. (2015). ZINC 15–ligand discovery for everyone. *Journal of Chemical Information and Modeling*, 55(11), 2324–2337.

Su, M., Yang, Q., Du, Y., Feng, G., Liu, Z., Li, Y., & Wang, R. (2018). Comparative assessment of scoring functions: The CASF-2016 update. *Journal of Chemical Information and Modeling*, 59(2), 895–913.

Tao, X., Huang, Y., Wang, C., Chen, F., Yang, L., Ling, L., & Chen, X. (2020). Recent developments in molecular docking technology applied in food science: A review. *International Journal of Food Science & Technology*, 55(1), 33–45.

Trott, O., & Olson, A.J. (2010). AutoDock Vina: Improving the speed and accuracy of docking with a new scoring function, efficient optimization, and multithreading. *Journal of Computational Chemistry*, 31(2), 455–461.

Van Santen, J.A., Jacob, G., Singh, A.L., Aniebok, V., Balunas, M.J., Bunsko, D., & Linington, R.G. (2019). The natural products atlas: An open access knowledge base for microbial natural products discovery. *ACS Central Science*, 5(11), 1824–1833.

Xing, J., Kirby, B.J., Whittington, D., Wan, Y., & Goodlett, D.R. (2012). Evaluation of P450 inhibition and induction by artemisinin antimalarials in human liver microsomes and primary human hepatocytes. *Drug Metab Dispos*, 40(9), 1757–64. doi:10.1124/dmd.112.045765. Epub 2012 Jun 7.

Yang, S.Y. (2010). Pharmacophore modeling and applications in drug discovery: challenges and recent advances. *Drug Discovery Today*, 15(11-12), 444–450.

Yoshida, T., Maruyama, T., Miura, M., Inoue, M., Fukuda, K., Shimazu, K., & Shibata, H. (2018). Dietary intake of pyrolyzed deketene curcumin inhibits gastric carcinogenesis. *Journal of Functional Foods*, 50, 192–200.

14 Nanotechnology-Based Approaches Applied to Nutraceuticals in Connection with its Legal Aspects

Kavita Srivastava, Lily Srivastava,
Sachidanand Singh, Hiral S. Desai, and Tanvi Jain

14.1 INTRODUCTION OF NUTRACEUTICALS

In 1989, DeFelice combined the words "nutrition" and "pharmaceutical" to create the term "nutraceutical," which was first used to describe a food or component of a diet that has health benefits, such as the ability to prevent or treat disease (Kalra 2003).

A nutraceutical can be an ingredient in a food, such as omega-3 oil from salmon, or it can be a food that is naturally high in nutrients, such as spirulina, soy or garlic. They are additionally known as nutritional supplements, dietary supplements, and medical foods. It comprises isolated nutrients, nutritional supplements, designer nutrients that are genetically altered, herbal goods, and processed foods like cereal and soups. Due to their alleged safety and potential nutritional and therapeutic properties, they have attracted a lot of interest.

Nutraceuticals are utilised in pharmaceutical formulations, such as capsules, tablets, liquids, or drops, and offer physiological effects. They are based on food as well as herbal or other natural items. All of these properties are primarily intended to enhance health and lower the chance of illness. Over time, nutraceuticals have proven a number of positive impacts on human health, including the treatment of arthritis, inflammation, diabetes, cholesterol, and a number of other illnesses (Paolino et al. 2021).

Unfortunately, while being all-natural, nutraceuticals have numerous limitations and shortcomings. Poor targeting, poor solubility, low permeability, rapid metabolism, and other difficulties may be present in nutraceuticals. Due to these drawbacks, researchers have been motivated to discover and develop new methods for improving the bioavailability, pharmacokinetics, and efficacy of these drugs (Asghar et al. 2018).

Furthermore, the use of nanotechnology emerges as a promising method for improving the stability, bioavailability, absorption, and controlled release of nutrients and nutraceuticals, thereby enhancing health benefits. Effective encapsulation and

 DOI: 10.1201/9781003392934-14

skillful delivery and release from a nanoformulation are examples of potential benefits of applying nanotechnology to nutraceuticals. Additionally, research is ongoing to boost the absorption and therapeutic potential of nutraceuticals by encapsulating them in biodegradable, ecologically friendly nanocarriers. In order to ensure safety and efficacy when used to manage health disorders, particularly for individuals who are ineligible for a standard pharmaceutical therapy, the nano-nutraceutical formulations represent a helpful and promising technique (Durazzo et al. 2020).

When nano-nutraceuticals are produced and used, there is yet another challenge. Through the water, air, and soil, nanomaterials constantly are at risk of getting into the food chain. Cell death, cell membrane breakdown, and DNA damage could all result from this. There hasn't been much focus in in-vivo research to date on the effects of nano nutraceuticals on the health of humans and animals.

Utilizing these nanotechnologies can therefore significantly improve food production and product quality, which will benefit human health and wellbeing if handled and properly regulated (Nile et al. 2020). Therefore, factors like efficiency, quality, and safety should be taken into account. However, more research is still needed on the regulatory front regarding nano-nutraceuticals. This chapter aims to present a fair assessment of the opportunities and advantages that nanotechnology can be predicted to offer to the food industry, as well as any potential risks connected to these novel materials and applications. Additionally, it expresses concern about significant social and legal issues.

14.2 NUTRACEUTICALS AND ITS BENEFITS

Due to their numerous positive effects, nutritional supplements have been used to treat and prevent a wide range of illnesses, including diabetes, obesity, cancer, inflammation, hypertension, and other cardiovascular diseases. Some nutraceuticals are utilised in the treatment and prevention of steatosis, including silymarin, curcumin, docosahexaenoic acid, vitamin E, choline, and phosphatidylcholine. Numerous nutritional supplements, including curcumin, gallic acid, caffeine, and others, also have antioxidant and anti-aging properties. Fish oils high in PUFA1 improve brain functioning and lessen the risk of coronary cardiovascular disorders. Because of the anticancer effectiveness of nutraceuticals, many of its constituents, including pomegranate, curcumin, and epigallocatechin gallate, are used to treat many cancers, including prostate cancer, breast cancer, and other types of cancer (Helal et al. 2019). The natural nutraceuticals are listed in Table 14.1. Incorporating these nutraceuticals into one's diet may help promote overall wellness and prevent chronic diseases.

14.3 NEED FOR NOVEL NUTRACEUTICAL DELIVERY METHOD

Nutraceuticals have been proven to have fewer toxicity and adverse effects when used to treat diseases and symptoms. They can increase resistance to various diseases and promote good health. However, because the majority of studies have been in vitro, it is now necessary to develop and identify oral delivery methods that can survive in a daily setting (Ting et al. 2014). Oral administration of nutraceuticals is practical and cost-effective for patients with chronic diseases.

TABLE 14.1
Lists of Various Natural Nutraceuticals and their Advantages

Nutraceutical	Active Ingredient	Pharmacological Property	Reference
Natural Honey	**Sugar**	**Antimicrobial, Antioxidant, In treatment of eye diseases, Ulcers**	Ajibola et al. 2012
Red yeast rice,	**monacolin k**	**Dyslipidaemia**	Cimaglia, et al. 2019
citrus peel	**phenolic compounds**	**Antioxidant, diabetes, hypertension**	Singh et al. 2020
Fatty fish	**Omega-3 PUFAs**	**cardiovascular diseases, bipolar depression, asthma, and diabetes.**	Bowen et al. 2016
Cloves	**Eugenol**	**antiseptic, antioxidant, antimutagenic, anticancer effect**	Jaganathan and Supriyanto 2012
Traditional Chinese Medicine (TCM)	**Polysaccharide**	**Anticancer**	Chang 2002
Green tea	**Epigallocatechin Gallate (EGCG)**	**Antioxidative, hypolipidemic effects**	Hong et al. 2014

However, due to their complex chemical compositions, their biological availability is limited. The gastrointestinal tract (GI) encounters more difficulties in absorbing nutraceuticals due to various human body conditions. The rapid absorption of these components through the intestine's active metabolism leads to changes in their chemical composition and bioactive properties (McClements and Li 2010).

Various delivery techniques have been developed to improve bioavailability. Nanotechnology offers novel methods to improve biorecognition, immunogenicity, nonspecific toxicity, pharmacodynamics, pharmacokinetics, and effectiveness of nutraceutical properties. Nano-based formulation approaches have improved the bioavailability and absorption of drugs orally. They also improve the therapeutic properties of nutraceuticals and bio-accessibility/bioavailability of natural bioactive substances or extracts (Asghar et al. 2018). However, it is crucial to note that the substance used in delivery systems must be generally recognized as safe (GRAS) to avoid harmful side effects like toxicity and physical injury (Pouton 2000).

14.4 NANOTECHNOLOGY AS A PROMISING, NOVEL TOOL FOR NUTRACEUTICAL DELIVERY

Nanotechnology is a branch of science, technology, and engineering that operates at the nanoscale, ranging from 1 to 100 nanometres. These particles are more easily absorbed into the body, providing greater health benefits with smaller doses. Nanotechnology is an exciting and rapidly developing area of research and development, with the potential to enhance safety and quality of life, ultimately improving human health (Javeri 2016).

14.5 POTENTIAL USES OF NANOTECHNOLOGY IN NUTRACEUTICALS

Nanotechnology has the potential to improve the flavor, absorption, and bioavailability of nutritional supplements and nutraceuticals. Nanosized ingredients and additives, such as vitamins, antioxidants, and preservatives, can be used to create functional food products. For example, green tea beverages containing nanoselenium can lower inflammation, combat free radicals, enhance the immune system, and reduce cancer risk. Nanoencapsulation, a process that involves packing materials at the nanoscale, allows for controlled core release, longer shelf life, increased stability, simultaneous delivery of active ingredients, and pH-triggered controlled release. Nanodelivery systems incorporate functional elements like antioxidants, vitamins, carotenoids, probiotics, omega fatty acids, preservatives, peptides, proteins, carbohydrates, and lipids. Nanoliposomes and nano-cochleates are promising lipid-based carriers for antioxidants. Nanoliposomes also offer controlled and targeted distribution of nutraceuticals, enzymes, minerals, vitamins, additives, and antimicrobials (Mozafari et al. 2008).

14.6 NANO FORMULATIONS USED IN NUTRACEUTICALS

Nanoformulations in nutraceuticals include nanoemulsions, liposomes, solid lipid nanoparticles (SLNs), nanostructure lipid carriers (NLCs), nanospheres and nanocapsules, pH-responsive formulations, nano-hydrogel, composite colloidal nanoparticles, self-assembly nanoparticles, and dendrimers (Singh et al. 2022). The potential use of nano-formulation in the delivery of nutraceuticals is briefly described in Table 14.2.

14.7 LIMITATIONS OF NANOMATERIALS IN NUTRACEUTICALS

Advancements in nanoparticles (NPs) in diagnostics, engineering, medication, and nutraceutical delivery have a negative impact on the environment and must be carefully evaluated. The exposure of which plays a crucial role in interactions between NPs, macromolecules, and organelles, potentially harming cells. Therefore, careful evaluation is necessary to mitigate their negative environmental impact. Cell death, genotoxicity, immunotoxicity, oxidative stress, and cytotoxicity are all possible effects of NPs. One of the most often utilised nanoparticles (NPs) in the food business is TiO_2 nanoparticles. TiO_2 nanoparticles are used as anti-caking agents and antimicrobial plastic packaging. Most in vitro experiments using TiO_2 nanoparticles reveal elevated amounts of DNA breaks, and in some experiments, oxidised DNA lesions (Magdolenova et al. 2014).

14.8 GLOBAL ASPECTS ON REGULATION OF NANOTECHNOLOGY IN NUTRACEUTICALS

To guarantee the safety of the nanofood products now on the market, regulatory guidance offers safe pathways for makers, importers, and users to follow. Each stage of creating, processing, packaging, and consuming food products containing

TABLE 14.2
Overview of the Potential Application of Nano-Formulation in the Delivery of Nutraceuticals

Nutraceuticals	Pharmacological Activity	Nanoformulation	Reference
β-Carotene	improving vision and treating vitamin A deficiency	Nanoemulsion	Luo et al. 2017
curcumin	Antioxidant	Polymeric nanoparticles in conjugation with chitosan	Hu et al. 2018
Black Soybean Seed Coat Extract (BSSCE)	antioxidant activity	pH-responsive chitosan film	Wang et al. 2019
Curcumin	antioxidant	Composite-colloidal nanoparticles	Sun et al. 2017
Omega-3 PUFAs	colorectal cancer, reduce the level of lipids in serum	Solid Lipid Nanoparticles	Serini et al. 2018
Rutin	antioxidant, anti-inflammatory, anticancer, antiviral, hypolipidemic	Nanostructured-Lipid Carriers (NLCs)	Babazadeh et al. 2016
Genistein	antioxidant, anti-inflammatory	Enzymatically synthesized dextran nanoparticles	Semyonov et al. 2014
Acylethanolamides	prevention or treatment of alcohol dependence syndrome, alcohol poisoning, and pathological intoxication.	Nanocapsules,	Orío et al. 2017
Oleuropein, tyrosol, hydroxytyrosol	antioxidant activities	Liposome	Larussa et al. 2017
Resveratrol	Anti-cancer	Solid Lipid nanoparticles, Nanostructure Lipid Carriers	Neves et al. 2016

nanoparticles should take health and safety considerations into account. However, there is no unique law that is applicable everywhere that addresses the regulatory implications of using nanomaterials in industries that deal with food. In addition, several nations have no laws at all governing the evaluation of the safety of nanoproducts. The primary challenges restricting the potential market of nanoproducts created via the quickly developing technology are a lack of standards for correct handling and an inadequate understanding of assessing risk for the environment and human health. Need of time, before being approved for usage, food additives and substances created using nanotechnology must pass a safety evaluation.

14.8.1 The United States

The US Department of Agriculture first addressed nanotechnology in the food and agriculture industries in 2003 (U.S. DOA 2003). The FDA is responsible for regulating new technology in food applications, while the EPA identified six common industrial nanomaterials for research. In 2016, the FDA published draft guidance on submitting notifications for new dietary ingredients (USFDA 2014a).

According to Section 402(f) of the FD&C Act (21 U.S.C. 342(f)), a dietary supplement that contains a new dietary ingredient is deemed adulterated unless it has been presented to the Food and Drug Administration (FDA) with evidence that the ingredient has been used as a dietary supplement for a period of time sufficient to establish its safety prior to marketing. It is mentioned that the document containing safety data is evaluated by the FDA within 75 days of the anticipated marketing date for new dietary ingredients (NDI) in the US (USFDA 2014b). If more safety information is needed to ensure the safe use of the NDI, the FDA may request it from the producer. Guidelines about the notification process and information needs are available. The FDA states that modified traditional foods and food additives, including those utilising nanotechnology, must be assessed as NDI. All food and substances in nanoform must therefore be regarded as NDI. NMs used in new dietary supplements are assessed according to the current regulations, but specific premarket review (i.e., registration) procedures may need more information on safety or efficacy, as appropriate (USFDA 2015). In order to avoid confusion when determining whether food or food ingredients are NMs eligible for NDI process approval, the FDA recommends producers share information with the agency on safety issues before marketing a product (USFDA 2015).

14.8.2 Canada

Health Canada and the Canadian Food Inspection Agency have established standards for nanomaterials in nutraceuticals, using the current regulatory system. They recommend addressing nanotechnology-specific issues through pre-submission meetings, discussing intended use, manufacturing processes, characterization, physicochemical properties, and toxicological, eco-toxicological, and metabolic information. This will help ensure the safety and efficacy of nanomaterials in nutraceuticals. (Health Canada 2011).

14.8.3 Europe

An exclusive regulatory framework for nanomaterials was developed by the European Union in 2004 in response to biosafety concerns regarding nanomaterials. The European Commission has created strategic action plans and entities for the uses of nanoscience and nanotechnology (Regulation (EU) No 257/2010).

The European Commission rule (Regulation (EU) No. 1935/2004) mandates that labels for products containing nanomaterials be required. The prospective risks of nanoparticles employed in industrial products were noted in "Guidance on the Risk Assessment of the Application of Nanoscience and Nanotechnologies in the Food and Feed Chain" published by the European Food Safety Authority (EFSA). Determining the physicochemical features, surface shape, chemical composition, and probable exposure levels of certain materials is also necessary for risk assessment (EFSA 2011).

According to European commission 2013 in "Proposal for a regulation of the European parliament and of the council on novel foods", all food ingredients that are comprised of engineered nanomaterials must be disclosed on the label of food products (European Commission 2013).

14.8.4 India

The Food Safety and Standards Act governs food safety in India (FSSAI). In 2007, the Indian government established the Mission on Nano Science and Technology (Nano Mission) to promote the field. The government established a Nanoregulatory Task Force to provide guidelines and best practices for safe handling of nanomaterials in research laboratories and industries. The guidelines are based on published publications by regulatory organizations such as the International Organization of Standard (ISO), Organization for Economic Cooperation and Development (OECD), National Institute for Occupational Safety and Health (NIOSH), Occupational Safety and Health Administration (OSHA). The Centre for Knowledge Management of Nanoscience and Technology (CKMNT) prepared the guidelines under the direction of the Nano Mission and Nanoregulatory Task Force. The document addresses potential risks and secure handling procedures of nanomaterials, ensuring societal benefits and environmentally friendly use. Comparing laws governing nutraceutical formulation in different countries is crucial for companies entering the global market, helping them understand regulatory requirements and comply with them. Table 14.3 presents a summary of the legal frameworks that each country has in place for the establishment of nutraceuticals.

14.9 CONCLUSION

This chapter discussed the rising interest of people in nutraceutical compounds obtained from naturally occurring sources, such as plants or food, as well as the significance of the positive effects of nutraceuticals on human health. Nutraceuticals' poor water solubility and physicochemical instability in environmental circumstances serve as the principal barriers to their usage. Nanotechnology has the potential to address each of these issues (Paolino et al. 2021). However, there is a need for more research in the advancement of nanotechnology, as well as access to potential environmental and health risks. The government of India is very supportive and has taken several initiatives to promote research in the field of nanotechnology as an example of 'Nanomission'. Furthermore, as developed nations like the United States and Europe have done, it is essential that Indian regulatory agencies establish procedures to evaluate the risks of nanoparticles in the food industry. The Indian government should also provide adequate funding and resources for the advancement of nanotechnology research in the food industry.

TABLE 14.3
Overview of the Laws Governing the Formulation of Nutraceuticals in Various Countries

Country	Regulatory Agency	Regulation	Online Resources	Provision and comment
USA	**Food and Drug Administration (FDA) & US-Environmental Protection Agency (US-EPA)**	**Federal Food, Drug, and Cosmetic Act (FFDCA)** **Federal Insecticide, Fungicide, and Rodenticide Act (FIFRA)**	1. https://www.fda.gov/regulatory-information/laws-enforced-fda/federal-food-drug-and-cosmetic-act-fdc-act 2. https://www.epa.gov/enforcement/federal-insecticide-fungicide-and-rodenticide-act-fifra-and-federal-facilities	**No specifications on nano-products in FFDCA of FIFRA**
Canada	**Canadian Food Inspection Agency (CFIA)** **Public Health Agency of Canada (PHAC)**	**Food and Drugs Act**	1. https://www.canada.ca/en/health-canada/services/drugs-health-products/nanotechnology-based-health-products-food.html 2. https://laws-lois.justice.gc.ca/eng/regulations/c.r.c.,_c._870/index.html	**Nano-products are regulated under existing legislation but No nano specific regulatory framework**
EU	**European Commission (EC)** **European Parliament and Council**	1. **Regulation on the provision of food information to consumers (1169/2011)** 2. **Regulation on plastic food contact materials and articles (10/2011)** 3. **Regulation on active and intelligent materials and articles (450/2009)** 4. **The biocidal products regulation (528/2012)** 5. **The cosmetic products regulation (1223/2009)**	1. https://eur-lex.europa.eu/LexUriServ/LexUriServ.do?uri=OJ:L:2011:304:0018:0063:en:PDF#:~:text=matter%20and%20scope-,1.,functioning%20of%20the%20internal%20market. 2. https://eur-lex.europa.eu/LexUriServ/LexUriServ.do?uri=OJ:L:2011:012:0001:0089:en:PDF 3. https://eur-lex.europa.eu/LexUriServ/LexUriServ.do?uri=OJ:L:2009:135:0003:0011:EN:PDF 4. https://eur-lex.europa.eu/legal-content/EN/TXT/PDF/?uri=CELEX:32012R0528	**These legislations have nano specific provisions. But no exclusive NM legislation** **EU taking the initiative to regulate nanoproducts.**

(Continued)

TABLE 14.3 (Continued)
Overview of the Laws Governing the Formulation of Nutraceuticals in Various Countries

Country	Regulatory Agency	Regulation	Online Resources	Provision and comment
		6. **Registration, Evaluation, Authorization and Restriction of Chemicals (REACH) regulation (1907/2006)**	5. https://health.ec.europa.eu/system/files/2016-11/cosmetic_1223_2009_regulation_en_0.pdf 6. https://eur-lex.europa.eu/LexUriServ/LexUriServ.do?uri=OJ:L:2007:136:0003:0280:en:PDF	
Australia and New Zealand	**Food standards Australia New Zealand (FSANZ)**	**Australian New Zealand Food Standards Code**	1. https://www.foodstandards.gov.au/code/Pages/default.aspx 2. http://www.nicnas.gov.au/communications/issues/nanomaterials-nanotechnology/nicnas-regulatoryactivities-in-nanomaterials 3. http://www.foodstandards.gov.au/consumer/foodtech/nanotech/pages/default.aspx	**Amended FSANZ Application Handbook to support new food regulations to manage risks from nanoproducts.** **The first regulatory program for "industrial nanomaterials" was introduced by the National Industrial Chemicals Notification and Assessment Scheme (NICNAS)**
China	**Ministry of Agriculture Ministry of Health**	**Food Safety Law of China**	1. http://en.nim.ac.cn/ 2. http://en.nim.ac.cn/division/overview/924	**National Centre for Nanoscience and Technology (NCNST) and the commission on nanotechnology standardization**
Japan	**Ministry of Health, Labour and Welfare**	**Food Sanitation Law**	1. http://www.mhlw.go.jp/english/policy/health-medical/food/index.html 2. http://www.jetro.go.jp/en/reports/regulations/	**No NM-specific legislation**
India	**Food Safety and Standards Authority of India**	**Food Safety and Standards Act (2006)**	1. https://fssai.gov.in/upload/uploadfiles/files/Nutraceuticals_Regulations.pdf	**DST Nano mission has come up with safe handling of NMs in workplace and industry.**

There is a need for better environmental risk and life cycle assessment, as well as defined sustainability goals, in the governance of technical innovation in the field of nanotechnology.

REFERENCES

Ajibola, A. et al. (2012). Nutraceuticals values of natural honey and its contribution to human health and wealth. *Nutrition & Metabolism*, 9, 61.

Asghar, A., Randhawa, M.A., Masood, M.M. et al. (2018). Nutraceutical formulation strategies to enhance the bioavailability and efficiency: An overview. In A.M. Grumezescu, and A.M. Holben (eds.) *Role of Materials Science in Food Bioengineering*, 329–352. Academic Press.

Babazadeh, A. et al. (2016). Novel nanostructured lipid carriers as a promising food grade delivery system for rutin. *Journal of Functional Foods*, 26, 167–175.

Bowen, K.J. (2016). Omega-3 fatty acids and cardiovascular disease: Are there benefits *Current Treatment Options in Cardiovascular Medicine* 18(11), 69.

Chang, R. (2002). Bioactive polysaccharides from traditional Chinese medicine herbs as anticancer adjuvants. *The Journal of Alternative and Complementary Medicine*, 8(5), 559–565.

Cimaglia, P. et al. (2019). Effectiveness of a novel nutraceutical compound containing red yeast rice, polymethoxyflavones and antioxidants in the modulation of cholesterol levels in subjects with hypercholesterolemia and low-moderate cardiovascular risk: The NIRVANA study. *Frontiers in Physiology*, 10, 217.

Durazzo, A. et al. (2020). An updated overview on nanonutraceuticals: Focus on nanoprebiotics and nanoprobiotics. *International Journal of Molecular Science*, 21(7), 2285. doi: 10.3390/ijms21072285. PMID: 32225036; PMCID: PMC7177810.

EFSA (2011). Scientific Opinion: Guidance on the risk assessment of the application of nanoscience and nanotechnologies in the food and feed chain. *EFSA Journal*, 9(5), 2140–2176.

European Commission (2013). Proposal for a regulation of the European parliament and of the council on novel foods. COM (2013) 894 final. https://eur-lex.europa.eu/legal-content/EN/TXT/?uri=CELEX%3A52013PC0894 (accessed December 25, 2022)

Health Canada, (2011). Nanotechnology-based health products and food. http://www.hc-sc.gc.ca/dhp-mps/nano-eng.php. (accessed January 3, 2023)

Helal, N.A. et al. (2019). Nutraceuticals' novel formulations: The good, the bad, the unknown and patents involved. *Recent Patents on Drug Delivery & Formulation*, 13(2), 105–156.

Hong, Z. et al. (2014). Improving the effectiveness of (-)-epigallocatechin gallate (EGCG) against rabbit atherosclerosis by EGCG-loaded nanoparticles prepared from chitosan and polyaspartic acid. *Journal of Agricultural and Food Chemistry*, 62(52), 12603–12609. https://eur-lex.europa.eu/LexUriServ/LexUriServ.do?uri=OJ:L:2010:080:0019:0027:EN:PDF (accessed December 23, 2022)

Hu, Q. et al. (2018). Biocompatible polymeric nanoparticles with exceptional gastrointestinal stability as oral delivery vehicles for lipophilic bioactives. *Food Hydrocolloids*, 89, 386–395.

Jaganathan, S.K., & Supriyanto, E. (2012). Antiproliferative and molecular mechanism of eugenol-induced apoptosis in cancer cells. *Molecules*, 17(6), 6290–6304.

Javeri, I. (2016). Application of "nano" nutraceuticals in medicine. In R.C. Gupta (ed.) *Nutraceuticals*, 189–192. Academic Press.

Kalra, E.K. (2003). Nutraceutical-definition and introduction. *American Association of Pharmaceutical Scientists*, 5(3), E25. https://doi.org/10.1208/ps050325

Larussa, T. et al. (2017). Oleuropein decreases cyclooxygenase-2 and interleukin-17 expression and attenuates inflammatory damage in colonic samples from ulcerative colitis patients. *Nutrients*, 9, 391.

Luo, X. et al. (2017). Fabrication of beta-carotene nanoemulsion-based delivery systems using dual-channel microfluidization: Physical and chemical stability. *Journal of Colloid and Interface Science*, 490, 328–335.

Magdolenova, Z., et al. (2014). Mechanisms of genotoxicity. Review of recent in vitro and in vivo studies with engineered nanoparticles. *Nanotoxicology*, 8, 233–278

McClements, D.J. and Li, Y. (2010). Review of in vitro digestion models for rapid screening of emulsion-based systems. *Food and Function*, 1(1), 32–59.

Mozafari, M.R.et al. (2008). Nanoliposomes and their applications in food nanotechnology. *Journal of Liposome Research*, 18 (4), 309–327.

Neves, A.R. et al. (2016). Nanoscale delivery of resveratrol towards enhancement of supplements and nutraceuticals. *Nutrients*, 8(3), 131.

Nile, S.H. (2020). Nanotechnologies in food science: Applications, recent trends, and future perspectives. *Nano-Micro Letters*, 12(1), 45.

Orío, O.L. et al. (2017). Compositions for the prevention and/or treatment of alcohol use disorders. WO2017178682A1. https://patents.google.com/patent/WO2017178682A1/en

Paolino, D. et al. (2021). Nanonutraceuticals: The new frontier of supplementary food. *Nanomaterials(Basel)*, 11(3), 792.

Pouton, C.W. (2000). Lipid formulations for oral administration of drugs: Non-emulsifying, self-emulsifying and 'self-microemulsifying' drug delivery systems. *European Journal of Pharmaceutical Sciences: Official Journal of the European Federation for Pharmaceutical Sciences*, 11, S93–S98.

Semyonov, D. et al. (2014). Enzymatically synthesized dextran nanoparticles and their use as carriers for nutraceuticals. *Food & Function*, 5(10), 2463–2474.

Serini, S. et al. (2018). Omega-3 PUFA loaded in resveratrol-based solid lipid nanoparticles: Physicochemical properties and antineoplastic activities in human colorectal cancer cells in vitro. *International Journal of Molecular Science*, 19(2), 586.

Singh, A.R. et al. (2022). Nanotechnology-based approaches applied to nutraceuticals. *Drug Delivery and Translational Research*, 12(3), 485–499.

Singh, B. et al. (2020). Phenolic composition, antioxidant potential and health benefits of citrus peel. *Food Research International*, 132, 109114.

Sun, C. et al. (2017). Preparation, characterization and stability of curcumin-loaded zein-shellac composite colloidal particles. *Food Chemistry*, 228, 656–667

Ting, Y. et al. (2014). Common delivery systems for enhancing in vivo bioavailability and biological efficacy of nutraceuticals. *Journal of Functional Foods*, 7, 112–128.

US DOA. (2003). *"Nanoscale Science and Engineering for Agriculture and Food Systems: A Report Submitted to Cooperative State Research, Education and Extension Service."* Washington, DC: Department of Agriculture (2003).

US FDA, (2014a). New dietary ingredients in dietary supplements—background for industry. https://www.fda.gov/food/new-dietary-ingredients-ndi-notification-process/new-dietary-ingredients-dietary-supplements-background-industry (accessed November 15, 2022.

US FDA (2014b). Label claims for conventional foods and dietary supplements. https://www.fda.gov/food/food-labeling-nutrition/label-claims-conventional-foods-and-dietary-supplements. (accessed November 15, 2022).

US FDA (2015). FDA's approach to regulation of nanotechnology products. https://www.fda.gov/science-research/nanotechnology-programs-fda/fdas-approach-regulation-nanotechnology-products.(accessed November 16, 2022).

Wang, X. et al. (2019). Preparation and characterization of antioxidant and pH-sensitive films based on chitosan and black soybean seed coat extract. *Food Hydrocolloids*, 89, 56–66.

15 Role of Nutraceuticals in Maintaining Oral and Periodontal Health

Garima Singh, Ashish Thakur, Dheeraj Chitara, and Prashant Kumar

15.1 INTRODUCTION

Dental caries and periodontal disease rank among the world's most common and significant health issues. The multifactorial disease known as periodontitis is influenced by the complex and soft tissues, microbial colonisation (with or without invasion), inflammatory reactions, and adaptive immune responses.

Our ability to understand the vital protective functions in the tissues has been hampered by the complexity of the local tissue components, which include bacteria and their products and nearly all facets of host defence mechanisms. Additionally, the complexity of these components has repeatedly shown that host destructive factors may be the disease's primary causative factors. Non-surgical and surgical therapy for periodontal disease are standard treatment options. These methods focus primarily on mechanical debridement and are frequently combined with antibiotics (Gupta 2011). Antimicrobial medications that cause gastrointestinal side effects owing to broad-spectrum antibiotics, bacterial resistance, and allergic responses may be needed to treat certain disorders or their consequences. Because of this, numerous authors have suggested alternate treatments that can deliver positive outcomes without harming the patient. Probiotics are non-pathogenic living microorganisms that improve the host's health when given in sufficient quantity through food or dietary supplements (Maria Seminario-Amez et al. 2017).

Maintaining oral and periodontal health is difficult today because of the numerous risk factors for periodontal disease, including alcohol, stress, smoking, genetics, diabetes, and hormonal changes (such as menopause or pregnancy). This is further complicated because periodontal disease can also be a risk factor for several chronic diseases. It is widely acknowledged that periodontitis is inextricably linked to several chronic conditions, including rheumatoid arthritis, inflammatory bowel disease, type 2 diabetes mellitus (DM2), and cardiovascular disorders. Consequently, the connection between oral health and systemic health is gaining attention (Alfonso Varela-López et al. 2018).

A new diet health paradigm that emphasises the advantages of diet has recently begun to emerge. People's fundamental eating habits have changed due to their

DOI: 10.1201/9781003392934-15

adopted lifestyles. The use of junk food has multiplied, causing several ailments brought on by inadequate nutrition. Obesity is currently acknowledged as a significant global problem. Heart disease, followed by cancer, osteoporosis, arthritis, and many other conditions, is the leading cause of mortality in most developing nations globally. Consumers are looking for complementary or alternative helpful items because they are fed up with current medications' pricey, high-tech, disease-treating approach. The new class of natural goods known as nutraceuticals blurs the distinction between food and medicine (Adelaja and Schilling 1999). Although individuals have used nutraceuticals for a long time, only recently have they begun to show promise based on scientifically validated nutritional and medicinal evidence (Dillard and German 2000). The future development of novel food products is made possible by the nutraceuticals of both animal and plant origin. Nutritional research is currently concentrating on analysing foods for their ability to protect against and prevent disease instead of unfavourable characteristics, including the number of microorganisms, additives, fats, and inorganic contaminants (Kaur and Kapoor 2001). This chapter focuses on the overall idea and health-promoting effects of different nutraceuticals that may be added to the diet. Thus, this editorial provides information about these nutraceuticals and outlines their many functions in treating periodontal and oral illnesses.

15.2 WHAT ARE NUTRACEUTICALS?

The term "nutraceutical" is a combination of "nutrition" and "pharmaceutical." Nutraceuticals are foods or components of foods that significantly alter and sustain the normal physiological function necessary to keep healthy humans alive. The present demographic and health trends are the main drivers of the global nutraceutical market's expansion. Dietary fibre, prebiotics, probiotics, polyunsaturated fatty acids, antioxidants, and other diverse kinds of herbal/natural foods are some food products used as nutraceuticals. These nutraceuticals help combat some of the biggest health problems of the era, including overweight, coronary heart disease, malignancy, osteoporosis, joint problems, diabetes mellitus, and cholesterol. Overall, the term "nutraceutical" has ushered in a new era of medicine and health, one in which the food industry has evolved into a field focused on research. Stephen De Felice, the founder of the Foundation for Innovation in Medicine (FIM), Cranford, NJ, developed the phrase "nutraceutical" from the words "nutrition" and "pharmaceutical" in 1989 (Maddi et al. 2007). A food (or component of food) that offers medical or health benefits, such as the prevention and treatment of a disease, is referred to as a nutraceutical in De Felice's definition. Nutraceuticals, on the other hand, are described by Health Canada as "a product derived from foods but offered in the form of pills, or powder (potions), or other therapeutic forms, not normally associated with foods." Products containing nutraceuticals are produced by the herbal and dietary supplement market, the food industry, the pharmaceutical manufacturers, and the recently integrated pharmaceutical/ agribusiness/ nutrition conglomerates. It could include isolated nutrients, herbal products, nutritional supplements, diets, and processed meals like cereals, soups, and beverages that have been genetically modified (Malik 2008).

The majority of therapeutic aspects are covered by nutraceuticals, including the treatment of diabetes, depression problems, osteoporosis, elevated blood pressure, high cholesterol levels, depression, cold sores, sleep disorders, digestive issues, and the prevention of some cancers (Pandey et al. 2010; Sami Labs 2002). Herbal/natural goods, dietary supplements, and functional foods are the three primary areas of the nutraceutical industry, according to Rishi and Hathcock (Rishi 2006; Hathcock 2001). Herbal/natural items and dietary supplements are two of these that are expanding the fastest. The global market for dietary supplements increased to $74.7 billion in 2007 from $46.7 billion in 2002. (BCC Research). USA, the UK, and Japan are the top three nations with nutraceutical markets (BCC Research) (Lipi Das et al. 2012).

Compounds obtained from fruits and vegetables are the most often utilised nutraceuticals. They frequently contain substances with antioxidant or anti-inflammatory qualities that are said to offer defence against long-term conditions like osteoporosis, cancer, diabetes, and cardiovascular disease. Flavonoid plant pigments like anthocyanins from berries, flavanols from dark chocolate, polyphenols like resveratrol from red grapes, and catechins from tea and quercetin are examples of widely used nutraceuticals. The active catechol in green tea extract, EGCG, commonly thought to be responsible for green tea's antioxidant benefits, has metabolites that may increase oxidative stress and have been linked to liver damage. The nutraceutical flavonoids that have been the most thoroughly investigated are the soy-derived isoflavones genistein and daidzein, as well as the daidzein metabolite equol (Kumar et al. 2022).

Although the form in which they are provided may be the same, nutraceuticals are different from dietary supplements and other food supplements according to their definition (e.g., pills, tablets, capsules, or liquid). The following list of key differences can be distilled: (i) Nutraceuticals are intended for use as a conventional food or as an item of meal or diet; (ii) Nutraceuticals are active substances extracted from vegetal (as phytocomplexes) or animal origin food concentrated and administered in a suitable pharmaceutical form; (iii) Scientific evidence has substantiated the effectiveness of nutraceuticals; (iv) nutraceuticals are intended for use as a conventional food or as an item of meal or diet. (v) Food supplements are formulations, frequently multicomponent, micronutrient based, comprising dietary elements, such as vitamins, minerals, amino acids, or other botanical or dietary compounds, but are not expressly designed to prevent and/or treat a health concern; (vii) Food supplements, probiotics, and/or herbal products do not necessarily need to possess a clinically proven efficacy on a specific health condition but can help to prevent illness or provide micronutrients as an integral part of a diet (Antonello Santini and Ettore Novellino 2017).

15.3 TYPES OF NUTRACEUTICALS

The use of nutraceuticals is expanding quickly and is well-received by the public due to their all-natural origin. Although they cannot wholly replace pharmaceuticals, some pathological conditions can be prevented and treated with the help of nutraceuticals. The worldwide study has concentrated on the mechanism of action, safety, and clinical data of nutraceuticals produced from either plant or animal foods. These therapeutic agents do not advertise themselves as drug alternatives but instead aim to avoid metabolic syndrome, a group of illnesses that include type 2 diabetes mellitus, cerebrovascular accident (CVA), and cardiovascular disorders. Humans have used nutritious herbal food, nutritional supplements, and nutraceuticals to substitute or do away with radiation therapy or chemotherapy due to an overwhelming desire for natural healthcare, which has significantly increased the cost of hospital treatment (Berger et al. 1996).

The use and efficacy of numerous herbal products are generally denoted by the word "nutraceutical" (Zeisel 1999). Herbal products, vitamins, protein substances, minerals, fat, fibre, and amino acids are examples of the "nutritional elements" items. The nutritional components of dietary meals can be obtained in many forms, including tablets, capsules, soft gels, gel caps, suspensions, emulsions, beverages, and powders. They can also be collections, isolates, or concentrates. Vitamin B complement is one of the nutritional meal supplements that is typically sold in pill form. Examples of nutraceuticals used in human health include tumour treatment, vitamin E, vitamin D, soy, green tea, selenium, and lycopene. This topic aims to study the function and views of nutraceuticals on an individual's health from various viewpoints, including analytical elements, clinical trials, efficacy studies, and positive effects on health problems.

Various nutraceuticals are classified according to multiple factors as fatty acids, proteins, vitamins, minerals, carbohydrates, spices, dietary fibre, probiotics, prebiotics, polyunsaturated fatty acids, polyphenols, amino acids, antioxidants, antimicrobial, antidiabetic, analgesics, anti-inflammatory, carotenoids, dairy-based components, nutritional lipids, oils, phytochemicals, plant extracts, peptides, and soy-based substances and these are all considered to be components of nutraceuticals The nutraceuticals can be divided into two categories. Nutraceuticals that are either (1) potential or (2) established nutraceuticals (Lipi 2012) (Figure 15.1).

15.3.1 Functional Ingredients

Traditional food items that have been enhanced with a substance that has the potential to improve human health are often referred to as functional foods. Functional food ingredients have been used after conferring with clinical expertise and understanding. They live a better lifestyle and have more robust survival techniques. Eating functional foods is preferred to taking medication as a tablet or

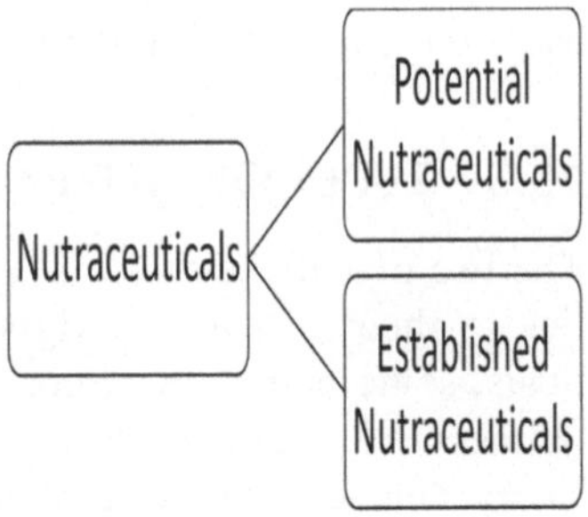

FIGURE 15.1 Types of nutraceuticals divided into two classes.

liquid. Occasionally, complementary extra nutrients are covered, such as vitamin D in milk. Functional foods are "normal foods which include components or materials that provide a specified scientific or physiological advantage, separate from a just nutritional effect," as per the Canadian Health Organisation. Japan holds that all beneficial ingredients must be present and occurring in their herbal form in place of a tablet, capsule, and powder consumed in the food plan occasionally or daily and should modify a biological system in order to prevent/control disease or disorder-like situations (Halsted 2003).

15.3.2 Medicinal Food

Clients do not receive therapeutic or clinical foods as a chip consequence. Medical nutrition, in the eyes of the Food & Drug Administration, is defined as "formulated, to be fed on or administered internally under the supervision of a physician and which is meant for the particular nutritional control of a disease or circumstance for which unique dietary requirements, based on recognised scientific ideas, are established by way of medical evaluation." The clinical food ingredients satisfy the nutritional requirements of individuals identified or observed exposed to specific pollutants and are fed orally or via a feeding tube. These ingredients are subject to FDA regulation and are approved by scientific consensus (Chandra et al. 2022).

15.4 DIET SUPPLEMENTS AND DIETARY FIBRES

The term "dietary supplement" should only be used to refer to specific substances used in the treatment or prevention of deficiencies, or when a steady supply of a nutrient is needed (for example, glucose in glycogen storage disease to prevent hypoglycaemia), or when a missing enzyme is substituted (e.g., lactase in lactose intolerance, pancreatic enzymes).

Saturated palmitic acid, stearic acid, monounsaturated oleic acid, polyunsaturated linoleic acid, and linolenic acids are essential, necessary fatty acids for human nutrition. Arachidonic acid, eicosatetraenoic acid, and docosahexaenoic acid are the fatty acids of freshly manufactured, safe, affordable, and sustainable plant origins (Wu 2005) (Figure 15.2).

15.4.1 Amino Acids

Amino acids are anti-inflammatory, immunomodulatory, and antioxidant capabilities significantly influence these processes (Lawrence et al. 2018). These are needed in protein biosynthesis and many other processes. For instance, L-arginine is necessary for the growth of infants, young children, and pregnant ladies and for the production of nitric oxide, agmatine, urea, creatine, and polyamines. Additionally helpful, it has antiproliferative and antihypertensive effects on the smooth muscles of the blood vessels. Glutamate is essential for metabolic stress, burn damage, muscle atrophy, weight loss, and other infections with low plasma levels. It has been demonstrated that increasing the number of amino acids in staple foods like rice, wheat, corn, and various flora helps patients and lowers the death rate.

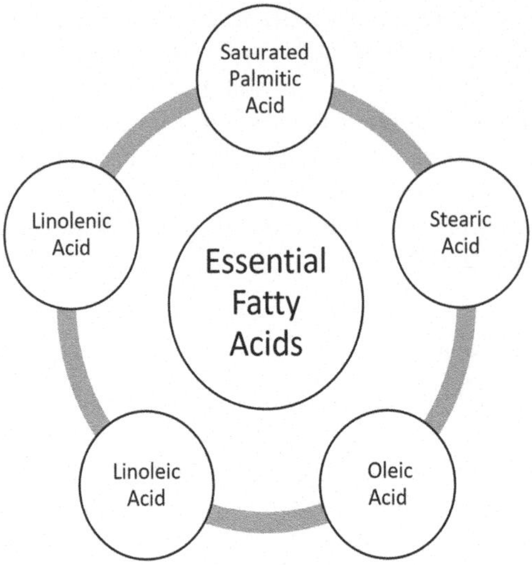

FIGURE 15.2 The essential fatty acids that are considered as nutraceuticals.

15.4.2 Dietary Fibre

Dietary fibre is any meal or, more specifically, any plant material that is not degraded by digestive tract enzymes but rather is digested by gut bacteria. Non-starch polysaccharides (NSP), such as cellulose, hemicellulose, gums, pectin, lignin, resistant dextrins and starches, make up the majority of dietary fibres. Fruits, oats, barley, and beans are foods high in soluble fibre. Dietary fibres are carbohydrate polymers with a degree of polymerisation of at least three in the small intestine that is neither digested nor absorbed. Dietary fibres can be classified into two types based on how much soluble in water: 1. Insoluble dietary fibre (IDF), which comprises celluloses, some hemicelluloses and lignins and is only partially fermented in the colon. 2. Soluble dietary fibre (SDF) comprises colon-fermented glucans, pectin's, gums, mucilage's, and hemicelluloses. IDF and SDF molecules are referred to as non-starch polysaccharides together (NSP) (Lipi 2012).

15.4.3 Selenium

Selenium is a crucial trace element that plays a role in thyroid hormone metabolism regulation, controlling the redox state of cells and protecting against the toxicity of reactive oxygen species. The highest-known source of selenium is Brazil nuts; one ounce has about 200 mcg. Humans have suffered significant health consequences as a result of its shortage, including Keshan's disease, a potentially deadly cardiomyopathy (disease of the heart muscle) that affects young girls and children. The antioxidant selenoproteins or seleno enzymes glutathione peroxidase and thioredoxin reductase play a significant role in selenium metabolism. Among the reactive oxygen species (ROS) and reactive nitrogen species (RNS), which include superoxide, hydrogen peroxide, hydroxyl radicals, nitric oxide, and peroxynitrite, glutathione peroxidase plays a critical role in preventing oxidative damage to cells. Selenium's antioxidant properties help maintain a healthy immune system and prevent cardiovascular problems (Stranges et al. 2006).

15.4.4 Polyunsaturated Fatty Acids (PUFA)

PUFAs are also "essential fatty acids" since they are necessary for the body to operate and are obtained from food. Omega-3 (n-3) and omega-6 (n-6) fatty acids are the two subgroups of PUFAs. The three primary omega-3 fatty acids are docosahexaenoic acid, eicosapentaenoic acid, and -linolenic acid (DHA). ALA comes before EPA and DHA. Fish oils and fatty fishes like mackerel, salmon, herring, trout, and bluefin tuna are the principal sources of EPA and DHA. Flaxseed, soybeans, canola, some nuts (including walnuts), and red and black currant seeds are the primary sources of ALA (Lipi 2012).

15.4.5 Prebiotics

Prebiotics are food components that alter the gut microbiota's composition or metabolism to positively affect the host. Specifically, fructose-based oligosaccharides that occur naturally in food or are added are short-chain polysaccharides with distinctive chemical structures humans cannot digest. Prebiotic use typically encourages the growth of Lactobacillus and Bifidobacteria in the gut, which aids metabolism. Fruit and vegetable sources of fructooligosaccharides include chicory roots, bananas, tomatoes, and alliums. Raffinose and stachyose, present in beans and peas, are two other examples of these oligosaccharides (Arora et al. 2022).

Prebiotics have anti-tumour qualities, the ability to neutralise toxins, the ability to increase lactose tolerance, the activation of the intestinal immune system, and the ability to reduce constipation, blood lipids, and blood cholesterol levels, among other health advantages (Lin et al. 1989).

15.4.6 Probiotics

A probiotic is a live microbial feed supplement that, when given to an animal in sufficient proportions, benefits the host by balancing the bacteria populations in the animal's intestines (Food and Agricultural Org. 2001). Bacteria from the following types typically make up probiotics:

- Lactobacilli such Lactobacillus acidophilus, L. casei, L. delbrueckii subsp. bulgaricus, L. brevis, and L. cellobiosus.
- Gram-positive cocci such Enterococcus faecalis, Streptococcus salivarius subsp. thermophilus, and Lactococcus lactis
- Bifidobacteria like B.bifidun, B.adolescentis, B.infantis, B.longum, and B. thermophilum.

Probiotics come in many forms, including powder, liquid, gel, paste, granules, capsules, and more.

Gastrointestinal issues like lactose intolerance, severe diarrhoea, and G.I. side effects from antibiotics are typically treated with specific probiotics. There is evidence that taking probiotics lowers the chance of developing systemic diseases like allergies, asthma, cancer, urinary tract, and cancer infections (Lenoir-Wijnkoop et al. 2007).

15.5 PHYTOCHEMICALS

Primary and secondary metabolites found in plants exhibit and perform various functions. Simple sugar, carbohydrates, nucleic acids, lipids, and amino acids are some of the fundamental metabolites crucial to mobile strategies. Secondary metabolites are employed as a deterrent and under pressure. Plants develop and expand particular variations of secondary metabolites helpful to humans and other living organisms. They call them "plant herbal items."

15.5.1 Carotenoids

Salmon, flamingos, goldfish, and autumn leaves are just a few examples of animals and plants that contain carotenoids. While "chlorophyll" has been removed from the leaves, only carotenoids and phenols remain. The numerous carotenoids found in bell peppers of different hues include: Alpha, beta, and gamma carotenoids are orange carotenoids. Astaxanthin and lycopene are red carotenoids. Zeaxanthin and lutein are two yellow carotenoids. The most beneficial 50 carotenoids for a human diet are absorbed into the bloodstream from the more than 600 carotenoids produced by plants. The carotenoids and a few others (but not lycopene or lutein) can be converted to vitamin A. According to studies on cells and animals, both beta-carotene and gamma-carotene are protective against liver and lung cancer. Carotenoids carry the highest concentration of lipid-rich (LDL) cholesterol particles into the bloodstream, where they bind to the most significant number of LDL receptors (Figure 15.3).

15.5.2 Lycopene

Red colours are also provided by lycopene, which is present in guava, tomatoes, watermelon, papaya, pink grapefruit, and papaya. It is a powerful antioxidant substance that lessens damage to DNA and proteins and provides better skin protection from ultraviolet light than -carotene. It prevents most cancers, lowers LDL cholesterol, and blocks insulin-like growth factors, which promote tumour growth (Figure 15.3).

15.5.3 Lutein

By utilising extraordinary resources, such as corn, avocados, and egg yolks, lutein creates a yellow colour in nature. It guards against colon cancer and treats eye conditions, including cataracts and macular degeneration. Its highest levels are kale, spinach, watercress, and parsley (Figure 15.3).

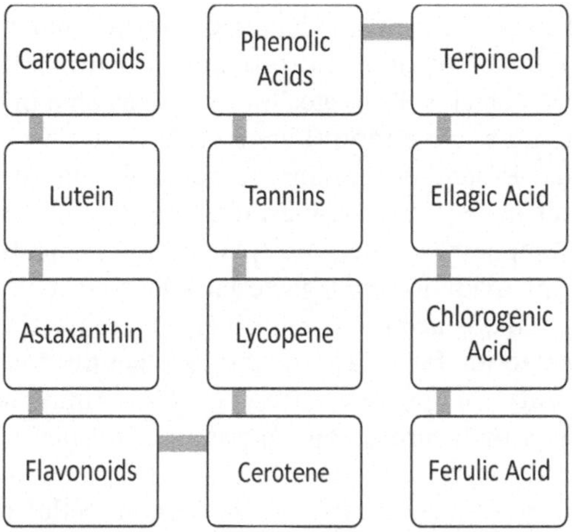

FIGURE 15.3 Various types of phytochemicals.

15.5.4 Astaxanthin

Salmon, shrimp, and crabs are given various colours by astaxanthin. Unlike any other carotenoid, it has strong antioxidant properties. Additionally, it enhanced T-cell production and cytokine, allowing it to pass the "blood-brain barrier" (BBB) and release vitamin C that has been wholly contained (Figure 15.3).

15.5.5 Flavonoids

Flavonoids (flavone-like) are chemical substances with antioxidant and anti-inflammatory effects present in dark chocolate and red wine but absent from white wine due to their distinct extraction methods. Ultrafiltration is occasionally employed to lessen astringency and bitterness in red wine, while fermentation is the preferred method of preparation or production. It is utilised by patients receiving chemotherapy and radiation therapy (Figure 15.3).

- **α-Carotene:** Due to the release of immunogenic cytokines (IL-1 and TNF-), α -carotene is ten times stronger and a more effective anticarcinogenic substance in assessment than β–carotene (Figure 15.3).
- **β-Carotene** can significantly increase LDL cholesterol and β-carotene content without affecting other carotenes. They can also increase the activity of natural killer "T-cells, β-cells, and N.K. cells," energise "DNA" mend enzymes, and grant better cornea protection against extremely-violet light than lycopene. β-Carotene is a much less active antioxidant but vital against singlet oxygen (Figure 15.3).
- **Tannins:** Tannins (polyphenolics), which give cranberries and pomegranates their acidic flavour, are used for tanning and protecting leather, as first observed in the 18th century A.D. It aids in the improvement and synthesis

of collagen when combined with vitamin C. By preventing germs (bacteria) from attaching to the partitions, it prevents UTI (urinary tract infection). Black tea, which contains 90% catechin and epicatechin in natural grapes, is available in its most active form (Figure 15.3).

- **Phenolic Acids:** Proanthocyanidins, resveratrol, and ellagic acid, which are also present in red wine, grape juice, and raisins and are especially abundant in cranberry juice, are phenolic chemicals that diminish LDL cholesterol oxidation and bacterial adhesion to tooth enamel and bladder lining cells, hence reducing urinary tract infections (UTIs), tooth decay, and the tooth fairy. The sugar-coat nature components reduce phenolic's ability to prevent sticking. Most malignancies produce phenolic acids, which turn dietary nitrate and nitrites into nitrosamines (Figure 15.3).
- **Terpineol:** In most cancer stages, the origin cellular architecture is retained, and terpineol gives carrots their distinctive flavour. They are chemical molecules not soluble in water and categorised as high-class secondary metabolites and hydrocarbon components by isoprene units. It is used to demonstrate cytotoxic and antibacterial properties (Iliopoulou et al. 2002) (Figure 15.3).
- **Ellagic Acid:** Ellagic acid is present in both strawberries and raspberries, but it is 50% more abundant in the latter. Ellagic acid lowers the risk of oesophagal and colorectal tumours by delaying the formation of DNA adducts, delaying stage 1, and enhancing the effects of phase 2 adjuvant therapy.
- **Chlorogenic Acid:** In addition to the ester of caffeic acid (also known as "hydroxyl cinnamic acid"), which reduces the mutagenicity of polycyclic aromatic hydrocarbons and exhibits intense antioxidant action, chlorogenic acid is also present in excessively high levels in blueberries, tomatoes, and bell peppers (Figure 15.3).
- **Ferulic Acid:** Whole wheat, brown rice, oats, apples, artichokes, orange pineapple, and peanut seeds contain large amounts of ferulic acid within their cellular walls. As the predecessor of vanillin and anticancer agent in breast and liver cancer cases, its properties are employed as an antioxidant and anticancer (Figure 15.3).

15.6 MICRONUTRIENTS

There are various micronutrients like Carbohydrates, Vitamins, Minerals, Calcium, Iron, Zinc, and Fluoride.

15.6.1 Vitamins

Vitamins are micronutrients/food supplements crucial to our day-to-day lives for perfect health and act as an enzyme cofactor precursor in the metabolic pathway (Joao et al. 2020).

15.6.2 Minerals

Chemicals known as minerals are essential for the healthy growth and complete development of all living beings, including plants, animals, and humans. They safeguard the bodies against a variety of illnesses. Maintaining a special nutritious diet is essential for preventing significant diseases, including cancer, diabetes, digestive disorders, and cancer, by ensuring one consumes the proper amount of minerals (Kersting et al. 2001). The various types of micronutrients available in nature like Carbohydrates, Vitamin A, Vitamin B Complex, Vitamin C, Vitamin D, Vitamin E, Vitamin K, Calcium, Magnesium, Iron, Zinc, Fluoride.

15.7 IMPORTANCE OF ORAL HEALTH

The primary cause of adult tooth loss is oral and periodontal disease, which can result in severe functional, phonatory, and cosmetic difficulties (Isola 2020). According to data, there are now 3.5 billion people worldwide who have untreated dental caries, severe periodontitis, and oral illnesses. According to GLOBOCAN figures, the number of malignancies affecting the lips and oral cavity reached more than three lakhs in 2020. (Sung 2021). Nowadays, oral illness is a significant global public health issue. As awareness of the benefits of good oral health has increased, science and business have been motivated to study nutrients to prevent and care for dental problems, including isolated nutrients and components such as dietary supplements. The compounds from marine sources include protein and peptides, protein, -3 polyunsaturated fatty acids (PUFA), polysaccharides, polyphenolic compounds, enzymes, vitamins, and pigments. Numerous physiological effects of these compounds include anticancer, antioxidant, antiviral, and immunomodulatory effects. Shaikh et al. (Shaikh 2020) reviewed the use of marine-derived substances in dentistry, including chitosan, bio-adhesives, tissue regeneration gel, calcium hydroxyapatite, gypsum, and algal extracts. Ibrahim et al. (Ibrahim et al. 2018) discovered that marine bioactive compounds could protect tooth health by inhibiting the growth of Streptococcus mutants (S. mutans).

A person's oral health is crucial to their general health and quality of life. Oral health is described by the World Health Organisation (WHO) as "a state of being free from chronic mouth and facial pain, oral and throat cancer, oral infection and sores, periodontal disease, tooth decay, tooth loss, and other diseases and disorders that limit an individual's capacity for biting, chewing, smiling, speaking, and psychosocial well-being" (Petersen 2003). In recent years, as oral epidemiology has evolved globally, the primary oral disorders that affect people's lives are dental caries, periodontal disease, oral cancer, oral manifestations of HIV, oro-dental trauma, cleft lip and palate, and Noma (Petersen 2003).

Dental caries and periodontitis are thought to start and develop due to plaque in the mouth cavity. Plaque is a bacterial biofilm comprised of numerous bacteria, intercellular material, a tiny number of white blood cells, lost epithelial cells, and food particles that cannot be eliminated by water. According to the definition of the term used in dentistry, biofilms are microbial colonies of surface-attached cells encapsulated in a self-produced extracellular environment (Soto 2013). The oral microbiota in the oral cavity significantly impacts the onset and progression of oral disease. S. mutans, Actinomyces species, Treponema denticola, Tannerella forsythia, Bacteroides species, A. actinomycetemcomitans, Staphylococcus intermedius, Porphyromonas gingivalis, and Candida albicans are a few of the microorganisms that can cause oral diseases (Chugh et al. 2020). Additionally, factors like immune system deterioration or steroid use might upset the equilibrium of oral microorganisms and result in opportunistic infections. Opportunistic infections can be brought on by any process that lowers immunity or by steroid medication that upsets the oral bacterial equilibrium. A poor diet can also change the microbiome in the mouth, which can cause periodontitis and dental caries, among other oral disorders. Therefore, regular care and maintenance of the oral cavity are necessary to ensure oral health (Huang et al. 2021).

15.8 MAINTENANCE OF ORAL HEALTH

A mechanical oral hygiene assist is essential for maintaining dental health (Mariotti 1999). Brushing is the most critical and popular mechanical oral cleaning technique, yet it is ineffective for clearing plaque from the gingival sulcus of healthy teeth. As a result, using a toothbrush regularly needs to be supplemented by other methods of plaque removal. The daily regimen includes using mouthwash and chewing gum as oral cleaning tools, rinsing the mouth by force flushing, and preventing plaque from building up on the teeth. Oral disorders are treated with anti-inflammatory drugs such as triclosan, dextranase, menthol, and chlorhexidine; however, prolonged use of these drugs can have adverse side effects (Isola 2020). Sea 4 R Encias (seawater) oral rinse and 0.20% chlorhexidine were both evaluated by Calvo-Guirado et al. (Calvo-Guirado et al. 2020) for their efficacy. According to this study, saltwater mouthwash exhibited antibacterial activity comparable to chlorhexidine. Seawater mouthwash can lessen adverse effects like tooth discolouration and become a regular choice for preserving oral health despite chlorhexidine's superior clinical performance. The mechanical stimulation of chewing gum, mouthwash, and removal of plaque and dietary fermentable carbohydrates from the mouth, on the other hand, stimulates salivation in the mouth. Additionally, chewing gum's base is very sticky, which helps to remove plaque from the surface of the teeth. Although sugar-free chewing gum and brushing can significantly and marginally reduce plaque generation, gingivitis has not dramatically improved. Based on these traits, if substances are helpful and can withstand S. mutans, chewing gum may be a highly efficient means of distributing and retaining bioactive compounds, with possible anti-caries benefits. S. mutans strains [e.g., quercetin (Qt)] are added to chewing gum formulations. In addition to cleaning, it is believed that the essential role of diet, natural substances, and nutrition is also indirectly accountable for the well-being of periodontal tissues and the struggle against the resorption of alveolar bone. (Kose et al. 2016).

15.9 EFFECTS OF NUTRACEUTICALS ON ORAL AND PERIODONTAL HEALTH

The interaction between teeth, food, and bacteria causes dental caries, a common chronic illness. Streptococcus mutans and S. sobrinus are thought to be the primary bacteria, while numerous other kinds are also thought to be present. Caries has been broken down into three stages: adhesion of bacteria to the teeth, development of glycocalyx (a biofilm) from the deposition of plaque and the creation of a sticky branched glucan by the action of the bacterial enzyme glucosyl transferase (GTase) on sucrose. The bacteria in dental plaque continue to produce acid, which demineralises the teeth's enamel because they can digest carbohydrates in an acidic environment. (Hamilton-Miller 2001).

15.9.1 Effect of Tea on Dental Caries

Since tea leaves are high in fluoride, there is debate about whether drinking tea has any dental advantages. In many countries, the inclusion of fluoride in drinking water reduces the occurrence of dental cavities.

The main components of teas are polyphenolic catechins and theaflavins, which are well-recognised as bactericidal and inhibitory against Streptococcus spp. and can be found in green and black teas, respectively, as monomers or polymers. Green tea extract (20 mg/mL) has been observed to reduce the quantity of S. mutans from 107 to 102 after 3 minutes, while the lowest inhibitory concentration of tea polyphenols against cariogenic bacteria has been reported to be 0.25–1.0 mg/mL. At 50 g/mL or less, the monomeric catechins -epigallocatechin gallate (EGCG) and -epicatechin gallate (ECG), which are found in both green and black tea, was found to prevent streptococci from adhering to teeth (Wang et al. 2003). They cause aggregation, bind to the bacteria's surface proteins, and block the enzyme activity of glucosyl transferase. Both teas reduce plaque overall by inhibiting salivary and streptococcal amylase (Hamilton-Miller 2001). By preventing bacteria from adhering to and growing on the surface of teeth and streptococci from synthesising glucan, green tea, EGCG, and ECG have been found to suppress the growth of cariogenic bacteria. Additionally, it has been shown that the flavours of tea, indole, and delta-cadinene work together to suppress S. mutans. EGCG also prevents Porphyromonas gingivalis, the cause of periodontal disease, from growing and adhering to surfaces.

According to a theory, both black and green tea leaves can be utilised as a source of polyphenols with a slow release in the mouth to reduce caries (Lee et al. 2004). Tea extracts have been added to chewing gum and candies to lessen cavities and freshen breathing.

Halitosis is mainly brought on by foodstuff and bacterial proteins in the mouth that enzymes break down to produce volatile odorous sulphides, mainly methyl mercaptan. Tea catechins, especially EGCG, have a deodorising effect by effectively neutralising the methyl thio group of methyl mercaptan through a chemical process. The anti-GTase activity of proanthocyanidins, like the catechins in tea, has been examined in various plant sources, but catechin and epicatechin were found to have the maximum activity. Notably, the smaller molecular weight enzymatic metabolites of these two exhibited substantial GTase inhibitory action, indicating that human metabolites may be responsible for tea's activity rather than naturally occurring plant components (Mitsunaga 1999).

One of the most common oral health illnesses is periodontal disease, which encompasses several conditions, from gingivitis to periodontitis. In particular, periodontitis affects more than 60% of people over 65 and about half of adults over 30 in its mildest form. It is a disease marked not only by gingival inflammation but also by the loss of connective tissue attachment, which results in the resorption of alveolar bone and, subsequently, tooth loss. Although microbial biofilms are the leading cause of chronic periodontitis, numerous additional local and systemic variables might influence the illness (Nguyen et al. 2021).

It is a long-lasting inflammatory condition brought on by particular oral microbes. It is the primary reason for tooth loss due to the destruction of the alveolar bone and supporting periodontal ligament. Maintaining oral and periodontal health is difficult nowadays, mainly because periodontal disease can be a risk factor in and of itself for several chronic conditions. Other risk factors for periodontal disease include genetics, diabetes, hormonal changes related to pregnancy or menopause, alcohol, stress, smoking, and other drugs. It is widely acknowledged that several chronic diseases, including type 2 diabetes mellitus, cardiovascular conditions, inflammatory bowel disease, and rheumatoid arthritis, are linked explicitly to periodontitis. As a result, the connection between dental health and systemic health is gaining attention (López et al. 2018).

There is no doubt that oral microbes are essential for the pathogenesis of periodontal disease, but among the risk factors, nutrition constitutes a significant element that is frequently disregarded. Dietary factors are crucial for balancing oral bacteria and host response, which determines the beginning and course of periodontal disease. In the past, "healthy" dietary approaches have mainly concentrated on lowering the consumption of "undesirable" dietary components like sodium, refined carbohydrates, and saturated fats. However, there is now more emphasis on encouraging the consumption of "curative nutrients." This idea that "food or nutrient is a medicament" has prompted researchers to look for an increasing number of novel chemicals, ranging from dietary supplements to "nutraceuticals," to enhance human health and make us fitter and more resistant to disease. "nutraceuticals" refers to a class of compounds without a clear legal definition frequently offered as dietary supplements or additives to regular foods. According to Zeisel (Zeisel 1999), Nutraceuticals are dietary supplements that give a concentrated form of a biologically active food component in a non-food matrix to improve health. A dietary supplement is a product that contains one or more ingredients, such as a vitamin, mineral, herb, amino acid, concentration, metabolite, constituent, extract, or combination (López et al. 2018).

Scaling, root planning, and oral hygiene are the main methods used to manage periodontitis. The causal causes (plaque, microbial biofilm, and calculus) are also removed. Antibiotics are thought to be beneficial in cases with systemic involvement or severe illnesses. Original teeth with substantial bone loss periodontally can extend their usable lives by guided tissue regeneration (GTR) and bone grafting (Sheikh et al. 2015). Implant therapy can restore teeth lost due to significant and unchecked immune cell-induced periodontal and bone tissue deterioration. Immune cells' production of inflammatory substances destroys periodontal tissue. The presence of microorganisms at the site of periodontitis draws polymorphonuclear leucocytes. When bacterial antigens stimulate leucocytes, they release enzymes, defensins, and reactive oxidative species (ROS), which cause the pathogens to break down during phagocytosis (Khurshid et al. 2016). Because ROS are non-selective, they also harm healthy tissues. As a result, ROS causes DNA damage to normal cells during the inflammatory condition and encourages macrophages and monocytes to generate cytokines. Additionally, it has been proposed that ROS could activate osteoclasts, the bone-resorbing cells. Infected periodontal tissues have higher amounts of ROS than healthy tissues due to the breakdown of oxidative tissues.

The health of the periodontium is significantly influenced by a range of nutrients (Ritchie & Kinane 2003). There are two categories of nutrients: macronutrients and micronutrients. Micronutrients are food ingredients that the body needs in very minute or small amounts. The human diet's micronutrients have various antioxidant characteristics. Melatonin (Najeeb et al. 2016), vitamin A (carotenoids and -carotene), vitamin C (ascorbic acid), vitamin E (tocopherol), and glutathione are antioxidant micronutrients. According to studies, antioxidants may reduce the periodontal tissues' inflammatory response to ROS.

Along with water and oxygen, macronutrients such as minerals, proteins, carbs, and lipids are also necessary for considerable amounts. Periodontal disease and dental cavities have been linked to high carbohydrate intake (Hujoel 2009). For instance, a diet full of sugars promotes plaque development and, in response to poor oral hygiene, causes the beginning or aggravation of dental decay. Obesity and periodontal disorders have been linked, according to reports. Increased gingival bleeding in elderly patients has been linked to a higher body fat percentage. Conversely, it has been found that polyunsaturated fats (like omega-3) are suitable for periodontal health (Najeeb et al 2016).

15.10 ROLE OF VARIOUS NUTRIENTS IN MAINTAINING PERIODONTAL HEALTH

15.10.1 Carbohydrates

Bacteria, mucin, and glycoproteins form a biofilm called plaque that sticks to the oral cavity's surfaces (Nanci 2012). For a few days, plaque still adhered to teeth turns into calculus as it mineralises. Periodontal pathogens such as Porphyromonas gingivalis, Prevotella intermedia, Tannerella forsythia, and Treponema denticola may be able to live on the porous calculus. The leading cause of plaque formation is long-established to be sugar consumption. Compared to fructose and glucose, sucrose is more cariogenic (Frostell et al. 1991). Because bacteria ferment sugars and make acid; as a result, demineralisation of the tooth structure and dental caries are both caused by sugars. According to studies, lactose is less cariogenic than other sugars. Dental decay and sugar consumption frequency with amount were directly correlated in earlier research (Saido et al. 2016). Xylitol, a sugary alcohol made by hydrogenating xylose sugar, is an artificial sweetener used as a substitute for table sugars. Therefore, the oral and periodontal health of the broader population may be improved by reducing sugar while also employing scaling, root planing, and gums that include xylitol and maltitol.

15.10.2 Vitamins

The general well-being and proper operation of the body depend on vitamins. Similarly, different vitamins are necessary to keep periodontal and dental tissues healthy. Vitamin deficiencies in food lead to oral symptoms such as rickets and Scurvy.

15.10.2.1 Vitamin A

In order to preserve the health of epithelial cells, vitamin A, a fat-soluble vitamin, is necessary (Gunther 1976). Eggs, cod liver oil, carrots, capsicum, liver, sweet potatoes, broccoli, and green vegetables are dietary sources of vitamin A. A healthy person needs about 900 g per day. Deficiency causes retinal problems (such as night blindness and hyperkeratosis). Due to its ability as an antioxidant, vitamin A has been used as a supplement to periodontal therapy.

15.10.2.2 Vitamin B Complex

Vitamin B1 (thiamine), Vitamin B2 (riboflavin), Vitamin B3 (niacin), Vitamin B5 (pantothenic acid), Vitamin B6 (pyridoxine, pyridoxal, and pyridoxamine), Vitamin B7 (biotin), Vitamin B9 (folic acid), and Vitamin B12 are all members of the vitamin B complex family (cobalamins). B vitamins are essential for cell proliferation, repair, and metabolism. Dermatitis, paraesthesia, and oral manifestations such as angular cheilitis and glossitis indicate a vitamin B deficit. Vitamin B12 deficiency can result in gingival bleeding in addition to anaemia. Recent research by Zong et al. found a negative connection between serum vitamin B12 concentrations and the degree of periodontitis. (Zong et al. 2016). Additionally, smokers have been found to have lower serum levels of vitamin B9, which may contribute to periodontitis (Erdemir, Bergstrom 2007). B-vitamin complex supplementation has been found to hasten the healing of ulcers following periodontal flap surgery, according to Neiva et al. (Neiva et al. 2005).

15.10.2.3 Vitamin C

Collagen formation depends mostly on vitamin C (ascorbic acid), which also serves as a ROS scavenger to avoid oxidative damage. The condition brought on by a lack of vitamin C is known as Scurvy, and Sir Thomas Barlow first recognised it in 1883 (Barlow 1883). Periodontal signs of Scurvy include bleeding and swollen and sore gums, malaise, drowsiness, and skin patches. Scurvy can be treated and avoided with vitamin C supplementation (Camarena, Wang 2016). According to an in vitro investigation, local administration of magnesium salt containing vitamin C may lessen gingival fibroblasts' irritation caused by ROS and increase collagen synthesis (Tsutsumi et al. 2012). In a clinical experiment by Shimabukuro et al. (Shimabukuro et al. 2015), a dentifrice containing a magnesium salt containing vitamin C effectively reduced gingival inflammation.

Additionally, compared to regular dentifrice, the vitamin C-containing formulation showed noticeably better anti-ROS efficacy. Vitamin C may be used as coatings, gels, or both to increase the integration of dental implants into the bone and recover periodontal tissues following surgery because of its beneficial effects on periodontal health. Due to their powerful antioxidant properties, ascorbate molecules can assist smokers in slowing down the deterioration of periodontal tissues (Ritchie, Kinane 2003).

15.10.2.4 Vitamin D

The body needs vitamin D for a variety of vital processes. It increases the digestive tract's absorption of minerals like calcium, magnesium, iron, phosphate, and zinc. Vitamins D2 (cholecalciferol) and D3 are two crucial categories of vitamin D in humans (ergocalciferol). Clinical investigations have demonstrated that a vitamin D shortage in the diet causes periodontitis and a slowdown in the periodontium's recovery after surgery. Other clinical studies, however, have yet to discover any conclusive relationship between serum vitamin D levels and periodontal health (Lee et al. 2015). However, the link between serum vitamin D levels and the onset of disease was found to be inverse in those above the age of 60 years (Alshouibi et al. 2013). As a result, more research is needed to clarify the relationship between vitamin D insufficiency and adult periodontal health. Vitamin D supplementation has more noticeable local effects on periodontal tissues than systemic Delivery. For instance, coating dental implants with vitamin D3 may improve osseointegration with alveolar bone (Javed et al. 2016). Additionally, intraperitoneal injections of vitamin D3 have been demonstrated to speed up orthodontic tooth movement, allowing patients receiving bisphosphonate therapy to induce orthodontic tooth movement (Kale et al. 2004).

15.10.2.5 Vitamin E

Considered to be one of the essential extracellular antioxidants, vitamin E (tocopherol) is a fat-soluble vitamin. Poultry, meat, fish, nuts, seeds, and cereals are high in vitamin E (García-Closas et al. 2004). By preventing the free radical reaction, vitamin E maintains the membrane's structural integrity. As per a few studies, there are no significant differences in the plasma level of vitamin E between patients with periodontitis and orally healthy individuals (Slade et al. 1976). In contrast, a few studies found that vitamin E positively prevented inflammation and maintained periodontal health. In addition, patients with periodontal disorders have lower levels of vitamin E than healthy people. Smokers have lower levels of vitamin E in their alveolar fluid, which is consistent with an increase in oxidant generation during smoking (Pacht et al. 1986).

15.10.2.6 Vitamin K

Prothrombin and factors VII, IX, and X are only a few examples of the blood coagulation factors produced due to the production of proteins that are part of the vitamin K group (Shearer M.J., Newman 2008). Additionally, studies have shown that vitamin K synthesises proteins needed for the metabolism of bone, including osteocalcin and periostin (Coutu et al. 2008). Many foods contain vitamin K1, including kale, spinach, collard greens, and mustard. Since vitamin K1 can be converted to vitamin K2 by anaerobic bacteria in the gut, vitamin K2 deficiency is rare. However, consuming antibiotics may upset the equilibrium of gut micro-organisms, resulting in a vitamin K shortage. Therefore, coagulopathies may be seen if antibiotics are included in periodontal care for an extended period. Warfarin's anticoagulant effects can be reversed by vitamin K, a crucial pharmacological substance frequently given to haemodialyses patients (Elliott et al. 2007). Therefore, vitamin K can be utilised to treat any bleeding occurrences if periodontal therapy is given to individuals with kidney failure. A healthy person can get enough vitamin K from a regular diet; thus, vitamin K insufficiency is relatively uncommon. However, vitamin K deficiency needs to be assessed in patients with digestive disorders or those who have taken antibiotics for a long time (Hathaway 1993). Although vitamin K deficiency may result in gingival bleeding, a recent study by Aral et al. showed that vitamin K treatment could not reduce pro-inflammatory markers in the periodontium (Aral et al. 2015).

15.11 MINERALS AND TRACE ELEMENTS

Other than oxygen, carbon, nitrogen, and hydrogen, minerals are components individuals need for survival and performing their usual functions. For instance, an abundance of calcium, phosphorus, potassium, sulphur, salt, chlorine, and magnesium is typically needed. Trace minerals include iron, cobalt, copper, zinc, manganese, molybdenum, iodine, bromine, and selenium because they are needed in minor concentrations. Mineral deficiency can also affect periodontal health (Vander Velden et al. 2011).

15.11.1 Calcium

The proper operation of the body's systems and muscles depends on calcium. Furthermore, calcium is required to develop and maintain hard tissues like bone and teeth. Additionally, blood cells must operate for the same. Dietary sources of calcium include dairy products, leafy green vegetables, nuts, and seeds. Tetany, numbness, tingling in the hands, feet, and area around the lips, as well as cardiac rhythms, can result from hypocalcemia or a lack of calcium. Deficits in dietary calcium may also harm oral and periodontal health. Co-supplementing calcium and vitamin D is common and improves the outcomes of periodontal therapy (Garcia et al. 2011).

15.11.2 Magnesium

The development of bones, cell metabolism, and cell maintenance all require magnesium. Osteoporosis is a direct effect of a magnesium deficiency's interference with the parathyroid hormone. It has been demonstrated that magnesium supplements lower the risk of fractures in people with osteoporosis, illustrating their positive effects on bone health (Toba et al. 2000). However, doctors must exercise extreme caution when recommending magnesium supplements because too much of the mineral can adversely affect bone health and even raise bone mineral density. However, it is still unknown how dietary magnesium affects periodontal health. Only one study has indicated that diets high in magnesium benefit nonsurgical periodontal therapy (Staudte et al. 2012).

15.11.3 Iron

Haemoglobin and enzyme production are two of the critical purposes for which iron is needed. Iron is abundant in foods like red meat, spinach, fish (tuna and salmon), and legumes. Anaemia and associated symptoms are brought on by iron deficiency. Recurrent ulcers, pale mucosa, and mouth burn are all signs of anaemia in the mouth. According to a study, iron deficiency anaemia decreases antioxidant enzymes, which increases oxidative stress and worsens periodontal disorders (Chakraborty et al. 2014).

15.11.4 Zinc

Dietary zinc is mainly obtained from meals high in protein (Osis et al. 1972). Zinc is the trace mineral in the human body in the second-highest concentration after iron (Lansdown et al. 2007). Many processes that are regulated by enzymes require zinc as a cofactor. In particular, it controls the keratinocyte migration and auto-debridement mechanisms during wound healing (Mirastschijski et al. 2004). In addition to neutralising bacterial toxins, it also has an antioxidative action by scavenging ROS (Rostan et al. 2002). As a result, zinc plays a crucial role in periodontal dressings (Jentsch et al. 2016). Dietary zinc might be crucial for preserving periodontal health. It has been hypothesised that patients with type 2 diabetes mellitus who do not get enough zinc in their diet may experience deteriorating periodontal disease (Pushparani 2015). The antioxidant action of zinc due to Pushparani's systematic review has further confirmed its significance in avoiding diabetes-related periodontitis (Pushparani 2014). Therefore, the therapeutic effects of periodontal therapy may be enhanced by zinc supplementation (Kulkarni et al. 2014).

15.11.5 Fluoride

Fluoride has long been known to have anticarie properties (Maguire 2014). Fluorine prevents caries by forming fluorapatite, which strengthens enamel and cementum, and acts as an antibacterial agent by inhibiting bacterial growth and adherence (Seppa et al. 1993). Therefore, topical fluoride has been utilised as a prophylactic measure against dental cavities in dentifrices, gels, foams, and varnishes. Because of its valuable functions, fluoride has been added to several restorative materials, including glass ionomers. Even though toothpaste, mouthwashes, and foods high in fluoride can contain fluoride, these substances act as reservoirs that release and recharge fluoride into the oral cavity. Fluoride can be administered systemically with water, milk, and pills. The American Tooth Association (ADA) recommends against giving systemic fluoride supplements to children with a high risk of acquiring dental caries (Maguire 2014). Fluoride supplementation of 0.25 to 1 mg daily is indicated, depending on the amount of fluoride already present in the drinking water (ppm F) (American Academy of Paediatric Dentistry 2013). Additionally, fluoride administration may lessen the resorption of roots brought on by tooth movement during orthodontic treatment (Karadeniz et al. 2011).

Another food that is necessary for good oral health and is exceptionally rich in nutrients is green tea, which contains calcium, phosphorus, and fluoride (Khurshid et al. 2016).

15.12 CONCLUSION

Due to their potential for nutritive, safe, and therapeutic effects, nutraceuticals are presently gaining awareness. Various diseases can be prevented and treated with the use of nutraceuticals. They have become a crucial part of the diet for the average consumer due to the rise in lifestyle-related health issues. For the majority of health-conscious Indians, nutraceuticals are now their primary dietary supplement. Nutraceuticals (dietary supplements) are now widely used in the healthcare industry and come in various forms, such as pills, syrups, gums, and capsules. The coordinated and synergistic activity of nutrients and physiologically active substances is signalled as a potential health benefit. The usage of nutraceuticals is expanding quickly, and people accept them because they are all-natural. This interest is sparked by the need for fewer synthetic drugs, which encourages the industry to create and market new products with positive health claims. Although they cannot wholly replace medications, nutritional supplements can be a powerful, highly effective instrument for pathological condition therapy and prevention.

Oral illnesses can result in significant patient financial strain and decreased productivity by causing discomfort, poor function, and diminished quality of life. Therefore, dental health directly affects people's ability to lead regular lives. Recent studies in vitro and in vivo have demonstrated the critical function that marine bioactive constituents have in guarding against several oral health problems, such as dental decay, bad breath, and periodontitis.

Oral diseases are far more particular than systemic disorders, and the great majority of therapies include surgery and routine patient interaction with their blood, mucous, and gingival sulcus fluid. The aerosols and droplets created when patients have respiratory-transmitted diseases, including microorganisms in the mouth and nasopharynx, including mycobacterium TB, influenza, pneumonia virus, and other pathogens, can be extremely dangerous. Numerous persons receiving treatment for oral disorders may be impacted, particularly in the current COVID-19 pandemic. So maintaining good dental hygiene is crucial. Consumers also prefer foods and supplements with beneficial oral health properties due to the increasing understanding of maintaining dental health and avoiding oral diseases.

According to the literature evaluation, bacteriotherapy in the form of probiotics reduces the CFU counts of cariogenic microorganisms (S. mutans). Probiotics are quickly becoming an exciting area of oral medicine. This idea opens up new possibilities for the connection between diet and oral health. Probiotics are increasingly being used in dental care applications. There is mounting evidence that using probiotic strains now available can improve oral health.

In periodontology, vitamin D is essential because it synthesises proteins required for developing mucosal membranes. Establishing a physical barrier prevents germs from spreading into deeper tissues. Immune and epithelial cells begin to produce antimicrobial proteins, and non-specific immune responses are also triggered.

Vitamin D also contributes to a particular immunological response by reducing the damaging effects of chronic periodontitis. Additionally, it keeps the jawbone and systemic densities in balance. More study is required before vitamin D can be prescribed to treat periodontal disorders.

Vitamins and polyunsaturated fatty acids are antioxidants that either work naturally to scavenge free radicals or enhance the body's defence system.

As a result, this chapter considers using nutraceuticals to preserve periodontal and dental health. However, genetic predisposition and lifestyle diseases like smoking and excessive alcohol intake significantly affect a person's vulnerability to any disease. So, each person will react differently to nutraceuticals. When consumed within the appropriate Recommended Dietary intake, nutraceuticals have been shown to positively affect health and help people stay healthy in general.

REFERENCES

Adelaja, A.O., & Schilling, B.J. (1999). Nutraceutical: Blurring the line between food and drugs in the twenty-first century. *Mag Food Farm Resour* (14), 35–40.

Alshouibi, E.N., Kaye, E.K., Cabral, H.J., Leone, C.W., & Garcia, R.I. (2013). Vitamin D and periodontal health in older men. *J. Dent. Res.*, 92, 689–693.

American Academy of Pediatric Dentistry. (2013). Guideline on fluoride therapy. *Pediatr. Dent.*, 35, 165–168.

Aral, K., Alkan, B.A., Saraymen, R., Yay, A., Sen, A., & Önder, G.Ö. (2015). Therapeutic effects of systemic vitamin K2 and vitamin D3 on gingival inflammation and alveolar bone in rats with experimentally induced periodontitis. *J. Periodontol.*, 86, 666–673.

Arora, R., Trivedi, J., Mohapatra, S., & Kumar, P. (2022). Trends in probiotics on human health and industrial application. In: S.K. Nayak, B. Baliyarsingh, I. Mannazzu, A. Singh, & B.B. Mishra (eds) *Advances in Agricultural and Industrial Microbiology* Singapore: Springer. 10.1007/978-981-16-8918-5_13

Barlow, T. (1883). On Cases Described as "Acute Rickets", which are probably a combination of Scurvy and Rickets, the Scurvy being an essential, and the rickets a variable, element. *Med. Chir. Trans.*, 66, 159–220.

Berger, M.M., Spertin, F., & Shenkin, A. (1996). Clinical immune and metabolic effects of trace element supplements in burns, a double-blind placebo-controlled trial. *Clinical Nutrition*, 15 (2), 94–96.

Calvo-Guirado, J.L., Fernández Domínguez, M., Aragoneses, J.M., Martínez González, J.M., Fernández-Boderau, E., & Garcés-Villalá, M.A. (2020). Evaluation of new seawater-based mouth rinse versus chlorhexidine 0.2% reducing plaque and gingivitis indexes. A randomised controlled pilot study. *Appl Sci.*, 10, 982. doi: 10.3390/app10030982

Camarena, V., & Wang, G. (2016). The epigenetic role of vitamin C in health and disease. *Cell. Mol. Life Sci.*, 73, 1645–1658.

Chakraborty, S., Tewari, S., Sharma, R.K., Narula, S.C., Ghalaut, P.S., & Ghalaut, V. (2014). Impact of iron deficiency anaemia on chronic periodontitis and superoxide dismutase activity: A cross-sectional study. *J. Periodontal Implant Sci.*, 44, 57–64.

Chandra, S., Saklani, S., Kumar, P., Kim, B., & Coutinho, D.M.H. (2022). Nutraceuticals: Pharmacologically Active Potent Dietary Supplements. *BioMed Research International* Volume, (1-10) Article ID 2051017. 10.1155/2022/2051017

Chugh, P., Dutt, R., Sharma, A., Bhagat, N., & Dhar, M.S. (2020). A critical appraisal of the effects of probiotics on oral health. *J Funct Foods*, 70, 103985. doi: 10.1016/j.jff.2020.103985

Coutu, D.L., Wu, J.H., Monette, A., Rivard, G.E., Blostein, M.D., & Galipeau, J. (2008). Periostin, a member of a novel family of vitamin K-dependent proteins, is expressed by mesenchymal stromal cells. *J. Biol. Chem.*, 283, 17991–18001.

Dillard, C.J., & German, J.B. (2000). Phytochemicals: Nutraceuticals and human health. *J Sci Food Agric* (80), 1744–1756.

Elliott, M.J., Zimmerman, D., & Holden, R.M. (2007). Warfarin anticoagulation in hemodialysis patients: A systematic review of bleeding rates. *Am. J. Kidney Dis.*, 50, 433–440.

Erdemir, E.O., & Bergstrom, J. (2007). Effect of smoking on folic acid and vitamin B12 after nonsurgical periodontal intervention. *J. Clin. Periodontol.*, 34, 1074–1081.

Frostell, G., Birkhed, D., Edwardsson, S., Goldberg, P., Petersson, L., Priwe, C., & Winholt, A. (1991). Effect of Partial substitution of invert sugar for sucrose in combination with Duraphat treatment on caries development in preschool children: The Malmö study. *Caries Res*, 25, 304–310.

Food and Agricultural Org World Health Org. (2001). Health and nutritional properties of probiotics in food including powder milk with live lactic acid bacteria. http://www.who.int/foodsafety/publications/fsmanagement/probiotics/en/index.html

Garcia, M.N., Hildebolt, C.F., Miley, D.D., Dixon, D.A., Couture, R.A., Anderson Spearie, C.L., Langenwalter, E.M., Shannon, W.D., Deych, E., & Mueller, C. (2011). One-year effects of vitamin D and calcium supplementation on chronic periodontitis. *J. Periodontol.*, 82, 25–32.

García-Closas, R., Berenguer, A., Tormo, M.J., Sánchez, M.J., Quiros, J.R., Navarro, C., Arnaud, R., Dorronsoro, M., Chirlaque, M.D., & Barricarte, A. (2004). Dietary sources of vitamin C, vitamin E and specific carotenoids in Spain. *Br. J. Nutr.*, 91, 1005–1011.

Gunther, S. (1976). Vitamin A acid: Clinical investigations with 405 patients. *Cutis*, 17, 287–290.

Gupta, G. (2011). Probiotics and periodontal health. *Journal of Medicine and Life*, 4 (4), 387–394.

Halsted, H. (2003). Dietary supplements and functional foods: 2 sides of a coin. *The American Journal of Clinical Nutrition*, 77 (4), 1001S–1007S.

Hamilton-Miller, J.M.T. (2001). Anti-cariogenic properties of tea (Camellia sinensis). *J Med Microbiol*, 50, 299–302.

Hathaway, W.E. (1993). Vitamin K deficiency. *Southeast Asian J. Trop. Med. Public Health*, 24, 5–9.

Hathcock, J. (2001). Dietary supplements: how they are used and regulated. *J Nutr* (131), 1114–1117

Huang, Y., Jin, Z., Wang, Z.M., Qi, L.B., Song, S., Zhu, B.W., & Dong, X.P. (2021). Marine Bioactive compounds as Nutraceutical and functional food ingredients for potential Health care. *Frontiers in Nutrition*, 8, 686663. doi: 10.3389/fnut.2021.686663

Hujoel, P. (2009). Dietary carbohydrates and dental-systemic diseases. *J. Dent. Res.*, 88, 490–502.

Ibrahim, N.M., Alias, A., Noraini, N.N., Kamarudin, S.S., Li, A.R., & Hasan, M.K.N. (2018). Sea cucumber as inhibitor of bacterial adhesion in dental plaque: Would this be a possible reality? *Int J Stud Childwomen Elderly Dis.*, 4, 140–149.

Iliopoulou, D., Roussis, V., Pannecouque, C., De Clercq, E., & Vagias, C. (2002). Halogenated sesquiterpenes from the red alga Laurencia obtuse. *Tetrahedron*, 58, egori

Isola, G. (2020). Current evidence of natural agents in oral and periodontal health. *Nutrients*, 12, 585. doi: 10.3390/nu12020585

Javed, F., Malmstrom, H., Kellesarian, S.V., Al-Kheraif, A.A., Vohra, F., & Romanos, G.E. (2016). Efficacy of vitamin D3 supplementation on osseointegration of implants. *Implant. Dent.*, 25, 281–287.

Jentsch, H.F., Knöfler, G.U., Purschwitz, R.E., & Eick, S. (2016). Periodontal dressing as an adjunct after scaling and root planing—A useful preventive tool? *Oral Health Prev. Dent.* 14, 101–109.

Joao, C., Adriana, L., & Diana, P. (2020). A comprehensive review of the nutraceutical and therapeutic applications of red seaweeds (Rhodophyta). *Life*, 10 (3), article 19.

Kale, S., Kocadereli, I., Atilla, P., & Aşan, E. (2004). Comparison of the effects of 1,25 dihydroxycholecalciferol and prostaglandin E 2 on orthodontic tooth movement. *Am. J. Orthod. Dentofac. Orthop.*, 125, 607–614.

Karadeniz, E.I., Gonzales, C., Nebioglu-Dalci, O., Dwarte, D., Turk, T., Isci, D., Sahin-Saglam, A.M., Alkis, H., Elekdag-Turk, S., & Darendeliler, M.A. (2011). Physical properties of root cementum: Part 20. Effect of fluoride on orthodontically induced root resorption with light and heavy orthodontic forces for 4 weeks: A microcomputed tomography study. *Am. J. Orthod. Dentofac. Orthop.*, 140, e199–e210.

Kaur, C., & Kapoor, H.C. (2001). Antioxidants in fruits and vegetables-the millenium's health. *Int J Food Sci Technol* (36)7, 03–725.

Kersting, M., Alexy, U., & Sichert-Hellert, W. (2001). Dietary intake and food sources of minerals in 1 to 18 year old German children and adolescents. *Nutrition Research*, 21 (4), 607–616.

Khurshid, Z., Naseem, M., Sheikh, Z., Najeeb, S., Shahab, S., & Zafar, M.S. (2016). Oral antimicrobial peptides: Types and role in the oral cavity. *Saudi Pharm. J.*, 24(5), 515–524.

Kose, O., Arabaci, T., Yemenoglu, H., Kara, A., Ozkanlar, S., & Kayis, S. (2016). Influences of fucoxanthin on alveolar bone resorption in induced periodontitis in rat molars. *Marine Drugs*, 14, 70. doi: 10.3390/md14040070

Kulkarni, V., Bhatavadekar, N.B., & Uttamani, J.R. (2014). The effect of nutrition on periodontal disease: A systematic review. *J. Calif. Dent. Assoc.*, 42, 302–311.

Kumar, P., Rai, S., Verma, S.K., Prakash, P.S., & Chitara, D. (2022). Classification, mode of action and uses of various immunomodulators. In R.K. Kesharwani, R.K. Keservani, A.K. Sharma (eds) *Immunomodulators and Human Health*. Singapore: Springer. 10.1007/978-981-16-6379-6_1.

Lansdown, A.B., Mirastschijski, U., Stubbs, N., Scanlon, E., & Ågren, M.S. (2007). Zinc in wound healing: Theoretical, experimental, and clinical aspects. *Wound Repair Regen.*, 15, 2–16.

Lawrence, K.P., Long, P.F., & Young, A.R. (2018). Mycosporine – like amino acids for skin photoprotection. *Current Medicinal Chemistry*, 25 (40), 5512–5527.

Lee, H., Je, D., Won, S., Paik, D., & Bae, K. (2015). Association between vitamin D deficiency and periodontal status in current smokers. *Community Dent. Oral Epidemiol.*, 43, 471–478.

Lee, M-J, Lambert, J.D., & Prabhu, S. (2004). Delivery of tea polyphenols to the oral cavity by green tea leaves and black tea extract. *Cancer Epidemiol Biomarkers Prev*, 13, 132–137.

Lenoir-Wijnkoop, I., Sanders, M.E., Cabana, M.D., Caglar, E., Corthier, G., Rayes, N., Sherman, P.M., & Timmerman, H.M. (2007). Probiotic and prebiotic influence beyond the intestinal tract. *Nutr Rev*, 65, 469–489.

Lin, S.Y., Ayres, J.W., Wrinkler, W., & Sandine, W.E. (1989). Lactobacillus effects on cholesterol: In-vitro and in-vivo results. *J Dairy Sci*, 72, 2885–2899.

Lipi, D., Eshani, B., & Utpa, R. (2012). Role of nutraceuticals in human health. *Journal of Food Science and Technology*, 49(2), 173–183.

López, A.V., María D., Navarro-Hortal, Giampieri, F., Bullón, P., Battino, M., & Quiles, J.L. (2018). Nutraceuticals in periodontal health: A systematic review on the role of vitamins in periodontal health maintenance. *Molecules* 23, 1226. 10.3390/molecules23051226

Maddi, V.S., Aragade, P.D., Digge, V.G., & Nitaliker, M.N. (2007). Importance of nutraceuticals in health management. *Phcog Rev* (1), 377–379.

Maguire, A. (2014). ADA clinical recommendations on topical fluoride for caries prevention. *Evid. Based Dent.*, 15, 38–39.
Malik, A. (2008). The potentials of nutraceuticals. *Pharmainfo.net*, 6.
Maria, S.A., Jose, L.L., Albert, E.D., Raul, A.M., & Enric, J. (2017). Probiotics and oral health: A systematic review. *Med Oral Patol Oral Cir Bucal*, 2017 May 1; 22 (3), e282–e288. doi: 10.4317/medoral.21494. PMID: 28390121; PMCID: PMC5432076. http://www.medicinaoral.com/medoralfree01/v22i3/medoralv22i3p282.pdf
Mariotti, A. (1999). Dental plaque-induced gingival diseases. *Ann Periodontol*, 4, 7–17. doi: 10.1902/annals.1999.4.1.7
Mirastschijski, U., Haaksma, C.J., Tomasek, J.J., & Ågren, M.S. (2004). Matrix metalloproteinase inhibitor GM 6001 attenuates keratinocyte migration, contraction and myofibroblast formation in skin wounds. *Exp. Cell. Res.*, 299, 465–475.
Mitsunaga, T. (1999). Anticaries activity of bark proanthocyanidins. *Basic Life Sci*, 66, 555–573.
Najeeb, S., Khurshid, Z., Zohaib, S., & Zafar, M.S. (2016). Therapeutic potential of melatonin in oral medicine and periodontology. *Kaohsiung J. Med. Sci.*, 32, 391–396.
Nanci, A. (2012). *Ten Cate's Oral Histology: Development, Structure, and Function*; Mosby: St. Louis, MO, USA; London, UK, 411.
Neiva, R.F., Al-Shammari, K., Nociti, F.H., Jr., Soehren, S., & Wang, H. (2005). Effects of vitamin-B complex supplementation on periodontal wound healing. *J. Periodontol.*, 76, 1084–1091
Nguyen, T., Brody, H., Radaic, A., & Kapila, Y. (2021) Probiotics for periodontal health—Current molecular findings. *Periodontol 2000*, 87 (1), 254–267. doi: 10.1111/prd.12382.
Osis, D., Kramer, L., Wiatrowski, E., & Spencer, H. (1972). Dietary zinc intake in man. *Am. J. Clin. Nutr.*, 25, 582–588.
Pacht, E.R., Kaseki, H., Mohammed, J.R., Cornwell, D.G., & Davis, W.B. (1986). Deficiency of vitamin E in the alveolar fluid of cigarette smokers. Influence on alveolar macrophage cytotoxicity. *J. Clin. Investig.*, 77, 789–796.
Pandey, M., Verma, R.K., & Saraf, S.A. (2010). Nutraceuticals: New era of medicine and health. *Asian Journal of Pharmaceutical and Clinical Research*, 3, 11–15.
Petersen, P.E. (2003). The world oral health report 2003: continuous improvement of oral health in the 21st century – The approach of the WHO global oral health programme. *Commun Dent Oral Epidemiol*, 31 (1), 3–24. doi: 10.1046/j.2003.com122.x
Pushparani, D. (2014). Zinc and type 2 diabetes mellitus with periodontitis—A systematic review. *Curr. Diabetes Rev.*, 10, 397–401.
Pushparani, D.S. (2015). Serum zinc and β D glucuronidase enzyme level in type 2 diabetes mellitus with periodontitis. *Curr. Diabetes Rev.*, 11.
Rishi, R.K. (2006). Nutraceuticals: borderline between food and drug? *Pharma Rev*, 51–53.
Ritchie, C.S., & Kinane, D.F. (2003). Nutrition, inflammation, and periodontal disease. *Nutrition*, 19, 475.
Rostan, E.F., DeBuys, H.V., Madey, D.L., & Pinnell, S.R. (2002). Evidence supporting zinc as an essential antioxidant for skin. *Int. J. Dermatol.*, 41, 606–611.
Saido, M., Asakura, K., Masayasu, S., & Sasaki, S. (2016). Relationship between dietary sugar intake and dental caries among Japanese preschool children with relatively low sugar intake (Japan Nursery School SHOKUIKU Study): A nationwide cross-sectional study. *Matern. Child Health J.*, 20, 556.
Santini, A., & Novellino, E. (2017). Nutraceuticals in hypercholesterolaemia: An overview. *British Journal of Pharmacology* (174), 1450–1463.
Seppa, L., Forss, H., & Ogaard, B. (1993). The effect of fluoride application on fluoride release and the antibacterial action of glass ionomers. *J. Dent. Res.*, 72, 1310–1314.

Sami Labs—pioneer in nutraceuticals (Aug 05 2002). The Hindu Newspaper; Available from: http://www.hinduonnet.com/thehindu/ biz/2002/08/05/stories/2002080500040200.htm
Shaikh, H.S. (2020). Diverse application of marine components and bioactives in dentistry: a review. *World J Adv Sci Res.*, 3, 169–181.
Shearer, M.J., & Newman, P. (2008). Metabolism and cell biology of vitamin K. *Thromb. Haemost.*, 100, 530–547.
Sheikh, Z., Najeeb, S., Khurshid, Z., Verma, V., Rashid, H., & Glogauer, M. (2015). Biodegradable materials for bone repair and tissue engineering applications. *Materials*, 8, 5744–5794.
Shimabukuro, Y., Nakayama, Y., Ogata, Y., Tamazawa, K., Shimauchi, H., Nishida, T., Ito, K., Chikazawa, T., Kataoka, S., & Murakami, S. (2015). Effects of an ascorbic acid—Derivative dentifrice in patients with gingivitis: A double-masked, randomised, controlled clinical trial. *J. Periodontol.*, 86, 27–35.
Slade, E.W., Jr., Bartuska, D., Rose, L.F., & Cohen, D.W. (1976). Vitamin E and periodontal disease. *J. Periodontol.*, 47, 352–354.
Soto, S.M. (2013). Role of efflux pumps in the antibiotic resistance of bacteria embedded in a biofilm. Virulence. 4, 223–229. doi: 10.4161/viru.23724
Staudte, H., Kranz, S., Völpel, A., Schütze, J., & Sigusch, B.W. (2012). Comparison of nutrient intake between patients with periodontitis and healthy subjects. *Quintessence Int.*, 43, 907–916.
Stranges, S., Marshall, J.R., Trevisan, M., Natarajan, R., Donahue, R.P., Combs, G.F., Farinaro, E., Clark, C.L., & Reid, M.E. (2006). Effects of selenium supplementation on cardiovascular disease incidence and mortality: Secondary analyses in a randomised clinical trial. *Am J Epidemiol*, 163, 694–699.
Sung, H., Ferlay, J., Siegel, R.L., Laversanne, M., Soerjomataram, I., & Jemal, A. (2021). Global cancer statistics 2020: GLOBOCAN estimates of incidence and mortality worldwide for 36 cancers in 185 countries. *Cancer J Clin.*, 71, 209–249. doi: 10.3322/caac.21660
Toba, Y., Kajita, Y., Masuyama, R., Takada, Y., Suzuki, K., & Aoe, S. (2000). Dietary magnesium supplementation affects bone metabolism and dynamic strength of bone in ovariectomised rats. *J. Nutr.*, 130, 216–220.
Tsutsumi, K., Fujikawa, H., Kajikawa, T., Takedachi, M., Yamamoto, T., & Murakami, S. (2012). Effects of L-ascorbic acid 2-phosphate magnesium salt on the properties of human gingival fibroblasts. *J. Periodont. Res.*, 47, 263–271.
Vander Velden, U., Kuzmanova, D., & Chapple, I. (2011). Micronutritional approaches to periodontal therapy. *J. Clin. Periodontol.*, 38, 142–158.
Wang, H., Provan, G., & Helliwell, K. (2003). The functional benefits of flavonoids: The case of tea. *Phytochem Funct Foods*, 128–159.
Wu, M. Truksa, & Datla, N. (2005). Stepwise engineering to produce high yields of very long-chain polyunsaturated fatty acids in plants. *Nature Biotechnology*, 23, 1013–1017.
Zeisel, S.H. (1999). Regulation of nutraceuticals. *Science* 285, 1853–1855.
Zong, G., Holtfreter, B., Scott, A.E., Völzke, H., Petersmann, A., Dietrich, T., Newson, R.S., & Kocher, T. (2016). Serum vitamin B12 is inversely associated with periodontal progression and risk of tooth loss: A prospective cohort study. *J. Clin. Periodontol.*, 43, 2–9.

16 Nutraceutical Mediated AMPK Activation

Prospects and Molecular Executors

Aaysha Gupta and Sonam Chawla

16.1 INTRODUCTION

According to the federal Food, Drug, and Cosmetic Act (FFDCA), Nutraceuticals is a portmanteau term coined by Dr Stephen L. DeFelice from "Nutrition" and "Pharmaceutical" in 1989 (Lyons and Roche 2018; Santini et al. 2017; Di. Nicolantonio et al. 2022). According to Dr. Stephen, nutraceuticals are biologically herbal dietary components isolated from herbal and dietary supplements purported to postulate additional health benefits, in addition to availability of nutrition In food (Santini et al. 2017). It includes: vitamins, minerals, farmaceuticals, and biopharmaceuticals. Additionally, nutraceuticals are used to improve health and wellness, as an anti-ageing drug, chronic disease prevention, structural and functional support to the body, and also help to overcome pathophysiological conditions (Prasad et al. 2017). Furthermore, the key benefit of nutraceuticals is the activation of AMPK to maintain cellular homoeostasis (Lewis et al. 2022).

Heterotrimeric unit (αβϒ) of AMPK consists of 3 subunits which involve: catalytic alpha subunits (α1, α2), regulatory beta subunits (β1, β2), and Gamma subunits (γ1, γ2, and γ3). These structural subunits have their specific role in activity, specific mechanisms of AMPK, differential tissue localisation, and different functionality under different conditions (Yan et al. 2018; Yan et al. 2019). 5′AMP-activated protein kinase (AMPK) is an evolutionary conserved fuel-sensing serine-threonine kinase enzyme that plays a key role in energy homoeostasis. It gets activated in various cellular metabolism by regulating the AMP:ATP ratio. When AMPK gets activated by the breakdown of ATP synthesis, it stimulates glucose synthesis (via regulating insulin signalling pathways) together with fatty acid uptake and increased oxidation, inhibition of protein, and lipid synthesis (Aslam et al. 2022). This is why it is considered the "Energy Sensor of the Cell." Furthermore, AMPK involves the activation of various energy-producing pathways (Insulin signalling pathway, nutrient signalling pathway), similarly inhibition of energy-consuming pathways (glycogen synthesis inhibition) (Mihaylova and Shaw 2011).

 DOI: 10.1201/9781003392934-16

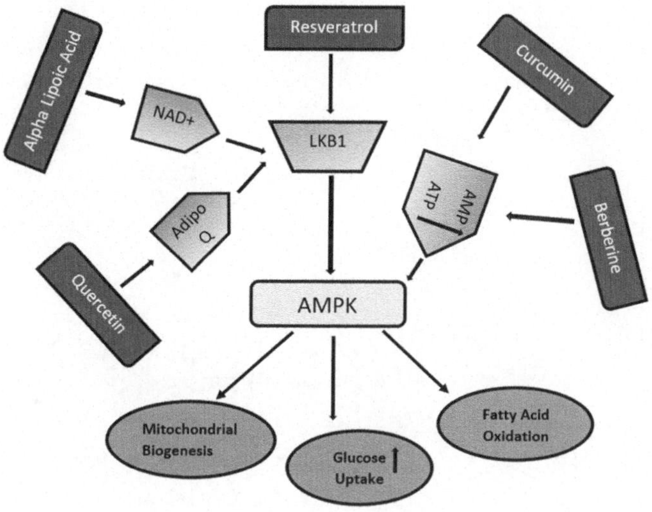

FIGURE 16.1 Illustration of AMPK activation by different nutraceuticals for improved cellular energy homoeostasis.

Additionally, nutraceuticals (such as; resveratrol, curcumin, berberine, epigallocatechin, alpha lipoic acid, and quercetin) are widely used when it comes to improving health conditions and maintaining cellular homoeostasis. Specifically, nutraceuticals are shown to activate AMPK through various mechanistic pathways and metabolism including; activation of energy-producing pathways, upstream kinases activation, protein phosphatases inhibition, mitochondrial biogenesis, lipid metabolism, and glucose metabolism (Valero T 2014; Herzig and Shaw 2018). Further, Figure 16.1 represents the activation of various AMPK through various nutraceuticals. In conclusion, this chapter outlines the AMPK-associated signalling pathways, activation of AMPK through various nutraceuticals to deal with metabolic disorders as well as clinical studies and their outcomes in order to provide proof of evidence for the beneficial effects of AMPK activation by various nutraceuticals.

16.2 AMPK SIGNALLING PATHWAYS

There are various molecules, targeting AMPK activation where AMP is found to be the most prominent molecule activating AMPK, represented in figure 17.2 (Ge et al. 2022). However, it is also activated by a biomolecule known as Liver Kinase B1 (LKB1). Another activator of AMPK is exercise which promotes the breakdown of ATP into AMP (Mihaylova and Shaw 2011). Thus, various other signalling cascades are involved in the activation of AMPK, and a few of them are discussed below (Figure 16.2):

16.2.1 Protein Metabolism and Autophagy

AMPK regulates the mTOR signalling pathway negatively, which is responsible for protein synthesis (Ge et al. 2022). Thus, AMPK activation suppresses protein

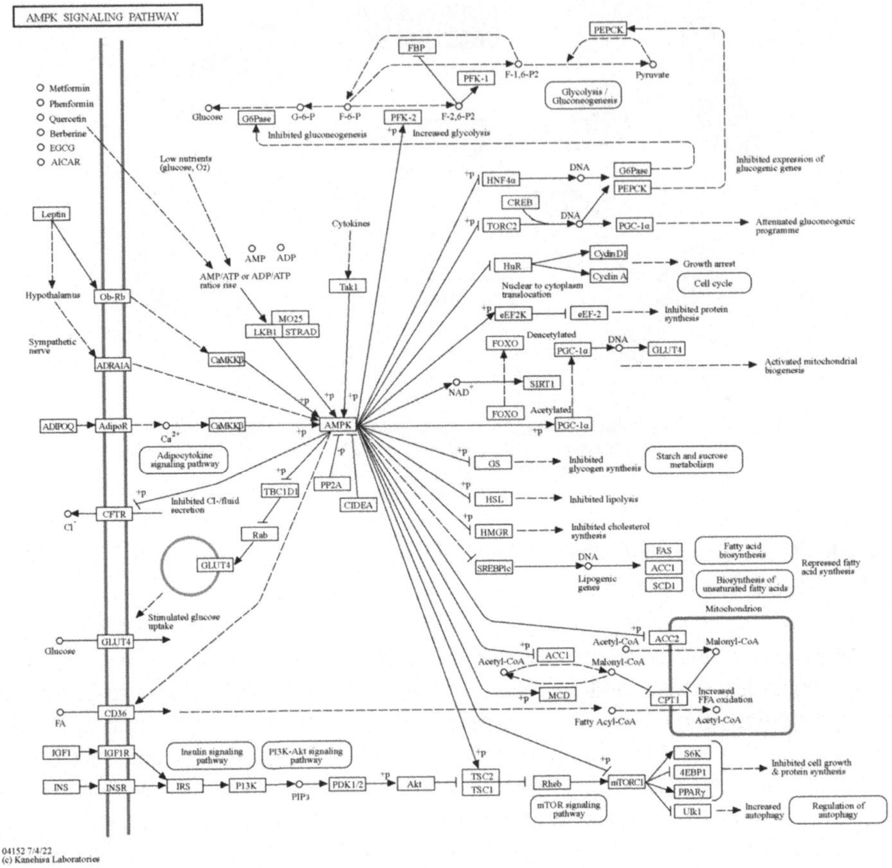

FIGURE 16.2 AMPK Signalling Pathways (KEGG Pathway Database: https://www.genome.jp/pathway/hsa04152)

synthesis. Additionally, AMPK activates ULK1 which is a very important protein responsible for macro autophagy thus promoting autophagy (Mihaylova and Shaw 2011).

16.2.2 Lipid Metabolism

AMPK activates adenosine triglyceride lipase (ATGL), a lipids homoeostasis regulator and the first enzyme needed for the release of fatty acids from the triglyceride molecule. Thus, basically activating fatty acid catabolism (Mihaylova and Shaw 2011; Zang et al. 2018; Shen et al. 2019). While promoting fatty acid catabolism, Acetyl CoA (ACC)inhibition by inhibiting synthesis of fatty acid is reported to be inhibited by AMPK. It also inhibits HMG-CoA reductase which is necessary for cholesterol synthesis. Thus, AMPK also plays a role in reducing cholesterol formation (Mihaylova and Shaw 2011).

16.2.3 Glycogen Metabolism

AMPK also inhibits glycogen synthase and thus inhibits glycogen synthesis. Another important function of AMPK at the cellular level is the activation of glucose uptake through GLUT4. Through activation of TBC1D1, glucose uptake via GLUT4 is triggered (Steinberg and Hardie 2022). This procedure promotes an insulin-sensitive cell to increase the uptake of glucose independent of insulin signalling. The uptake takes place through the AMPK-dependent pathway (Muraleedharan and Dasgupta 2021). This is what happens during exercise. Majorly, the increase in glucose uptake and glycolysis is triggered (Mihaylova and Shaw 2011).

16.3 NUTRACEUTICALS AND THEIR POTENTIAL TO ACTIVATE AMPK FOR MANAGEMENT OF METABOLIC DISORDERS

Nutraceuticals primarily activate AMPK (energy metabolism regulator) to exert their health benefits. During low energy states, AMPK gets activated to restore energy via regulation of major longevity pathways, including: insulin signalling pathways and nutrient sensing pathways. Several key nutraceutical attributes to activate AMPK are listed in Table 17.1 with their potential metabolic activity (Valero 2014).

16.3.1 Resveratrol

Resveratrol is a natural polyphenol of plants mainly grapes, peanuts, and berries. It exhibits various health benefits including; anti-inflammatory, antioxidative and can protect against the high risk of carcinogenic damage. The activating mechanism of AMPK by resveratrol is majorly involved in health benefits (Price et al. 2012).

Resveratrol mediated AMPK activation by several mechanisms including, increasing the ratio of AMP/ATP, which signifies the lower energy ratio, and thus, AMPK gets activated to increase glucose uptake and further increase energy level. Additionally, AMPK translocation promotion, inhibition of deacetylase activity of SIRT1, increasing levels of intracellular calcium, activation of upstream kinases (Liver Kinase B1(LKB1)), leads to activation of AMPK (Huang et al. 2019).

16.3.2 Alpha Lipoic Acid

Alpha lipoic acid (ALA) is an antioxidant. It is absorbed from the gastrointestinal tract rapidly. In the body, it dissolves in both water and fat (Zhou L and Cheng Y 2019). ALA includes food sources; yeast, meat, and vegetables. ALA from food, however, is not found to be highly productive in order to provide a noticeable increase in the free ALA body's level. In order to improve a variety of health conditions, some individuals take ALA supplements (Prieto et al. 2015). Supplemental ALA carries inconclusive scientific evidence for the health benefits. Reported data on ALA suggests that approximately 30–40% of an ALA supplement's oral dose is absorbed. Empty stomach ingestion of ALA results in better absorption (Jiang et al. 2013). ALA is a naturally occurring compound. At the cellular level, it serves vital functions, such as producing energy. Interestingly, a healthy human body mechanism is able to produce sufficient ALA needed for these purposes. Despite that fact, ALA supplements are found to be hotcakes for researchers (Targonsky et al. 2006).

16.3.3 Quercetin

Quercetin is a polyphenol-extracted plant flavanol and phytochemically belongs to the flavonoid group. Various fruits such as berries, leaves, seeds, grains, red onions, and kale contain significant amounts of quercetin. Quercetin with a bitter taste is also reported in dietary supplements, drinks, and foods as an ingredient. The most prevalent dietary flavonoid of Quercetin has an estimated daily intake of 25–50 milligrams. With optimum concentration. One study found that 79% more quercetin was found in organically grown tomatoes than in non-organically grown produce. In different kinds of honey from various plant sources, Quercetin is present (Singh et al. 2021; Alizadeh and Ebrahimzadeh 2021; Goyal and Aggrawal 2022).

Quercetin with poor bioavailability is highly variable in humans (0 to 50%) and has an expeditious half-life of 1–2 hours after consumption when in the form of food and dietary supplements. The biological effects predicted from *in vitro* research cannot be applied *in vivo* due to the rapid and thorough metabolism that quercetin undergoes after dietary consumption. (Alizadeh and Ebrahimzadeh 2021).

Quercetin, a protein kinase enzyme non-specific inhibitor, also stimulates the functions of a variety of proteins or inhibits them. By stimulating oestrogen receptors, Quercetin has also been reported for its female sex hormone-like(oestrogenic) activities. The binding IC50 values for quercetin are 1015 nM and 113 nM, respectively, and it activates both the alpha (ERa) and beta (ERβ) oestrogen receptors. Quercetin is hence approx. (9 times) selective to ERβ and around two to three orders of magnitude less active than the endogenous oestrogen 17β-estradiol. Quercetin, in cancerous breast cell lines of humans, has also been demonstrated to behave as a G protein-coupled oestrogen receptor agonist (GPER) (Wilkinson et al. 2015)

16.3.4 EGCG (Epigallocatechin Gallate)

Epigallocatechin-3-gallatechin, a catechin commonly referred to as epigallocatechin gallate (EGCG), is an epigallocatechin and gallic acid ester. Because of its ability to influence human health and illness, EGCG, is a highly prominent tea catechin classified as a fundamental science polyphenol (Cione et al. 2019). In several dietary supplements, EGCG is used. Orally administered EGCG has a poor absorption rate albeit with daily ingestion ~8–16 cups of green tea, leading to negative side effects such as severe nausea or heartburn. Blood epigallocatechin levels reach their highest approx 1.7 hours after ingestion. The ingested EGCG has a plasma half-life (1/2) of around 5–6 hours, although more than half of it is eliminated in urine during the course of 0 to 8 hours. The plasma levels of methylated metabolites are 8–25 times higher than those of unmetabolized EGCG and have predominantly longer half-lives (Agarwal R 2000).

TABLE 16.1
Different Nutraceutical Attributes to Activate AMPK are Listed with Their Source and Potential Metabolic Activity

Nutraceutical	Source	Mechanism of AMPK Activation	References
Resveratrol	Grapes, berries, peanuts	↑AMPK:ATP ratio, activates AMPK via SIRT1	Zhang F et al. 2017
Curcumin	Turmeric	Activates AMPK via liver kinase B1 (LKB1)	Qiao P. j et al. 2020
Quercetin	Onions, apples, berries	↑AMP:ATP ratio, AMPK activation via LKB1	Dhanya et al. 2017
EGCG	Green tea	↑AMP:ATP ratio, AMPK activation via LKB1	Murase et al. 2009
Berberine	Barberry, goldenseal	Activated AMPK via LKB1	Di. Nicolantonio et al. 2022
Alpha lipoic acid	Spinach, broccoli, and potatoes	ALA can ↑AMPK activation, ↑ cellular AMP:ATP ratio	Wang et al. 2010

High levels are present in dried green tea leaves (738.0 mg per 10 g), white tea (424.5 mg per 10 g), and smaller amounts of black tea (93.6 mg per 10 g)(Tadesse et al. 2015). Polyphenolic oxidation of catechins leads to their conversion in theaflavins and thearubigins during the black tea developmental process (Takemoto et al. 2018) (Table 16.1).

16.4 MOLECULAR EXECUTORS OF NUTRACEUTICAL-MEDIATED AMPK ACTIVATION

Nutraceuticals provide various molecules and their mechanistic pathways in order to activate AMPK. Additionally, some kinases and enzymes also lead to activation of AMPK. For example, certain nutraceuticals may activate AMPK by phosphorylating it using LKB1, mitochondrial ATP inhibition that triggers a cellular response, further leading to increased energy production through AMPK activation. Also, Modulation of signalling pathways(mTOR) activates AMPK (Bi L et al. 2021; Han et al. 2020).

16.4.1 LKB1

Tumour suppressor serine/threonine kinase LKB1 is a key upstream activator of AMPK. The alpha subunit of AMPK's activation loop has a particular threonine residue (Thr-172) that is directly phosphorylated by LKB1. Therefore, it results in the conformational change in AMPK and also phosphorylation of downstream pathways occurs (Bi L et al. 2021).

Additionally, LKB1, scaffold protein (STE20-related kinase adaptor protein), regulatory protein, and mouse protein 25(MO25) interaction-mediated cytoplasmic translocation of LKB1 in energy stress conditions results in activation of

AMPK. Whereas in a normal state, LKB1 lies in the nucleus of the resting cells (Gan and Li 2014).

Various nutraceuticals like resveratrol and curcumin results in AMPK activation and downstream metabolic pathways through LKB1(Lee and Lin 2018).

16.4.2 CaMKKβ(Calcium/Calmodulin-Dependent Protein Kinase Kinase β)

Serine/threonine-regulated kinase CaMKKβ consists of three domains, including: an N-terminal kinase domain, a C-terminal regulatory domain, and several intermediary domains. These domains play a key role in the identification of substrates and also in their regulation. The activity of CaMKKβ is majorly regulated by various mechanisms, including: Regulatory protein interaction, post-translational modification and phosphorylation, and subcellular localisation (Tokumitsu and Sakagami 2022; Sun et al. 2018).

CaMKKβ is the activator of CaMKKβ I, CaMKKβ IV, and AMPK (Tokumitsu and Sakagami 2022). Various physiological pathways promote the activation of AMPK via CaMKKβ, including the formation of memory and learning, energy balance regulation, and differentiation of neurons (Roesler et al. 2014).

Various nutraceuticals have been shown to activate AMPK and downstream metabolic pathways by CaMKKβ, such as; resveratrol, EGCG, and quercetin.

16.5 CLINICAL STUDIES ON NUTRACEUTICAL-MEDIATED AMPK ACTIVATION AND THEIR OUTCOMES

This clinical study is based on nutraceutical-mediated AMPK activation. Clinical studies have reported the nutraceuticals' potential for activation of AMPK. One such study has shown the effects of resveratrol(nutraceutical) in obese adult human participants. The investigation showed that resveratrol increased AMPK activity through the activation of AMPK, leading to enhanced insulin sensitivity and decreased body weight (Baur et al. 2006). Similarly, numerous nutraceuticals and their clinical studies have been curated and tabulated in Table 16.2. These clinical studies suggest that nutraceuticals have a positive impact on AMPK activation. In addition, clinically safe studies are warranted to understand the efficacy of these nutraceuticals along with the exploration of new potential nutraceuticals.

16.6 CONCLUSION AND IMPLICATIONS FOR NUTRACEUTICALS USAGE IN THE MANAGEMENT OF METABOLIC DISORDERS THROUGH AMPK ACTIVATION

With age advancement and changing lifestyles, individuals are silently moving towards a deteriorating healthspan and increasing disorders such as obesity, diabetes, and elevated blood pressure, etc. These disorders further give rise to ageing-associated diseases including, frailty, cardiovascular diseases. and Alzheimers, etc. In order to hinder the prevalence of these diseases, nutraceuticals are widely used to activate the additional hallmark of ageing (AMPK).

TABLE 16.2
Clinical Trials Testing the Efficacy of the Nutraceuticals in the Activation of AMPK

Nutraceutical	Study Design	Participants	Outcomes	References
Resveratrol	Randomised study, double-blind, placebo-controlled trial	11 obese adults	AMPK activity increased	Timmers et al. 2011
Curcumin	Study was a randomised, double-blind, placebo-controlled trial	117 obese adults	Increased AMPK activity	Panahi et al. 2016
Quercetin	Study was a randomised, double-blind, placebo-controlled trial	60 obese adults	Zhu et al.2019	Zhu et al. 2019
Berberine	Study was a randomised, double-blind, placebo-controlled trial	116 adults (type 2 diabetes)	Increased AMPK activity	Yin et al. 2008
Omega-3 fatty acids	Study was a randomised, double-blind, placebo-controlled trial	30 adults (metabolic syndrome)	Increased AMPK activity	Ferramosca et al. 2016
Cinnamon	Study was a randomised, double-blind, placebo-controlled trial	66 adults (type 2 diabetes)	Increased AMPK activity	Akilen et al. 2010
Ginsenosides	Study was a randomised, double-blind, placebo-controlled trial	40 obese adults	Increased AMPK activity	Jin et al. 2018
Ginger	Study was a randomised, double-blind, placebo-controlled trial	70 obese adults	Increased AMPK activity	Salaramoli et al. 2022

In conclusion, the utility of nutraceuticals and activation of AMPK, has been established to improve various metabolisms, including lipid metabolism, glucose metabolism, insulin sensitivity, as well as potential neuroprotective effects. Clinical trials of various nutraceuticals have demonstrated their beneficial activity towards various metabolic and ageing-associated disorders. Furthermore, AMPK activation by nutraceuticals can be used as a promising avenue to identify a possible intervention of longevity-associated diseases and also can be used to identify new therapeutics for metabolic disorders including abdominal obesity, atherogenic dyslipidemia, and elevated blood pressure.

REFERENCES

Agarwal, R. (2000). Cell signaling and regulators of cell cycle as molecular targets for prostate cancer prevention by dietary agents. *Biochem Pharmacol*, 60(8), 1051–1059.

Akilen, R., Tsiami, A., Devendra, D., & Robinson, N. (2010). Glycated haemoglobin and blood pressure-lowering effect of cinnamon in multi-ethnic Type 2 diabetic patients in the UK: A randomized, placebo-controlled, double-blind clinical trial. *Diabetic Medicine*, 27(10), 1159–1167.

Alizadeh, S.R., & Ebrahimzadeh, M.A. (2021). Quercetin derivatives: Drug design, development, and biological activities, a review. *Eur J Med Chem.*, 229, 114068

Aslam, M., & Ladilov, Y. (2022). Emerging role of cAMP/AMPK signaling. *Cells.*, 11(2), 308.

Baur, J.A., Pearson, K.J., Price, N.L., Jamieson, H.A., Lerin, C., Kalra, A., Prabhu, V.V., Allard, J.S., Lopez-Lluch, G., Lewis, K. et al. (2006). Resveratrol improves health and survival of mice on a high-calorie diet. *Nature*; 444(7117), 337–342.

Bi, L., Ren, Y., Feng, M., Meng, P., Wang, Q., Chen, W., Jiao, Q., Wang, Y., Du, L., Zhou, F., Jiang, Y., Chen, F., Wang, C., Tang, B., & Wang, Y. (2021). HDAC11 regulates glycolysis through the LKB1/AMPK signaling pathway to maintain hepatocellular carcinoma stemness. *Cancer Res*, 81(8), 2015–2028.

Cione, E., La, Torre. C, Cannataro, R., Caroleo, M.C., Plastina, P., & Gallelli, L. (2019). Quercetin, epigallocatechin gallate, curcumin, and resveratrol: From dietary sources to human microRNA modulation. *Molecules*, 25(1), 63.

Dhanya, R., Arya, A.D., Nisha, P., & Jayamurthy, P. (2017). Quercetin, a lead compound against Type 2 diabetes ameliorates glucose uptake via AMPK pathway in skeletal muscle cell line. *Front Pharmacol*, 8, 336.

Di. Nicolantonio, J.J., McCarty, M.F., Assanga, S.I., Lujan, L.L., & O'Keefe, J.H. (2022). Ferulic acid and berberine, via Sirt1 and AMPK, may act as cell cleansing promoters of healthy longevity. *Open Heart*, 9(1), e001801

Ferramosca, A., Conte, L., & Zara, V. (2016). A krill oil supplemented diet suppresses hepatic steatosis in high-fat fed rats. *PLoS ONE*, 11(5), e0156689.

Gan, R.Y., & Li, H.B. (2014). Recent progress on liver kinase B1 (LKB1) expression, regulation, downstream signaling and cancer suppressive function. *Int J Mol Sci.*, 15(9), 16698–16718.

Ge, Y., Zhou, M., Chen, C., Wu, X., & Wang, X. (2022). Role of AMPK mediated pathways in autophagy and aging. *Biochimie*, 195, 100–113.

Goyal, A., & Agrawal, N. (2022). Quercetin: A potential candidate for the treatment of arthritis. *Curr Mol Med.*, 22(4), 325–335.

Han, D., Jiang, L., Gu, X., Huang, S., Pang, J., Wu, Y., Yin, J., & Wang, J. (2020). SIRT3 deficiency is resistant to autophagy-dependent ferroptosis by inhibiting the AMPK/mTOR pathway and promoting GPX4 levels. *J Cell Physiol*, 235(11), 8839–8851.

Herzig, S., & Shaw, R.J. (2018). AMPK: guardian of metabolism and mitochondrial homeostasis. *Nat Rev Mol Cell Biol*, 19(2), 121–135.

Huang, Y., Zhu, X., Chen, K., Lang, H., Zhang, Y., Hou, P., Ran, L., Zhou, M., Zheng, J., Yi, L., Mi, M., & Zhang, Q. (2019). Resveratrol prevents sarcopenic obesity by reversing mitochondrial dysfunction and oxidative stress via the PKA/LKB1/AMPK pathway. *Aging (Albany NY). 2019*, 11(8), 2217–2240.

Jiang, T., Yin, F., Yao, J., Brinton, R.D., & Cadenas, E. (2013). Lipoic acid restores age-associated impairment of brain energy metabolism through the modulation of Akt/JNK signaling and PGC1α transcriptional pathway. *Aging Cell*, 12(6), 1021–1031.

Jin, X., Jin, H.R., Ji, X.Y., & Ye, W.C. (2018). Ginsenoside Rg3 improves lipid metabolism and insulin sensitivity in obese rats via the AMPK signaling pathway. *Acta Pharmacologica Sinica*, 39(1), 120–128.

Lee, S.W., & Lin, H.K. (2018). A new mechanism for LKB1 activation. *Mol Cell Oncol.*, 5(3), e1035691.

Lewis, Luján, L.M., McCarty, M.F., Di, Nicolantonio J.J., Gálvez, Ruiz J.C., Rosas-Burgos, E.C., Plascencia-Jatomea, M., & Iloki, Assanga S.B. (2022). Nutraceuticals/drugs promoting mitophagy and mitochondrial biogenesis may combat the mitochondrial dysfunction driving progression of dry age-related macular degeneration. *Nutrients*, 14(9), 1985.

Lyons, C.L., & Roche, H.M. (2018). Nutritional modulation of AMPK-impact upon metabolic-inflammation. *Int J Mol Sci*, 19(10), 3092.

Mihaylova, M.M., & Shaw, R.J. (2011). The AMPK signalling pathway coordinates cell growth, autophagy and metabolism. *Nat Cell Biol*, 13(9), 1016–1023.

Muraleedharan, R., & Dasgupta, B. (2022). AMPK in the brain: Its roles in glucose and neural metabolism. *FEBS J*, 2247–2262.

Murase, T., Misawa, K., Haramizu, S., & Hase, T. (2009). Catechin-induced activation of the LKB1/AMP-activated protein kinase pathway. *Biochem Pharmacol*, 78(1), 78–84.

Panahi, Y., Hosseini, M.S., Khalili, N., Naimi, E., Majeed, M., Sahebkar, A., & Amirian, M. (2016). Effects of supplementation with curcumin on serum adipokine concentrations: A randomized controlled trial. *Nutrition*, 32(10), 1116–1122.

Prasad, S., Gupta, S.C., & Tyagi, A.K. (2017). Reactive oxygen species (ROS) and cancer: Role of antioxidative nutraceuticals. *Cancer Lett.*, 387, 95–105.

Price, N.L., Gomes, A.P., Ling, A.J., Duarte, F.V., Martin-Montalvo, A., North, B.J., Agarwal, B., Ye, L., Ramadori, G., Teodoro, J.S., Hubbard, B.P., Varela, A.T., Davis, J.G., Varamini, B., Hafner, A., Moaddel, R., Rolo, A.P., Coppari, R., Palmeira, C.M., de Cabo, R., Baur, J.A., & Sinclair, D.A. (2012). SIRT1 is required for AMPK activation and the beneficial effects of resveratrol on mitochondrial function. *Cell Metab*, 15(5), 675–690.

Prieto-Hontoria, P.L., Pérez-Matute, P., Fernández-Galilea, M., López-Yoldi, M., Sinal, C.J., Martínez, J.A., & Moreno-Aliaga, M.J. (2015). Effects of alpha-lipoic acid on chemerin secretion in 3T3-L1 and human adipocytes. *Biochim Biophys Acta*, 1861(3), 260–268

Qiao, P., Ma, J., Wang, Y., Huang, Z., Zou, Q., Cai, Z., & Tang, Y. (2020). Curcumin prevents neuroinflammation by inducing microglia to transform into the M2-phenotype via CaMKKβ-dependent activation of the AMP-activated protein kinase signal pathway. *Curr Alzheimer Res*, 17(8), 735–752.

Roesler, R., Brunetto, A.T., Abujamra, A.L., & Brunetto, A.L. (2014). Emerging roles of CaMKKβ/AMPK signaling in memory and learning. *Frontiers in Aging Neuroscience*, 6, 359.

Salaramoli, S., Mehri, S., Yarmohammadi, F., Hashemy, S.I., & Hosseinzadeh, H. (2022). The effects of ginger and its constituents in the prevention of metabolic syndrome: A review. *Iran J Basic Med Sci*, 25(6), 664–674.

Santini, A., Tenore, G.C., & Novellino, E. (2017). Nutraceuticals: A paradigm of proactive medicine. *Eur J Pharm Sci*, 96, 53–61.

Shen, B., Zhao, C., Wang, Y., Peng, Y., Cheng, J., Li, Z., Wu, L., Jin, M., & Feng, H. (2019). Aucubin inhibited lipid accumulation and oxidative stress via Nrf2/HO-1 and AMPK signalling pathways. *J Cell Mol Med*, 4063–4075.

Singh, P., Arif, Y., Bajguz, A., & Hayat, S. (2021). The role of quercetin in plants. *Plant Physiol Biochem*, 166, 10–19.

Steinberg, G.R., & Hardie, D.G. (2022). New insights into activation and function of the AMPK. *Nat Rev Mol Cell Biol*:41580-022-00547

Sun, B., Ou, H., Ren, F., Huan, Y., Zhong, T., Gao, M., & Cai, H. (2018). Propofol inhibited autophagy through Ca2+/CaMKKβ/AMPK/mTOR pathway in OGD/R-induced neuron injury. *Mol Med.*, 24(1), 58.

Tadesse, A., Hymete, A., Bekhit, A.A., & Mohammed, S.F. (2015). Quantification of total polyphenols, catechin, caffeine, L-theanine, determination of antioxidant activity and effect on antileishmanial drugs of Ethiopian tea leaves extracts. *Pharmacognosy Res*, 7(Suppl 1), S7–S14.

Takemoto, M., & Takemoto, H. (2018). Synthesis of theaflavins and their functions. *Molecules*, 23(4), 918.

Targonsky, E.D., Dai, F., Koshkin, V., Karaman, G.T., Gyulkhandanyan, A.V., Zhang, Y., Chan, C.B., & Wheeler, M.B. (2006). alpha-lipoic acid regulates AMP-activated protein kinase and inhibits insulin secretion from beta cells. *Diabetologia*, 49(7), 1587–1598.

Timmers, S., Konings, E., Bilet, L., Houtkooper, R.H., van de Weijer, T., Goossens, G.H., Hoeks, J., van der Krieken, S., Ryu, D., Kersten, S. et al. (2011). Calorie restriction-like effects of 30 days of resveratrol supplementation on energy metabolism and metabolic profile in obese humans. *Cell Metabolism*, 14(5), 612–622.

Tokumitsu, H., & Sakagami, H. (2022). Molecular mechanisms underlying Ca2+/Calmodulin-dependent protein kinase kinase signal transduction. *Int J Mol Sci.*, 23(19), 11025.

Valero, T. (2014). Mitochondrial biogenesis: Pharmacological approaches. *Curr Pharm Des*, 20(35), 5507–5509.

Wang, Y., Li, X., Guo, Y., Chan, L., & Guan, X. (2010). Alpha-lipoic acid increases energy expenditure by enhancing adenosine monophosphate-activated protein kinase-peroxisome proliferator-activated receptor-gamma coactivator-1alpha signaling in the skeletal muscle of aged mice. *Metabolism*, 59(7), 967–976.

Wilkinson, A.S., Taing, M.W., Pierson, J.T., Lin, C.N., Dietzgen, R.G., Shaw, P.N., Gidley, M.J., Monteith, G.R., & Roberts-Thomson, S.J. (2015). Estrogen modulation properties of mangiferin and quercetin and the mangiferin metabolite norathyriol. *Food Funct*, 6(6), 1847–1854.

Yan, Y., Zhou, X.E., Xu, H.E., & Melcher, K. (2018). Structure and physiological regulation of AMPK. *Int J Mol Sci*, 19(11), 3534.

Yan, Y., Zhou, X.E., Novick, S.J., Shaw, S.J., Li, Y., Brunzelle, J.S., Hitoshi, Y., Griffin, P.R., Xu, H.E., & Melcher, K. (2019). Structures of AMP-activated protein kinase bound to novel pharmacological activators in phosphorylated, non-phosphorylated, and nucleotide-free states. *J Biol Chem*, 294(3), 953–967.

Yin, J., Gao, Z., Liu, D., Liu, Z., & Ye, J. (2008). Berberine improves glucose metabolism through induction of glycolysis. *American Journal of Physiology. Endocrinology and Metabolism*, 294(1), E148–E156.

Zang, Y., Fan, L., Chen, J., Huang, R., & Qin, H. (2018). Improvement of lipid and glucose metabolism by capsiate in palmitic acid-treated HepG2 cells via activation of the AMPK/SIRT1 signaling pathway. *J Agric Food Chem*, 66(26), 6772–6781.

Zhang, S., Gao, L., Liu, X., Lu, T., Xie, C., & Jia, J. (2017). Resveratrol attenuates microglial activation via SIRT1-SOCS1 pathway. *Evid Based Complement Alternat Med*, 2017, 8791832.

Zhou, L., & Cheng, Y. (2019). Alpha-lipoic acid alleviated 6-OHDA-induced cell damage by inhibiting AMPK/mTOR mediated autophagy. *Neuropharmacology*, 155, 98–103.

Zhu, L., Zhang, Y., Chen, Y., Zheng, X., & Chen, J. (2019). Quercetin intervention in AMPK/LOX pathways alleviates chronic kidney disease-associated endothelial dysfunction via autophagy enhancement. *Biochemical and Biophysical Research Communications*, 514(4), 1267–1273.

17 Agro-Food Waste, a Potential Bioresource for Nutraceuticals

Arpita Gupte, Anuja Kulkarni, Pratik Pawar, Smita Jadhav, and Anjali Kembhavi

17.1 INTRODUCTION

Agro-food waste, found at various stages of the food supply chain, deteriorates in nutritional quality. Growing demand for processed agricultural and food items has amplified waste generation, negatively impacting the environment and society. Recent studies (Faustino et al. 2019; Panzella et al. 2020; Vilas-Boas et al. 2021) have unveiled the potential of repurposing agro-food waste as a renewable source of bioactive compounds, prized for their health benefits and rheological properties.

The United Nations Food and Agricultural Organisations (FAO) report reveals higher agricultural production losses in developing nations, while economically stable regions experience greater consumer and retail food waste. Approximately 14% of harvested and retail food is lost, constituting 17% of global food waste. Most agro-based waste is seen in oil crops, roots, tubers (around 26%), and fruits and vegetables (about 22%), as reported by FAO. Cereals, root crops, fruits, vegetables, and oilseeds contribute 30%, 40%, and 20% to global annual food waste, respectively (FAO). Due to alarming environmental repercussions, waste disposal poses significant financial and ecological concerns, prompting global efforts to find alternative recycling and repurposing methods.

Food and agro-waste harbour biologically active compounds useful for producing nutraceuticals and functional foods (Dini I. 2021). Extracting these compounds depends on their chemical nature, functional properties, source, and intended application.

This chapter addresses the use of agricultural and food waste as a resource for nutraceuticals.

17.2 TYPES OF AGRO-FOOD WASTE

Agro-food waste is broadly categorised as agricultural waste and food processing waste. The agricultural waste comprises raw agricultural residues such as leaves, straw, seeds, stalks, bagasse, etc., as shown in Figure 17.1. Besides fruits and vegetables, oil crops, cereals, pulses, tuber roots, meat, and animal products are the primary contributors to food wastage and nutrient loss. The processing waste obtained during food growing and

DOI: 10.1201/9781003392934-17

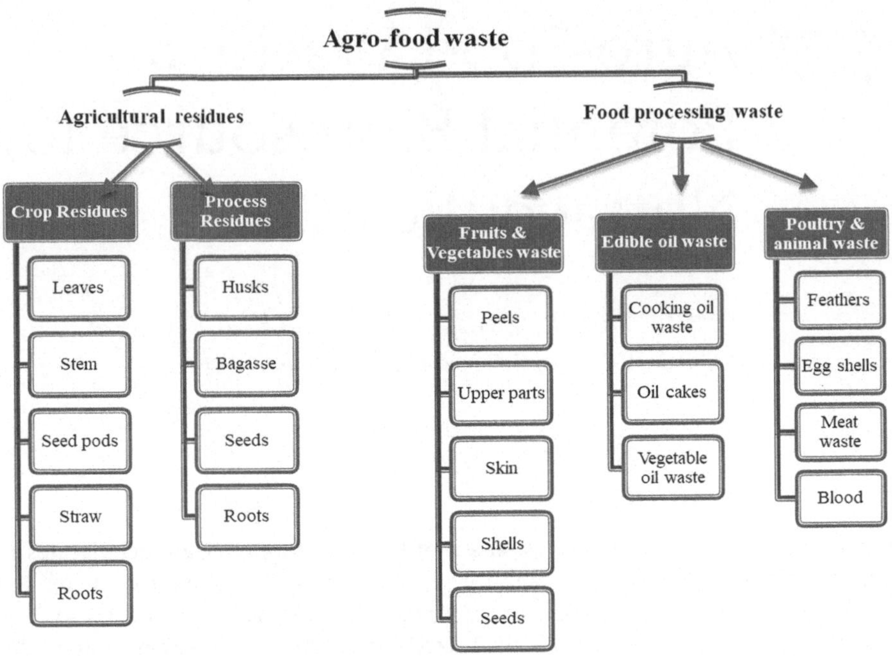

FIGURE 17.1 Types of Agro-food waste.

processing can be either in solid forms or liquid, slurry forms. Food industry waste also includes animal-derived wastes from meat, seafood, and dairy products.

Figure 17.2 shows the total waste produced (in 1000 tonnes) and the ratio percentage of the waste generated per amount of production in different food sectors (Baiano A. 2014). The majority of the waste generated comes from milk processing and the fruits-vegetable sector, which accounts for around 400k and 279k tonnes respectively.

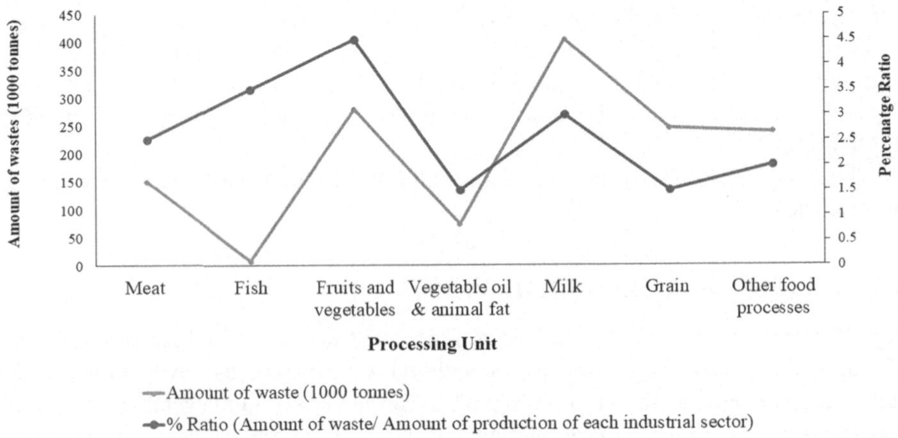

FIGURE 17.2 Waste generated in different food processing sectors.

This is followed by the processing of grain and other food products which generates around. The ratio of the waste generated per amount of product is also highest in the case of fruit and vegetable processing. Higher ratios for waste generated per amount of product are also observed in the milk and fish processing sectors as compared to others.

Agro-food wastes have been extensively used as feed for animals, as fertilisers, and even as biofuels. Several researchers have identified potential bioactive compounds which can be used for formulating nutraceutical products and functional food from agro-food wastes.

17.3 NUTRACEUTICALS

Nutraceuticals, sourced from agricultural and food origins, offer health benefits, especially in disease prevention and management. These bioactive compounds, found abundantly in fruit and vegetable by-products like citrus peels and grape pomace, serve as valuable assets for food, biotechnology, and pharmaceutical sectors. Researchers are exploring their potential in addressing cancer and cardiometabolic risks, with a focus on polyphenols, including anthocyanins and flavonols, renowned for their antioxidant properties. Additionally, they contribute to promoting cardiovascular health (Chopra et al. 2022).

17.4 NUTRACEUTICALS FROM FRUIT WASTE/ BY-PRODUCTS

Apples (Malus domestica): Apples, recognised for their antioxidant and phenolic content, generate apple pomace as a by-product, rich in dietary fibre and valuable compounds (Zhang et al. 2021). These by-products find applications in the food, biotechnology, pharmaceutical, and cosmeceutical industries, offering texture enhancement, antioxidant properties, and skincare benefits.

Bananas: Banana by-products, including peels, stems, and pulp, are often discarded but contain valuable bioactive compounds. They find applications in various industries, including food, biotechnology, pharmaceuticals, and cosmeceuticals, offering health benefits and contributing to waste reduction. Banana peels, in particular, are rich in dietary fibre, vitamins, minerals, and bioactive compounds (Gupta et al. 2022).

Citrus: Citrus, a widely cultivated fruit, generates by-products such as peels, pulp, seeds, and juice sacs. These by-products are often discarded but contain valuable compounds like dietary fibres, vitamins, flavonoids, and essential oils. They find applications in various industries, including food, biotechnology, pharmaceuticals, and cosmetics, offering potential health benefits and waste reduction (Panwar et al. 2021).

Grapes: Grapes yield valuable by-products with versatile applications, including grape pomace, grape seed oil, grape juice concentrate, and grape molasses. These by-products find use in the food, biotechnology, and pharmaceutical industries, offering health-promoting properties (Andrade et al., 2019).

Mango: Mango by-products, including peel, seed, and kernel, are rich in bioactive compounds, offering nutraceutical benefits. They have diverse applications in the food and cosmetics sectors, producing dietary fibre, edible oil, and skincare ingredients. The pharmaceutical and biotechnology industries also benefit from their biological activities (Kaur et al. 2022).

Plum, Peach, and Apricot: By-products of plum, peach, and apricot, packed with bioactive compounds, enhance foods like jams and baked goods. They hold pharmaceutical potential with antioxidant and anti-inflammatory properties and find biotechnological applications. Additionally, they offer cosmetic benefits (Munekata et al. 2022).

17.5 NUTRACEUTICALS FROM VEGETABLE WASTE

Beetroot: Beetroot by-products encompass pulp, molasses, leaves, and juice, with versatile applications. In the food industry, beetroot powder enhances colour, while pectin serves as a natural thickener, and molasses acts as a sweetener. Pharmaceutical uses involve antioxidants and anti-inflammatory properties, while the biotechnology and cosmeceutical industries benefit from their diverse applications (Puligundla & Mok 2021).

Carrots: Carrot by-products, including juice, pomace, puree, and oil, find utility in various industries. Carrot juice, rich in vitamins and minerals, offers potential health benefits. Carrot pomace enhances baked goods and serves as livestock feed, and carrot puree is used in infant food and snacks. Carrot oil finds applications in cosmetics for skincare (Rodrigues et al. 2022).

Cauliflower: Cauliflower by-products, including leaves, stems, meal, and juice, are valuable in the food, pharmaceutical, biotechnology, and cosmeceutical sectors. Cauliflower leaves and stems are rich in nutrition and biologically active compounds. Cauliflower waste serves as a sustainable biofuel feedstock, and cauliflower juice is abundant in phytochemicals and antioxidants (Sharma et al. 2021).

Garlic: Garlic by-products, such as peel, stem, bulb waste, and scape, have diverse applications, including natural food preservation, product quality improvement, antioxidant enhancement, antifungal properties, wound healing, cardiovascular disease management, biotechnology, and cosmeceuticals. (Ahmed & Wang 2021).

Onion: Onion by-products, including skin, waste, juice, and oil, serve multiple purposes, including natural dyes, animal feed, herbal teas, dietary supplements, flavouring agents, preservatives, food colourants, hair care products, and pharmaceuticals (Sagar et al. 2022).

Tomato: Tomato by-products, including pomace, seeds, skins, wastewater, and vines, have applications in enhancing nutritional value, producing natural colourants and antioxidants, biofuels, biofilms, irrigation, and value-added products in the food, pharmaceutical, biotechnology, and cosmeceutical industries (Trombino et al. 2021).

17.6 MARINE (FISH AND FISH PROCESSING WASTE)

Approximately 25% of global fish catch is wasted, leading to substantial annual fish waste (Mohanty et al. 2020). Valuable fish oil is extracted from this waste through solvent methods, including supercritical fluid extraction for omega fatty acids (Monteiro et al. 2018). Fish waste meal contains diverse proteins, with ongoing development of extraction techniques, including enzymatic and chemical hydrolysis for protein hydrolysates and bioactive peptides (Im et al. 2022).

17.7 ANIMAL, POULTRY, AND DAIRY PROCESSING WASTE

Animal husbandry, slaughterhouses, dairies, and poultries generate significant waste, including animal parts, flesh, blood, collagen, and bioactive proteins. Various protein recovery methods were compared, including keratin extraction from animal hair and bone minerals (Cassoni et al. 2018). Technologies like membrane-based whey protein recovery and enzyme-chemical hydrolysis are explored to yield saccharides and lactic acids.

17.8 OPTIMISING NUTRACEUTICAL RECOVERY FROM AGRO-FOOD WASTE: CHALLENGES AND STRATEGIES

In the recovery of nutraceuticals from agro-food waste, downstream processing is vital for economic viability. Critical factors like limited mass transfer and emulsion formation are often underestimated, and extracting hydrophobic molecules remains a challenge. Evaluating "Energy Returned on Energy Invested" (EROEI) is imperative for sustainability. Efficiency, cost-effectiveness, product quality, and scalability are essential, with concurrent recovery methods streamlining operations, conserving energy, and reducing solvent use (Pawar et al. 2019). Collaborative efforts, waste conversion, efficient logistics, and education are indispensable. A circular economy necessitates policies and waste management optimisation. Policies and guidelines for nutraceutical manufacturing are needed to navigate global regulatory variations, compliance, genotoxicity assessments, contamination cheques, and traceability challenges.

REFERENCES

Ahmed, T., & Wang, C.K. (2021). Black garlic and its bioactive compounds on human health diseases: A review. *Molecules*, 26(16), 5028.

Andrade, M.A., Lima, V., Silva, A.S., Vilarinho, F., Castilho, M.C., Khwaldia, K., & Ramos, F. (2019). Pomegranate and grape by-products and their active compounds: Are they a valuable source for food applications?. *Trends in Food Science & Technology*, 86, 68–84.

Baiano, A. (2014). Recovery of biomolecules from food wastes — A review. *Molecules*, 19, 14821–14842.

Cassoni, A.C., Freixo, R., Pintado, A.I.E., Amorim, M., Pereira, C.D., Madureira, A.R., & Pintado, M.M.E. (2018). Novel eco-friendly method to extract keratin from hair ACS sustain. *Chem. Eng.*, 6, 12268–12274.

Chopra, A.S., Lordan, R., Horbańczuk, O.K., Atanasov, A.G., Chopra, I., Horbańczuk, J.O., … & Arkells, N. (2022).

Dini, I. (2021). Bio discarded from waste to resource. *Foods*, 10, 2652.

Faustino, A.M., Veiga, M., Sousa, P., Costa, E.M., Silva, S., & Pintado, M. (2019). Agro-food byproducts as a new source of natural food additives. *Molecules*, 24, 1056.

Gupta, G., Baranwal, M., Saxena, S., & Reddy, M.S. (2022). Utilization of banana waste as a resource material for biofuels and other value-added products. *Biomass Conversion and Biorefinery*, 1–20.

Im, S.T., Kang, N., Kim, J. et al. (2022). Antioxidant and anti-hyaluronidase activities of taurine-enriched enzymatic hydrolysates prepared from turbo cornutus, a by-product of fish processing in Jeju Island. *Fish Sci*, 88, 509–517.

Kaur, B., Panesar, P.S., Anal, A.K., & Chu-Ky, S. (2022). Recent trends in the management of mango by-products. *Food Reviews International*, 1–21.

Mohanty, B., Swain, S., Hauzoukim, & Swain, S. (2020). A review on fish processing wastes generation in India and its further utilization prospects into different value added compounds.

Monteiro, A., Paquincha, D., Martins, F., Queirós, R.P., Saraiva, J.A., Švarc-Gajić, J., Nastić, N., Delerue-Matos, C., & Carvalho, A.P. (2018). Liquid by-products from fish canning industry as sustainable sources of ω3 lipids. *J. Environ. Manage.*, 219, 9–17

Munekata, P.E., Yilmaz, B., Pateiro, M., Kumar, M., Domínguez, R., Shariati, M.A., … & Lorenzo, J.M. (2022). Valorization of by-products from Prunus genus fruit processing: Opportunities and applications. *Critical reviews in food science and nutrition*, 1–16.

Panwar, D., Saini, A., Panesar, P.S., & Chopra, H.K. (2021). Unraveling the scientific perspectives of citrus by-products utilization: Progress towards circular economy. *Trends in Food Science & Technology*, 111, 549–562.

Panzella, L., Moccia, F., Nasti, R., Marzorati, S., Verotta, L., & Napolitano, A. (2020). Bioactive phenolic compounds from agri-food wastes: An update on green and sustainable extraction methodologies. *Front. Nutr.*, 7, 60.

Pawar P.P., Odaneth A.A., Vadgama R.N., & Lali, A.M. (2019). Simulataneous lipid biosynthesis and recovery for oleaginous yeast-Yarrowia lipolytica. *Biotechnology for Biofuels*.

Puligundla, P., & Mok, C. (2021). Valorization of sugar beet pulp through biotechnological approaches: recent developments. *Biotechnology Letters*, 43(7), 1253–1263.

Rodrigues, J.P., Liberal, Â., Petropoulos, S.A., Ferreira, I.C., Oliveira, M.B.P., Fernandes, Â., & Barros, L. (2022). Agri-food surplus, waste and loss as sustainable biobased ingredients: A review. *Molecules*, 27(16), 5200.

Sagar, N.A., Kumar, Y., Singh, R., Nickhil, C., Kumar, D., Sharma, P., … & Tarafdar, A. (2022). Onion waste based-biorefinery for sustainable generation of value-added products. *Bioresource Technology*, 362, 127870.

Sharma, M., Usmani, Z., Gupta, V.K., & Bhat, R. (2021). Valorization of fruits and vegetable wastes and by-products to produce natural pigments. *Critical Reviews in Biotechnology*, 41(4), 535–563.

Trombino, S., Cassano, R., Procopio, D., Di Gioia, M.L., & Barone, E. (2021). Valorization of tomato waste as a source of carotenoids. *Molecules*, 26(16), 5062.

Vilas-Boas, A.A., Pintado, M., & Oliveira, A.L.S. (2021). Natural bioactive compounds from food waste: Toxicity and safety concerns. *Foods*, 10, 1564.

Zhang, F., Wang, T., Wang, X., & Lü, X. (2021). Apple pomace as a potential valuable resource for full-components utilization: A review. *Journal of Cleaner Production*, 329, 129676.